UNDERSTANDING DEEPER DEVELOPMENTAL NEEDS

UNDERSTANDING DEEPER DEVELOPMENTAL NEEDS

Holistic Approaches for Challenging Behaviors in Children

Adam Blanning, MD

Lindisfarne Books | 2017

2017
Lindisfarne Books
An imprint of Anthroposophic Press / SteinerBooks
610 Main St., Great Barrington, MA
www.steinerbooks.org

Many of the English translations of Rudolf Steiner's quotations used here have been edited for gender-inclusive and more current use of language.

Design: Jens Jensen

Published with generous support from the
Waldorf Curriculum Fund

LIBRARY OF CONGRESS CONTROL NUMBER: 2017950620

ISBN: 978-1-58420-950-8 (paperback)
ISBN: 978-1-58420-951-5 (eBook)

Contents

This book is dedicated
to all the children

With loving thanks
to my family of faithful companions
and joyful collaborators

Introduction

It is always possible to start looking with new eyes. The perspectives presented in this book seek to enrich our approach to child observation and child development. These new insights can come by learning to recognize the child as a dynamic being—one who can be understood fully only through incorporating functional, sensory, and spiritual perspectives—for statistical measurements and physical attributes are not enough. This kind of an expanded lens comes through striving to appreciate the child on multiple levels. Such a holistic perspective can, in turn, help to clarify many present-day questions, for it broadens the context of our consideration by encouraging us to focus not only on why a particular behavior is happening but also on the questions "What stands behind this concern?" and "What is the child trying to accomplish with this behavior?" Those questions are the first steps on the pathway that will allow us to develop individualized therapeutic tools and experiences.

Such an expanded lens also allows us to look further back into the past to see what has been the child's pathway up until now and to help us see where the child needs to be guided in the future. The broader context of before, now, and after teaches us to think not just in problems or diagnoses, but also in living processes. This is possible because there are predictable, archetypal patterns in the way children learn and grow, both in body and spirit.

A wider lens brings new tools, but it also inevitably challenges some of our habits. It forces us to rethink prevalent modern assumptions about pediatric development and learning. This broadly integrative orientation—which acknowledges the child not as a being defined by the physical body, but rather as a being trying to find expression through the body—requires that we develop a more patient method of observation. We are looking not just to see the surface characteristics of an individual child, but also to see through those characteristics to acknowledge the unique individuality of that child. We have to learn to ask with real interest, "Who are you?" Our second question becomes "How can I help you to best unfold your full capacities?" The focus shifts, placing emphasis not only on current measures of growth and maturation but also on consciously finding future pathways for healthy development.

Here we explore this different way of looking from both pedagogical (educational) and medical orientations, which are, in fact, wonderfully complementary. There is a danger in both fields to understand the child with too limited a view. As an initial example, we can look at how one might use the standardized measures related to different developmental milestones.

These milestones are familiar, abbreviated measures of maturation, such as knowing at what age a child usually crawls (nine months) or how a child generally speaks by age two (using two- to three-word sentences). These milestones provide a set of measures that can be quickly assessed and recorded. Through brief inquiry one receives information about whether a child is meeting the expected milestones or falling behind in one or more developmental areas, such as gross motor, fine motor, speech, and socialization. With time pressures and the push for evermore standardized assessment there is the risk of overreliance on such abbreviated measures. This exemplifies a much broader and increasingly prevalent shift in medical thinking, one that becomes so committed to finding and defining objective facts that it regularly risks confusing those measures with the capacities they are trying to signify. Then an encounter with a child becomes less about really seeing who this child is and more about making sure that the child meets a checklist: "If the checklist items are met, then the job is done." These brief measures are really only meant to be screening tools, but they become our de facto lens if we do not consciously look to see past them.

This kind of abbreviation extends well beyond just screening measures, however. For that same kind of thinking now also extends into the process of actual diagnosis and treatment. Very often primary emphasis is placed on objectively recognizing and defining the names and qualities of development—healthy or imbalanced—with the belief that this naming will give us greater mastery and control. It is a process that perhaps started with a desire to look deeper, to understand better, but it regularly lands us in a place of black-and-white categorization. As an example: "Does this child have ADHD?" We risk having such an assessment of academic struggle center solely on whether or not a child fits into the diagnostic criteria for attention deficit hyperactivity disorder (ADHD). We may then be better able to name something, but not necessarily any more skilled at knowing what to do with those diagnoses. Certainly the numbers of new diagnoses that have come forward through revisions of the Diagnostic and Statistical Manual of Mental Disorders seem to outpace the number of non-pharmacologic supports we usually offer to children.

At a certain fundamental level, we are in real danger of losing our appreciation of the distinction between content (facts and names) and capacities (processes). Content and capacity are, of course, linked, but we must remember to look past the generalizations and connect back to the living processes and capacities that stand behind them.

The kind of narrowed or hardened thinking that most highly prioritizes statistical measures has now also found its way into many educational models. When this happens, teaching turns to focus almost exclusively on the conveying of content, the teaching of facts. Why would this be a concern? Well, let us look at the good aspects of this kind of learning. Teaching identifiers (names) and abbreviations for complicated processes is certainly an essential part of education. Factual content needs to be included. It helps us to quantify, quickly communicate, and categorize. Factual content also conveniently provides a means for assessing someone's familiarity with a particular topic, which is what we do with most testing. It gives us a quick measure for learning. This is where we must be very careful, however—for through so much emphasis on factual content, we increasingly equate measures (tests) with the learning processes that stand behind them. An undue emphasis on facts has created pressures that cause many teachers to decide to "teach to the test"—advocating that if we increase reading scores on standardized exams, we have succeeded in creating more capable and competent learners. A great deal of classroom time then focuses on the content of the test, not on the learning process itself.

Prioritizing measures and abbreviations over more dynamic interaction and experience leads to a short-term and hollow sense of security. Pushed too far, however, it results in a self-deceptive illusion. We believe that we are better and smarter because we diagnose more or test more, but in the process, we are losing connection with the actual health and life we are trying to foster. In an age where information is given such priority and power, there is a growing shift toward accepting virtual abbreviations as true representations and sometimes even preferring them over real experiences. That change is insidious and threatens to deaden our relationship with real life.

Incorporating a more holistic view of the human being helps us to avoid that danger because it constantly challenges us to remember that specific measures are only a snapshot of a process come to rest. The human being is more than a statistically defined set of behavioral characteristics and physical measurements. What then stands behind our physicality? How do we begin to think differently?

One answer, as has already been suggested, is to focus more on capacities. Observing and accurately describing capacities changes our thinking. Working to understand capacities is more complicated than looking at content because it deals with living processes. We find that our descriptive language necessarily shifts from an emphasis on nouns to an emphasis on verbs and adjectives.

How can we judge if someone is capable? We usually turn to a test, to a rote skill that can be learned—like a specific mechanical movement (e.g., jumping with two feet off the ground). Jumping to get two feet off the ground is a very specific kind of activity, but does it really adequately help us understand a child's capacity for healthy movement? A living capacity means that we are able to move beyond certain examples and exercise a skill in newly evolving ways. A process develops that stands above any specific application. For example, it is possible when gaining some fluency in a foreign language to have a dream and not be able to recall the language spoken. This is a true experience. People conversed in the dream—that much is remembered—and information was shared, but what was shared exists beyond specific words. In the morning, the content of the dream then has to be translated out of the realm of experience into the vocabulary of a particular language (whichever language seems most appropriate in that moment). It is also a familiar experience that once someone has learned to speak several languages, it becomes easier to acquire new, additional languages. That person's capacity to think and to communicate has become alive in a way that is not dependent on one specific language's vocabulary but can simultaneously find specific expression in many different vocabularies. Then a real capacity for language has been developed.

Some people are born with a particular capacity—be it musical or mathematical, memory, or social—which seemingly exists before any factual content is given to fill it. When someone has this kind of innate capacity, we recognize it because the gift of the skill is far advanced beyond what should have developed out of any specific instruction. It already existed from early in life, it seems, and such children are simply waiting for the right tools to be able to express it. Such innate capacities feel a little mysterious because they seem to have carried that capacity with them into life. But the development of a capacity before it has met any specific application happens on many levels and in all children. Process comes first and then flows down into content and expression we can physically observe.

The reverse flow can be experienced, in which working through a specific set of content helps us strengthen a new capacity. Content then flows upstream to awaken a new understanding. It develops through repetition and variation, so that in time people reach the point where they know instinctively what to do without having to go through a careful process of analysis. That shows a level of mastery. Within such persons there has now grown a living activity (think of master athletes or poets, counselors, or musicians) so flexible that they can respond directly to what the moment calls for. That upstream path receives a lot of attention—perhaps because we feel that we can control it, but that is actually not the way most development happens. We do not learn to walk by having someone move our feet or learn to speak by doing articulation exercises. Instead, there first emerges an awakened process—the drive to be upright or the drive to communicate—that will then be practiced until it can be physically manifest. Every growing child lives in a world of emerging, burgeoning capacities more universal than any specific content. It is the marvelous process seen in children in all parts of the world and in all cultures. The place where this living capacity originates is in a functional and also spiritual physiology.

Looking to understand this realm of emerging processes brings new possibilities for remedying challenges like aggressive behaviors, learning disabilities, ADHD, and Asperger's syndrome (all of which are examined in this book). To understand how we can work with capacity, we must look at the whole child. In the process we learn about many good, encouraging supports and activities that can be offered.

This book therefore has two primary goals and two ways in which it can be used. The first method is to provide descriptions that awaken and deepen our understanding of capacity and help us see how it relates to the spiritual aspects of the human being. That pathway is presented through the first three sections of the book, which outline vast developmental movements that are best understood through what are described as constitutional polarities. They are explored in depth with the hope that the reader will find in them not just a set of content but also the possibility to really live into them as developmental movements.

The second way to use this book is to focus on a specific problem—be it bullying, inattention, memory problems, or sensory-seeking behaviors—and then relate that specific behavior or problem back to the constitutional polarities. These symptom sections are inserted throughout the discussions and find heavier emphasis in the later portions of the text. The fourth section brings these two worlds closer together by developing a kind of differential diagnosis for attention and memory challenges. It is natural and necessary to breathe back and forth between the two approaches, between capacity and challenge, for ultimately one cannot be fully understood without the other. Understanding capacities helps us put many different facts of behavior in a broader context, while starting with a specific behavior helps lend practical application and assistance to the children with whom we are working.

At the end of the book are two appendices, which include additional perspectives and tools for approaching these processes from a biographical and then a medical perspective. The practice of anthroposophic medicine and the role of a school doctor lie very close to the pedagogical and therapeutic work of teachers and therapists. Remedy guides are included in order to show how the continuity of anthroposophic insight and observation supports children from many sides, though the actual selection and prescription of constitutional remedies should be done only by trained physicians and other qualified medical providers.

Part One

The Polarity of Integration: Between Heaven and Earth

Chapter 1

Building a Spiritual Concept of the Human Being

To gain a full understanding of children's experience we need to incorporate perspectives that extend beyond just the physical substance of the body. The goal is not to replace rigor of observation with a kind of mystical abandonment, however. It is to look toward functional, emotional, and spiritual aspects of the human being in a scientific way. Anthroposophy (from the Greek meaning "wisdom of the human being") offers a methodology for understanding these processes that live in the realm of capacity. Anthroposophic knowledge comes out of the work of Rudolf Steiner and provides a pathway for systematically coming to recognize and observe the spiritual aspects of the human being. Steiner described this path of knowledge as "Spiritual Science," a body of knowledge that is accessible to anyone who can approach it without prejudice and who is willing to develop greater powers of thought.

The spiritual processes Steiner described as part of the human being are related to four different "members": the physical body, the etheric body, the astral body, and the "I." They correlate with many other ancient and traditional conceptions of the human being and include the distinction between the body (made up of the physical body and the etheric), the soul (the astral body), and the spirit (the "I"). A brief overview of the differing qualities and activities of these spiritual members is presented here, although the reader new to these descriptions will benefit greatly by exploring Steiner's descriptions of them in his introductory works and in other secondary anthroposophic literature.[1] Much of the discussion in this book assumes that the reader has basic familiarity with the threefold human being (of nerve–sense system, rhythmic system, and metabolic–limb system) and the fourfold human being (physical, etheric, astral, and "I").

Study of the physical body dominates modern scientific thought. Most pedagogical and medical considerations arise out of thinking that most strongly connects to the physical facts of the world. This approach trains our thinking to work in a materialistic fashion (relating to the "theory that physical matter is the only or fundamental reality and that all being and processes or phenomena can be explained as manifestations or results of matter"[2]). Conceptions of health and illness based only on physical matter view the human being as an intricate, complicated machine, one that needs to be influenced or manipulated to maintain good health. Through an emphasis on objective parameters (by definition, those things that can be judged without taking into consideration the unique circumstances or experiences of an individual), statistical measures of physiology receive the greatest attention: weight, cholesterol and glucose levels, imaging results, and so on. These abbreviated measurements shed light with regard to the physical aspects of our body, but they can limit our thinking process.

There is a certain fatalism inherent in materialistic views of the body as a complex machine, because in time every machine stops functioning well and those breakdowns create disease. The ultimate breakdown of the machine is death. Materialistic medicine and therapy therefore focus on mechanical fixes for the body's machinery so that we can live longer (through placement of coronary artery stents, surgery to remove an appendix, or radiation of cancer cells, for example). The same materialistic thinking has now taken us from an organ level (which we can see with the naked eye) to the cellular level, with pharmaceutical drugs specifically developed to block or manipulate aspects of cellular physiology. These drugs are designed to function on a smaller, subtler level, but it is still a very mechanical way of working. If we make our view even finer, we come to the realm of gene therapy—the intentional manipulation of our DNA structure—where we seek to make submicroscopic but still mechanical changes in the structure of our physical body. All of these tools, whether working on the organ, the cellular, or the genetic level, focus on the structural foundations of life, which are all aspects of the physical body. It is true that the physical body is essential and easily identified, but it is not the sole origin of our existence as human beings.

If we can be open to expanding our considerations beyond the physical body, we find more proactive forms of therapy that move beyond working to fix what has become broken. This openness is especially important for children, since they are still building their "machines" and they are not yet fully manifest. It is hard to mechanically fix something that has not yet come forward. We instead need a way to look at how we can promote healthy unfolding.

If we return to the realm of capacity (that which lives in the realm of process and has not yet come to rest in a manifest physical fact), we start to think in sequences and changes in time. We enter the realm of dynamic change. To do this, we have to recognize that in addition to the physical body there is an etheric body, which provides the possibility for growth, change, and regeneration in time. We also learn that there is an astral body, which awakens capacities for sensing activity, for feeling, and for the creation of specialized form. Finally, we learn to identify yet another distinct aspect, the "I," which brings the possibility for morality, for intention, and for self-conscious awareness. These four members of the human being—physical, etheric, astral, and "I"—are present for the infant, the child, and the adult, though with differing activity and emphasis depending on the specific stage of life.

The forming of these four members of the human being is perhaps more easily understood if we look at the times when their cooperative work changes most dramatically. These changes occur when the four members release from each other in the dying process and when they gather together again in preparation for birth and early childhood. It is the "I," the spiritual core of our individuality, that provides constancy through these transitions.[3] We begin with all four present and then subtract them away, leaving only the physical. Then we reverse the process and see how they come together in preparation for birth.

During normal waking life all four members (physical, etheric, astral, and "I") are present and active within the human being. It is their mutual interaction that defines the activity and experience of waking life.

The innermost spiritual kernel, or core, of our individual existence is called the "I" because we can say "I" only with reference to ourselves. The "I" cannot be substituted or switched with another person. Our "I" is unlike the "I" of any other person on the earth. The "I" is unique—the most essential part of our existence as an individual human being. Our sense of individual style, of distinctive expression, of immunity are all connected to the "I." Our most beautiful human activities—to be self-conscious, self-improving, and moral, beyond pleasure or desire—are made possible by our "I."

Not all of our waking life includes the activity of our "I." There are times when our consciousness is clouded or limited—through intoxication with alcohol or drugs, through psychiatric imbalance, through cognitive decline or dementia—and our behaviors become much more reactionary and primal. We then do not act out of a deeply developed sense of self but rather from the realm of emotions and drives. In these situations the "I" largely is absent from consciousness, and we live in a sensing state ruled by the astral body. We act more like an animal. All animals (in terms of their spiritual physiology) lead a threefold existence, with a physical body, etheric body, and astral body but no "I." There is no individualized conception or experience of self for an animal. This more instinctive, emotionally directed state comes for a human being when the "I" is blocked from its rightful engagement with the other three members. It is, in fact, the presence of an "I" that distinguishes the human being from the animal world. It is quite possible to spend much of our daily life in a reactionary or habitual mode of activity, but our deeper moments of true humanity are possible only through the engagement of the "I."

The presence and activity of the astral body and its differentiation from the etheric body can be seen when we look at the physiology of sleep. Whenever we are sensing—either the surrounding environment or our own body—the astral body is present, but in sleeping activity we become essentially only a twofold being (made up of the etheric and physical bodies). In sleep the "I" and the astral body release. During deep sleep we live only within the activity of the physical body and the etheric body. Dreaming marks a transitional state, in which the astral body rejoins the physical and etheric enough to convey some sensing and feeling experience from the outside but has not yet established a fully wakened connection with the environment. If we fall back into deep sleep, the astral body again leaves. Deep sleep, without the presence of the astral body, is a state of true rest and regeneration. We share this regenerative state with the plant world, for a plant lives only in this twofold interweaving of physical and etheric activities. The plant does not carry capacities for either sensing (astral) or self-conscious ("I") activity. Such an unconscious, regenerative state is appropriate for the human being for a certain length of time, but if that state continues inappropriately and the "I" and astral body are not able to enter back in, a person enters into a coma. The possibility for conscious sensing of and reaction to the environment is then gone, and the human being becomes much more like a plant. In older medical terminology, this lowered level of consciousness was even referred to as a "vegetative" state.

Death comes if we go still a step further, so that the etheric body and its forces release from the physical body. Such a separation is not an instantaneous process but happens over the course of about three days. Immediately after death there is usually still some hint of vitality, a disconcerting experience when we see a loved one in this state who looks as though that one might still take a deep breath. By the third day the body looks very different. It is clearly a husk. Only the physical substance remains. Left to itself, the physical body becomes subject to the gravitational and mechanical laws of the surrounding world. The etheric body preserves and renews the physical body, but without the etheric body the physical body cannot sustain itself and begins to break down. Death can be understood as the state when the physical body—fully independent from the etheric—truly becomes a machine and breaks down. The qualities of the fourfold human being are briefly summarized in table 1.

Table 1: Qualities of the fourfold human being

Members of the Human Being	Level of Consciousness	Main Quality and Process	Relation to the Natural World
"I"	Fully wakeful activity	Intentional, moral, and self-conscious capacities	Human being ("I," plus astral body, etheric body, and physical body)
Astral body	Dreaming activity	Sensing, emotional, and reactive activities	Animal world (astral body, plus etheric body and physical body)
Etheric body	Deep sleep	Processes of growth and generation	Plant world (etheric body and physical body)
Physical body	Death	Substantive qualities of quantity, color, and density	Mineral world or physical matter (physical body alone)

In a child all four members are striving to find the right ways to work cooperatively. They must collaborate for us to function as human beings. When their interweaving is interrupted, blocked, or too one-sided, we see patterns of developmental challenge. Different categories of challenge—motoric, moral, attentional, or behavioral—correspond to different imbalanced interactions of the four members. In severe chronic illness and advanced old age, we can see how the four members gradually release from their full cooperative activity, but for children we are looking not so much at a dissolution of their mutual activity as at an incomplete meeting.

Let us now therefore trace the pathway for the gathering of the four members as a preparation for birth, so that we can begin to see how blockages or incomplete interactions arise. It is a complex process, and when we incorporate these other members of the human being the birthing process must be seen as much longer. It extends beyond the labor of delivery, even beyond the nine months of pregnancy.

The way that the four members come together is determined by what children bring as their spiritual heritage from previous experience (carried in the astral body and "I") and by what they encounter as the hereditary stream in the earthly realm (carried in the physical body). We only receive the physical body from our parents. The rest we bring with us from other realms.

The different pathways for this gathering become more evident when we study constitutional polarities. There are certain archetypal capacities a child needs to unfold in the course of development, but there is great variation as to whether they are too big or too small or happen too fast or too slow. Development rarely follows a straight line, so a more useful way of looking at development is not merely to say whether things are present or absent, but instead to ask if a process leans too far in either one direction or the other. There is always some arbitrariness in defining a threshold of normal and abnormal. (If only six of seven required criteria are met, does that mean there is no problem?) Learning about the extremes of a process within a spectrum of development helps us to understand the developmental physiology of all children.

Our individual inclinations help to define who we are. There are several overarching patterns we observe as polarities of behavior:

- First, in relation to movement and whether a child moves with either too much gravity or too much levity
- Second, with respect to the speed of development and whether it progresses so fast that it does not have time to mature or unfolds so slowly and deliberately that it holds us back
- Third, in our experience of relating to the world around, whether we are too open and vulnerable or too closed and therefore cut off

In much the same way that temperament has been recognized as an innate quality already present at birth,[4] so do these constitutional types become fundamental influences on our path of individual growth and development.

Thinking in polarities allows us to look at developmental variations in a more dynamic way. We are able to identify a child's imbalanced inclinations and challenges (falling toward one side of a polarity) and at the same time also be guided toward the proper therapeutic gesture (which usually can be found by moving toward the other side of the polarity). For example, if a process is too fast, proper therapeutic support comes by protecting and slowing such children. Similarly, when children engages only superficially with those around them, a therapeutic activity will help them shift their attention to find real interest in the world. "Healthy" and "unhealthy" change from classifications of black and white to a consideration of whether children fall on one side of the polarity or the other. We then appreciate that healthy development is defined best as having an inclination one way or the other, while being flexible enough not to be defined or limited by it.[5] For the majority of children, these constitutional qualities are experienced simply as shades of personality (quiet or talkative, shy or curious, deductive or inductive thinkers) but are not strong enough to rigidly define behavior. At the extremes come the deeper challenges of development.

It has been nearly one hundred years since these polarities were introduced. Perhaps as a result, the relationship to Steiner's original descriptions has sometimes become rather superficial. As we move further away from the time of Steiner's original presentations, it is all the more essential that we continually strive to reenliven them. We need to look for their practical application in the world. After all, Steiner described the polarities because of processes he was immediately experiencing in the children around him. The descriptions of the polarities in this book do refer back to the traditional names used—such as feebleminded and maniacal, large-headed and small-headed, epileptic and hysteric—but they are placed within the context of three larger developmental gestures—integration, differentiation, and connection. Thinking in verbs helps us remember that working with the polarities is really learning to observe unfolding processes.

Steiner recognized the dangers of trying to describe dynamic spiritual processes with fixed words. He himself often coined new terms to try to reflect the living nature of things, a process that is much easier in the German language. In the medical literature he used the word *albuminizing,* referring to the physiologic process that stands behind the activity of the amorphous protein in the blood (albumen) and which he contrasted with a forming, clotting process (antimonizing). Steiner also created numerous compound terms like nerve–sense-system and metabolic–limb-system in an attempt to translate a spiritual process into modern language. One of Steiner's greatest gifts is his ardent striving to find and create language and descriptions flexible enough to adequately reflect living processes. He spoke of these living thought pictures as imaginations, which shift and change in time.

To learn to observe such living processes, we have to become curious about what is happening for a child, including just before and just after a particular behavior. We also need to know the archetypal developmental stages of childhood to see what processes must be in place for additional capacities to healthily unfold. Each of the three main developmental movements we explore here are distinct, but they do follow a kind of natural progression. The process of what we call integration, which involves the meeting of the spiritual and the earthly streams, must come as a primary task. It involves learning to really feel at home in the body. Then, once this process has achieved a certain completeness and maturation, out of integration (a claiming of the body) comes differentiation. With differentiation we develop more specialized organ function and nerve activity and new capacities for thought, memory, and independent activity. Then the third process, connection, brings us into new and striking association with other people and with the world around us. Connection evolves out of and depends upon the successful physiologic foundations laid down through integration and differentiation. We discuss these processes as broad developmental movements, working through this progression.

These developmental windows find particular emphasis at different times of life. The process of integration stands as the foundational developmental mandate of the first seven years, the process of differentiation emerges with the change of teeth and continues on through the grades (up to age fourteen), while conscious experiences of connection (and disconnection) with the outside world play the greatest role in adolescence and early adulthood (until age twenty-one). While these polarities show a healthy and archetypal chronological emphasis, all three processes are, in fact, happening all of the time. The very young child is still, on a more primitive level, finding the method for proper connection with the outside world (which is strongest in adolescence), and the adolescent must work to really feel at home and inhabit the physical body (which changes through growth spurts and sexual development). As fully grown adults, we, too, must work continuously to reenliven and refine these three processes, though we perhaps experience them more on the level of conscious steps of inner growth than as global steps of physiologic development.

Fortunately, the first primary steps in early life unfold without our needing to consciously guide and direct them ourselves. We are carried through a whole process of preparation and encounter. The first steps along that path involve meeting and finding connection with our body.

Chapter 2

The Polarity of Integration: Between Heaven and Earth

We have to work to feel at home in our physical body. This is not a sure thing. In fact, it is always a challenging task to fully penetrate the physical body. That penetration is the main developmental mandate of the first seven years of life.

During that seven-year span we are tasked with making a home in the "model" body we receive from our parents. Why is it a model? Because it is not yet something we have really made our own. The physical body of a newborn infant is beautiful and wise beyond words—think of the incredible processes of growth that occur, of the extraordinary architecture of the organs of respiration, circulation, digestion, and movement that already exist when children are born. Those processes are there, but in many ways children do not yet know how to use them except in very elementary ways. They provide, almost independently, the main activities of children's physiology without having to learn how to orchestrate them. Infants do not have to figure out how to digest in order to eat, how to breathe, or how to sleep; these just happen instinctively. Such gifts provide an introductory foundation for being in the world, which in time will become more individualized and gradually more consciously guided.

This model body brings important hereditary influences to our life: what we look like; the coloring of our hair, eyes, and skin; our size, shape, growth patterns, disease inclinations, and genetics. These influences come from the genetic streams of the birth parents, which may or may not reflect the patterns of the adults the child will grow up with. With many different family structures (including single-parent households, blended families, international adoptions, and sperm and egg donors) a child may receive one hereditary, model physical stream and yet grow up in a very different social or cultural environment.

In earlier times this hereditary body, as a gift of the bloodline of our ancestors, had great importance and often carried with it rich instinctive knowledge, including cultural, agricultural, religious, and social wisdom. Many traditional cultures speak vividly about memories being passed down through the generations, even without an outward sharing or relating of those experiences. They were passed on as a kind of unconscious gift. That kind of innate wisdom lives in the hereditary stream. Certain physical qualities may indeed be very important for the tasks of a particular child's life, and a child may look to be born into a family line of great musicians, artists, or philosophers. Think of multiple generations of musical composers, actors, inventors, or athletes, and it is easy to understand how being born into a body that can help a child accomplish a specific task would be a great gift. We are told by Steiner that the preparation for a specific incarnation—to come into a particular weaving of hereditary streams—may be planned for in the spiritual world for as many as thirty generations before the actual birth of a child.[6]

The giving of a model body continues today, though it perhaps does not play the same dominant role as in previous millennia or even as in previous centuries. We are gradually, globally moving away from a reliance on strict, cohesive, cultural norms and instead moving toward a more wakeful, individualized consciousness. There is now such a meeting and mixing of racial, religious, and ethnic streams that it frequently becomes difficult for people to strongly identify with any one ethnic or cultural stream. For all of these reasons it is increasingly important for us not only to look at the physical, hereditary qualities of a child but also to recognize that there is an individuality who is coming into this body, working to come into a life.

There is significant preparation for the child's meeting of the model body, which happens before birth in the spiritual world. For when we speak about the different "members" of a child, we must recognize that these more spiritual elements also had an existence and a home before the child was born. The "I," the astral body, and the etheric body come together in a threefold activity before they unite with the hereditary, physical body. They bring different activities and qualities that weave together in a completely unique way for each individual. The majority of developmental challenges arise out of an imbalanced interaction in the coming together of the four members. Sometimes that discordance is necessary because one aspect of an incarnation, of a coming life, has been given greatest priority and necessitates acceptance of other, less ideal conditions.

Our prebirth existence begins with the "I," which has already been described as the uniquely human, innermost spiritual aspect of an individuality. The "I" carries on a continuous existence, one that extends both before and after birth and is the aspect that continues from one lifetime to another. It finds its home within the spiritual world in the time between death and a new birth; at a specific point (called by Steiner the midnight hour) a decision is made to incarnate again into the earthly realm, and the long process of preparation for that new incarnation begins.[7] Something prompts that decision: the need to be on the earth at a specific time, to incarnate with a particular group of other individuals, or perhaps to experience a specific place on the earth. These are just a few of the largely unknowable karmic reasons that a child decides to incarnate. When this decision is made, parents have to be found. The reason and timing for incarnation may trump other considerations of finding the right hereditary, model body. According to Steiner, even in the best situations "there can never be complete harmony."[8] For this reason the taking on of a new physical body always carries an aspect of sacrifice. The spiritual and hereditary streams never fully match. As Steiner said, "Parents who will be exactly right for the germinal human being cannot always be found; all that can be done is to search for the most suitable.... This is the reason for the discord between soul and body in human beings."[9] Our core identity comes from the "I," but that spiritual kernel must find a home in a physical body. Then the physical garment of the body must be worked on in order to make it one's own. Because the "I" and the physical body have such different origins, great time and activity must be spent trying to find ways for them to work more congruously with each other. They really represent a polarity of heaven and earth.

The second spiritual member of the human being, the astral body, does, however, fit harmoniously with the "I." This is because with each incarnation the astral body is actually built anew, gathering the forces that will make possible our sensing and feeling activity in life. The forming of the astral body is orchestrated by the "I" "like iron filings scattered across a piece of paper," which then move in response to a magnet as "the irregularly distributed astral substance is attracted and arranged according to the forces which are in the soul and which correspond to what the soul has achieved in a previous life."[10] What we experienced in an outward way in a previous incarnation is transformed into a capacity or ability for the next incarnation.[11] This prior experience brings a formative knowledge for organ creation and activity in the coming lifetime. In other words, we come into life knowing how to do something in relation to what we have already worked through and experienced.

In this gathering, formative process, the astral body is already finely structured and individualized before physical birth, with many different structures that will eventually slip down into and re-form the physical organs that are originally given as part of the hereditary body.[12] The accumulated wisdom we bring with us through the "I" and astral body provides a living blueprint for what we will be able to accomplish as a human being. All of our organs—not simply as anatomic structures but as living centers for differentiated activity—arise out of the activity of the astral body.

The gathered knowledge that helps to form the structure of the astral body (gained through the depth and breadth of our experiences in previous incarnations) also helps guide us to find the best possible hereditary body, the one that will best match what we ourselves hope to unfold. We know how to look for the appropriate body based only on the wisdom that we already possess, so that it is very possible for an incarnating child to select a hereditary body that is incomplete or imbalanced. We do not know to look for what we do not yet know. Such an omission represents a pathway for a kind of karmic rebalancing, because we are then forced—through grappling for a lifetime with that deficit—to come to know what the missing capacity should really be. Steiner told us, "The existence of defective forces of heredity means that before conception there was a lack of knowledge of the human organization...if, in an earlier life, we neglected to develop interest in our surroundings or were prevented from doing so."[13] Over multiple incarnations each individual works through a whole repertory of challenges, resulting in a corresponding gathering and refining of capacities. In this way we continuously work to improve the form of our astral bodies through the cumulative wisdom held by the "I." There is, therefore, often a necessary but sometimes uncomfortable relationship between the hereditary and spiritual streams, as through karmic lawfulness we repeatedly choose a physical body that will force us to learn and experience what we do not yet know.

The third spiritual member of the human being, the etheric body, is also newly gathered in preparation for each incarnation. It could similarly be compared to the movement of iron filings in a magnetic field, because etheric substance is also gathered and oriented, but it is done by a being external to the human being. Where astral substance is gathered together in relation to the experiences carried by the "I" from the previous incarnation (such that the astral body and "I" complement each other), the etheric body is gathered out of the world ether by the spiritual beings who help guide particular cultural or ethnic groups, referred to by Steiner as "folk souls." This process is distinct from our bringing of the individual spiritual stream from a previous incarnation. If we are living in the same place as our ancestors, it helps for there to be some congruity between the ether body and the hereditary body we receive from our parents, but there may still be a mismatch between the "I" and the astral body on one side and the etheric body on the other. Steiner told us that this could stand as a source of "maladjustment and lack of satisfaction in life"[14] as the ethnic or cultural stream we are born into may or may not reflect who we are as spiritual beings, with a resultant restlessness and a longing to find one's "real" people.

Another potential challenge arises from this same gathering process for the etheric body, one in which the etheric and physical bodies do not unite fully. This can occur during the gathering of the etheric body, before the incarnating soul has actually met the physical body, when individuals are given a prevision of their coming life. It is a survey of what one's future life has in store.[15] When individuals have had unfortunate experiences in a previous life, they may experience a kind of shock at what is coming in future and will hesitate to unite with the physical body, which "holds back the soul from a complete incarnation."[16] With such an incomplete penetration, the hereditary body cannot be met and integrated properly into the activity of the spiritual members, with a resultant disconnect between the physical and etheric bodies. This can have profound ramifications for the way we are able to manifest our true individuality through the physical body, often resulting in significant developmental challenges.

From this overview of the coming together of the four members of the human being, it is easy to see that many potential hindrances lie in the process. It is essential to remember, however, that the process of building a fourfold human being is not complete at birth. In many ways it is just starting. If it were finished, then we would indeed be like a machine—most perfect as babies and then slowly falling apart. But child development is not a process that has already reached its peak early and then simply degrades. The first seven years of life are much more about working to claim the hereditary body so that true growth and learning can really begin to unfold in later years. The young child is occupied with transforming the physical body so that it will serve as the best possible vessel for meeting the experiences of later life. It is not given to us as a perfect vessel; it is only "relatively the best and the most suitable."[17] That fact should arouse in us the greatest possible compassion for the young child's struggle through the incarnation process and the greatest enthusiasm for trying to support its unfolding.

Chapter 3
Early Childhood as an Inflammation

Given the complex spiritual physiology of the coming together of the "I," the astral body, the etheric body, and the physical body, we may be tempted to think that the meeting of the spiritual and hereditary streams is totally unknowable. We might come to believe that it happens in far-off reaches, but this is not true. It is not carried out with dreamy abstraction; it is a real and practical part of the life of the small child. It is a "perpetual struggle" and an ongoing engagement as "the two elements fight each other."[18] At its most basic level this meeting is really a quest to grasp what is not yet "self" (the substance of the physical body) and to find ways to rework it. It parallels, as a larger developmental process, what is constantly carried out on an organ-specific level through our immune and digestive activities. At the boundaries of our skin, lungs, and gut, we assess what we want to take in and what to excrete. Even within the body, the physical substance of our bones, muscles, ligaments, blood, and organs is constantly being broken down and built anew. In this way we constantly renew our organism. In the young child this process is carried out in a more dynamic manner as the whole body, down to the baby teeth, must be totally reworked—the old, hereditary body excreted and the new individualized substance taking its place. Steiner describes this process as an essential developmental tasks for each child:

> We perpetually thrust something out of our body; an outward streaming, or centrifugal impulse, is always at work, casting the body off. The consequence is that the human body is completely renewed every seven or eight years.... The inherited body is used as a model; and according to whether the life of

> spirit and soul is strong or weak, it will either be in a position to proceed in a more individual way with the inherited form or be subject to the inherited form—in which case the soul will be compelled to shape the second body like the first, which was shaped by the parents.[19]

When the process happens successfully, the hereditary body is really transformed in the first seven years of life, so that it can then be properly inhabited. The way that this penetrating, sorting, and renewing process happens is for the "I" to weave all the way down with the astral body into the etheric body and then fully penetrate the physical body.

The four members of the human being can interact in different ways (as will be explored in later sections), but this full fourfold penetration stands behind all processes of loosening, transformation, and excretion. It underlies very important parts of our physiology. A very common example and expression of this fourfold weaving is inflammation.

Inflammation is a tool of the immune system, and it brings to visible expression the process of determining what is me and what is not me and also what needs to be destroyed and excreted and what needs to be reintegrated and made whole again. Whenever there is an inflammation in the body—whether it is a baby's cutting new teeth, influenza with high fever, or the painful red swelling around a splinter—all four members of the human being are active in that process. Inflammation was first recognized by the ancient Greeks, who defined it as the presence of four specific qualities—a definition that is still used in medical education today. The Greeks observed that the inflammatory process includes rubor (redness), tumor (swelling), dolor (pain), and calor (warmth). These qualities fit within the ancient Greek understanding of the four elements, with redness being a physical quality, swelling being a condition of fluid or water, pain related to air, and warmth being an expression of fire. Anthroposophically, we can similarly look at these same four qualities and recognize in them signatures of the four members: redness as a quality of the physical body, swelling related to the etheric body and the activity of bodily fluids, pain as an expression of the wakeful sensing of the astral body, and warmth as the primary tool of the "I" (see table 2). When all of those markers are present, we then know that a true fourfold interweaving is taking place. Knowing that an essential task of the first seven years of life is the healthy transformation of the hereditary body, it should come as no surprise that inflammatory illnesses, which include a strong warmth process (fever), are a vital part of the incarnation experience for the young child.

Table 2: The fourfold interweaving of the four members and the corresponding markers of the inflammatory process

"I"	Calor	Warmth
Astral	Dolor	Pain
Etheric	Tumor	Swelling
Physical	Rubor	Redness

In lectures to a group of young doctors, Steiner indicated that the classic inflammatory illnesses of childhood are important tools of incarnation. This fact is reaffirmed repeatedly in anthroposophic practice, since it is not at all unusual for parents or caregivers to recognize and report that children look physically different, or "dwell" differently in their body after a strong fever or inflammation. A new skill, a more sculpted face, or perhaps a more confident approach to the world is often reported as the positive result of a strong inflammation. When we recognize that inflammation properly belongs (as an essential developmental process) to the first seven years of life, methods for broadly preventing such strong inflammations (through vaccination) or suppressing them once they come (with fever suppressants, anti-inflammatories, or antibiotics) take on a different significance. For when inflammation is suppressed at all possible costs, a vital transformative window is lost, so that the hereditary body will have to be worked with in a different way. There are other ways to encourage and support the fourfold penetration of the "I" down to the hereditary body (described later), but none are quite so potent as the process of healthy inflammation, transformation, and excretion in childhood.

How this meeting of the spiritual and hereditary streams plays out during an inflammation varies from individual to individual. Different children have different incarnation challenges and as such get sick in different ways. Even when strongly exposed to an illness, not all children will contract the same illnesses, and the illness will not have the same severity in everyone who does get sick. There is individual variation, and the particular kind of illness or inflammatory pattern a child experiences can be instructive as to how the spiritual and hereditary streams are coming together in that particular individual. If there are challenges in fully claiming a part of the body (such as the ears, tonsils, and adenoids), then we may see that an inflammation is mounted over and over in an attempt to really penetrate those organs. Or, as alternatively described by Steiner, a particular imbalance may find resolution through a specific illness. He gave the example of scarlet fever and measles. He explained that when the spiritual activities (of the "I" and astral body) are too strong, we see scarlet fever as a balancing process. And when the hereditary body is dominant and resistant, then we see the inflammation of measles:

> Childhood illnesses are the expression of this fight.... When the second teeth appear, you can see how they push up against

> the first, how they still tussle with each other, and in this same way the whole second human being tussles with the first. But there is the supraearthly being within that second human and a foreign, earthly model in the first. These two work into each other and, if you truly observe this interaction, you can see how—if the inner human, who as a being of soul and spirit was present in pre-earthly existence, has too much the upper hand for a time, working into the physical very strongly and having to adjust itself, willy nilly, by dint of effort to the model—it damages the model by striking up against it everywhere, saying: I want to get this particular form out of you—then the fight expresses itself as scarlet fever. If the inner being is tender, so that there is a continuously shrinking back, a wish to model the ingested substances more in keeping with their own nature, and resistance is put up to the model, then the struggle expresses itself as measles.... If you form a true picture of an excessively strong working of the spirit and soul, the picture crystallizes into that of scarlet fever. A picture of too-feeble activity of the spirit and soul that wavers, in face of the model, becomes the picture of measles.[20]

When a child can be safely guided through these illnesses a certain harmonization of the four bodies is achieved. While both of these illnesses (scarlet fever and measles) are not commonly seen in Western nations today, we can appreciate that they have historically stood as important balancing tools and that while we usually think of illness as only a negative experience, inflammation is actually a fundamental tool for transformation. These inflammatory illnesses present themselves to help balance a process, and they should be looked at as possible solutions rather than just misfortunes. Illness and strong inflammation need, of course, to be treated with respect and proper medical supervision, but it is a loss when this pathway of inflammatory transformation is blunted or prevented without any awareness of the larger developmental consequences. It means that as those classic childhood illness experiences fade away from the life of small children, the task of guiding and supporting the child to really feel at home in the physical body must become a more consciously guided process. It is not such a leap to observe that imbalances that were previously worked through as inflammatory illnesses in past times are now finding a different but related expression in the behavioral and developmental challenges of the present age.

Chapter 4

Earthly and Cosmic Polarity

The weaving together of soul and spirit from one side and of the hereditary body from the other comes to observable expression in the form and function of the body. There is a fundamental relationship between the head and the incarnating spiritual stream (astral body and "I") on one side and between the hereditary body and the limbs on the other. This makes intuitive sense, because the sensing organs concentrated in the head tend to be quieter, receptive, and more removed from direct interaction or intervention in the physical objects of the world. The limbs, in contrast, are where we actively engage and meet the physical world in order to interact and exchange with it. Our digestion and metabolism carry out the same kind of interaction and exchange as the limbs, but through an inner meeting and transforming of the physical world. We can extend this observation into a physiologic principle: above in the head we receive, and below in the limbs we engage. Even our digestion follows this rule, with food and liquid coming into us through our head, brought down to the digestive organs, and then excreted back to the environment down below. Steiner characterized this polarity as the upper part and the lower part of the human being, and as the contrast between a receptive "nerve–sense system" and an active "metabolic–limb system." Both reveal consistent, but contrasting gestures not only in their function but also in their structural arrangement and even the architecture of the corresponding organs.[21]

Let us look at this contrasting physiology in even more detail. In his lectures to teachers at the founding of the upper school at the original Waldorf school, Steiner emphasized that it is a deception to believe that our head directs all of our activities in the world. He states that the head is only one pole of our physiology and is only really responsible for our perceptions—it does not help us move beyond merely taking in the impressions of the world around.[22] In those presentations Steiner emphasized that the role of the head during our lifetime is regularly overestimated and that "we really must get away from the materialistic view of the head that attaches too much importance to it. We need our head as a reflecting apparatus, no more."[23] Our sensing organs function as portals for the impressions of the outside world to come in. They live in the realm of receptivity. Taking things in, without changing them or reacting to them—a true reflecting process—belongs to the organs and activity of the head.

Steiner went on to say that "the functions of the head tear me away from the world. What I call seeing and hearing, what ultimately leads to the forming of ideas and mental images, cannot in this objective way impart itself to the world outside. My head is not part of that world; it is a foreign body on earth, a copy of what I was before I descended to earth.... We must learn to see the head as a picture of our prenatal spirit and soul organism."[24] The head physically expresses its relationship to our spiritual origin in its rounded form—a picture of the arching vault of the heavens, the cosmos above us. This nerve–sense pole is built by the spiritual heritage we bring with us into life through the "I" and the astral body. In the form and characteristics of the head we observe influences of the spiritual stream and the capacities that arose out of our previous experiences.

The limbs, in contrast, are active and committed to the physical world. They carry none of the head's and the senses' objectivity. The limbs instead accomplish the spirit's plunge into substance in order to shape it and make the physical world one's own. Through the limb physiology the human being is able to actively participate in the world and exert an influence on it. As the head is molded by the heavens, the limbs belong to the earth: "What we inherit enters the organism of our arms and legs. There we are our parents' children."[25] The hereditary stream and its model body find prominence in our metabolic–limb activity. How well we can take hold of the physical substance of the hereditary body determines both the form and function of the earthly/limb pole.

As a continuing examination of the head and limbs, Steiner tasked teachers during these lectures to work to recognize and help balance the spiritual and the hereditary streams in their students, in what would come to be known as the cosmic and earthly constitutional polarity:

> There is yet another essential and important task for you. Equipped with a sound understanding of the nature of the child, you must develop an eye for distinguishing the child with a predominant cosmic organization from the one with a predominant terrestrial/physical organism. The former will have a plastically formed head, the latter a plastically structured trunk and, especially, limbs.[26]

By learning to look at the sculptural quality of a child's body—looking not so much to see where the sculpting has been completed as to where it is still incomplete (still "plastic")—we begin to physically observe the weaving of the cosmic and the earthly. To avoid confusion, it is helpful to know that the German word *plastisch* cannot be entirely captured in a satisfactory way with the English word *plastic*. In this context it might be better if we substitute the word *moldable,* or *sculptable,* or even *doughy.* Such rounded, unsculpted tissue does naturally belong to early childhood. We expect an infant to be round and soft and know that that is healthy. Then, as a child grows and matures, the baby fat (which we can now also name as a kind of "plastic" tissue) diminishes. This sculpting process is usually not consistent in all parts of the body, so that when we still see quite sculptable tissue in one part of the body and emerging definition in another, it can tell us about the relative relationship of the spiritual and terrestrial streams.

In the "cosmic" child, who remains too much in the spiritual realm, the face and features remain soft and often are rounded. They keep the form of the heavens above. Like little cherubs, they are perhaps in the world but not yet really of the world. They are still living very much in the activity of the astral and "I" alone.

For the "earthly" child it is the limbs and trunk that remain unsculpted. The still unformed limbs have a different quality. They have a thickness and density, a bit like an unworked lump of clay. The limbs have not yet received their definition because the hereditary stream is particularly difficult to overcome. The limbs stay doughy, not so much because the child is unwilling to enter into them but because of an inability to adequately transform the model body. It is helpful to look for this quality, because sometimes when we are holding a child's hand or looking at his or her feet, we will be struck by how unformed or generic the limbs feel in comparison to what already seems like a well-individualized head or face. That is the sculptural relationship of the earthly child.

A still poorly transformed hereditary body influences not only the shape of the body but also the child's experience of that body. What remains untransformed cannot serve properly as a tool for the capacities brought by children through the spiritual stream and casts a shadow over children's experience of their body. Steiner included aspects of the associated soul state with his description of the sculptural qualities of the earthly and cosmic polarity:

> In the more earthly child, the hereditary forces are playing a major role; they permeate the entire metabolic–limb system in an extraordinarily strong way. Even when the child does not appear to be melancholic, there is, nonetheless, alongside the apparent temperament a nuance of melancholy. This is due to the child's earth nature, the "earthiness" in the child's being.[27]

The earthly child knows well what is left untransformed and feels its burden. The physical body, too dense, cannot be lifted into a full fourfold spiritual activity. The "clay" of the hereditary body feels like a weight, not easily penetrated and ensouled.

Steiner characterized the earthly pole in one additional way, which allows us to begin to think in therapeutic terms. He revealed that as soon as we identify an exaggerated influence of the hereditary stream, we can know its healthy balance by looking to the other pole (the spiritual stream). The most helpful process for an earthly child is to spiritualize the metabolic–limb system to help lift the child's incarnation experience away from the heaviness of the physical body. We can bring activity and encounters from the outside that help balance children's earthliness and instead lift them away from their melancholy:

> When we notice this [earthly] trait in children, we will do well by trying to interest them in music that passes from the minor mood to the major, from the melancholic strains of the minor to the major. Earthly children can be spiritualized by the movements of music and eurythmy. Children with a distinctly sanguine temperament and delicate melancholic features can easily be helped by painting. Even if such children seem to have but little talent for music or eurythmy, we should still try to develop the disposition for it that is certainly there. [28]

How do we define a "spiritualized" activity? Steiner gave the examples of music, painting, and eurythmy—all three artistic activities that bring the possibility for expression of archetypal beauty. Through them, one is able to imbue deeper feeling or nuanced meaning to what might otherwise be just a mechanical process (it is possible to play music, to paint a wall, or to move the body in very earthly ways). But the very fact that these activities can be spiritualized, enriched, and ensouled means that they help a child lift out of the experience of the world as a purely physical place.

All small children still carry within them echoes of their experiences in the spiritual world, and they look for their resonance in the physical world. The qualities inherent in a spiritualized activity (explored in greater detail in the next section) help to reassure earthly children that they are in the right place and doing the right thing.

Expression of a true spiritual archetype—whether through musical harmony, blended color, or artistic movement—helps children remember their origin in the spiritual world (which is still not far away and, on many levels, remains more familiar than the physical world for small children). Bringing truthful spiritual qualities into activities, not through contemplation or description but through active experience, shows children that the earthly body can indeed become a proper garment for their whole being—physical, etheric, astral, and "I." Such spiritualized activity soothes the melancholy of the earthly child, balancing what is otherwise felt to be an altogether mechanical and materialistic physical experience.

To summarize: the earthly constitution is recognized through an unsculpted, doughy quality of the limbs and trunk; through a melancholy that relates to the density of the physical body; and by an experience of health and relief brought through spiritualized activity. While all three elements are important, not all three will necessarily be clearly emphasized in every earthly child. In some children we may be most struck by the sculptable quality of the limbs and trunk and in others by the melancholy, but the discovery of one of these characteristics in a child should spur us to look for the other, perhaps subtler expressions as well.

If we now turn to the cosmic side of the polarity, there are several polar qualities related to a too spiritual imbalance. The first is a rounded, not yet sculpted head pole. The associated element of the soul—as a contrast to the melancholy—was not explicitly named by Steiner. Nonetheless, we can infer it through his therapeutic indications, that "care must be taken not to remain in the contemplative element but...to evoke moods, feelings, tension, curiosity that are again relaxed, satisfied, and so on."[29] In a cosmic child there is not so much the challenge of a heavy mood that permeates everything (as is seen with the earthly child's melancholy) but instead a kind of lack of feeling. The objectivity that defines the physiology of the nerve–sense pole comes to dominate the cosmic child's feeling life. Because of this lack of passion, the cosmic child's inclination is to not engage, to be rather noncommittal toward the activities and passions of the physical world. The cosmic child does not feel the strong pull of deep passions or feelings.

The therapeutic gesture for cosmic children, therefore, is to guide them increasingly into the earthly realm through the feeling life. The cosmic child needs to be enticed to notice the earthly realm. While artistry helps lift the density of the earthly child's limbs, strong feeling engages the cosmic child to pay more attention to the earth. Through feeling the cosmic child becomes engaged. Steiner recommended a curriculum that requires attentiveness: "A child with a distinctly pronounced head organism will benefit from subjects such as history, geography, and literary history."[30] For all three of these subjects, one has to pay attention for an extended period of time in order to understand a progression (history of literature) or relationship (geography). "But we must take care not to remain in the contemplative element,"[31] because remaining in a contemplative space accentuates the existing cosmic nature of the children, such that they will remain in a "waking–sleeping activity,"[32] in which the astral body and "I" remain largely outside the body.

Moving away from that contemplative stance is not always easy, for the cosmic child feels very comfortable staying in that dreamy consciousness and finds that having grand philosophical discussions without really committing to any firm plan or perspective feels wonderful. There are many such children today who love to have long discussions (really, narrations) about far-away galaxies or dinosaurs—things that cannot be immediately experienced in the physical environment around the child. By contrast, genuine strong feeling creates a bridge to the surrounding world that helps make the environment so interesting (with the limbs as part of that environment) that children cannot help but notice what surrounds them.

Every child—in fact, every human being—stands somewhere on the spectrum between cosmic nonengagement and earthly melancholy.

The earthly–cosmic polarity provides a basic tool for looking at foundational developmental orientation for any young child. We may ask: What is the starting point for children? Are they oriented toward the physical world and deeply influenced by the earth or still closely connected to the heavens and reluctant to truly engage? That small step, by itself, helps us begin to observe children in a new way. While this might seem abstract, expressions of this melancholy or superficiality are everywhere.

Steiner described the earthly and cosmic poles in the 1920s—almost one hundred years ago—but expressions of its imbalance are ubiquitous. It is not getting any easier to bring the spiritual and hereditary streams together. It seems that on many levels it is actually becoming more difficult for this integration to take place than it was in previous generations. There is certainly no shortage of melancholy in childhood; just consider the skyrocketing rates of pharmacologic treatment for depression in children. At the same time children are now also constantly surrounded by technological substitutes for real engagement and interaction. Those tools are good at fooling us into thinking that we are in contact, but they only add to the circumvention of a healthy feeling life (which is already the inclination for a cosmic child). Children live in the midst of this struggle between the spiritual and the physical, though at a very foundational level they are striving to find the right steps toward healthy development.

What was previously worked through with archetypal processes of acute inflammation (such as chickenpox) are being replaced by chronic behavioral or developmental inflammations. A process that used to happen quickly, without much conscious participation, has been replaced by much longer challenges that often extend over a whole biography. The call to more consciously cultivate a real medical and pedagogical understanding of how each child finds a healthy home in the body feels evermore urgent. Sharing and articulating an anthroposophic understanding of the importance of fever and inflammation in childhood is one significant task. Another is to explore all the different ways that a fourfold interweaving incarnation process can happen. The interweaving of the four members also stands behind other kinds of activity that can be consciously guided and supported. Steiner observed: "The ancient Greeks had this knowledge, but it got lost. They spoke of the crisis of an illness, of catharsis, and they spoke in the same way of the effects of a work of art and of education."[33]

If we shift to a detailed physiologic picture given by Steiner in 1923, we find a precise description of the working together of the four members in the human being and how their varied interaction stands behind all the different aspects of our body's physiology.[34] Steiner described how the fourfold interweaving of physical, etheric, astral, and "I" stands not only behind inflammation but also all processes of growth and of nourishment and the restorative activities of the metabolism. Those are perhaps not so surprising. We can see how an inflammatory process and a digestive process are related, as there is a similar breakdown and overcoming process in each. Then we learn an additional important fact, that this fourfold weaving is also what gives us the ability to move our limbs. Our movement and the use of our limbs also have to be woven in early childhood. Then comes a further step—the same fourfold process also stands behind our ability to morally navigate and sense the outer world. Our morality also has to be woven. This may sound like a strange linkage, but careful observation of children shows that these processes do indeed parallel one another. Inflammation, movement, and moral sensing all come about through the fourfold interpenetration of the "I" and the astral, etheric, and physical bodies. Out of this relationship come some important insights—we have multiple therapeutic windows for working to support this fourfold integration process. As a kind of therapeutic correlate, we can strive to therapeutically support one expression of this process by consciously cultivating richer activity in a related realm. Then consider what are perhaps two sides of this coin, two outgrowths of this relationship, namely:

- As the classic inflammatory illnesses of childhood are receding, challenges in the development of healthy movement and true moral sensing are understandably on the rise.
- When a child is deeply challenged—either in movement or in moral perception—the opportunity to experience and work through fevers or other inflammations without suppressing the process can be a potent developmental opportunity.[35]

Observing movement in children is a wonderful developmental tool for gaining understanding about the process of integration. Steiner gave very specific indications related to a polarity of movement, which we can expand into much broader process and gestures of therapeutic support.

Chapter 5

Seeing the Incarnation Process through Movement

Just as every child's incarnation pathway falls into either the cosmic or earthly constitution—leaning subtly or strongly toward density or superficiality—we can see the same dynamic expressed through movement. The activity of the limbs gives us another view into how a child is able to take hold of the heredity stream. There is, naturally, a spectrum of movement, which we can express in terms of either too little movement (so that sometimes nothing is accomplished) or excessive movement (which is superficial and directed by little, if any, intention). Infants and toddlers exhibit both patterns, because the integration of their movement is still very immature. They switch back and forth between still inertia and clumsy, fidgeting movement. Healthy motor development in the first years of life works to create a functional space between those two extremes.

Motor development can be measured quite precisely through watching the attainment of specific milestones as well as the overcoming of primitive reflex patterns. These steps indicate that the activity of the "I" and astral body have come down into the structures of the physical body. Then the movement capacities we bring with us from the spiritual stream unite with and individualize the early, instinctive movement patterns (reflexes) gifted to us through the hereditary body. Steiner described how early in life the astral body carries "an extraordinary number of organs."[36] With time and experience, these still wholly spiritual organs "gradually slip down into the brain and also penetrate the sense organs," so that by adulthood the organs of our physical body have completely taken in this "astral inheritance."[37] In a young child, especially an infant, the connection between the structures of the astral body and the organs of the physical body is still quite primitive, so that the astral body remains somewhat disconnected. Through repeated practice the primitive "ball" of the astral body becomes better integrated. Initially, however,

> the ball at once recovers its shape. No matter how forcefully the child kicks, while it does make impressions in the astral body, they do not last. However, more and more is retained in the astral body in proportion to the child's learning to speak and form mental pictures that are retained in memory. To the extent that the child speaks and develops memory, to that extent less and less is thrown back. Rather does one see how the movements which the child now makes—no longer kicking, but reasonable movements with the arms and legs and so on—are retained in the astral body.[38]

Another way of saying this might be that at the beginning of life there is indeed movement, but it is largely random or instinctive. Such movement is not well connected with the consciousness of the astral body or the intention of the "I," and it occurs almost independently. When the astral body and the limb movements are successfully bridged, a child becomes more and more able to carry out "reasonable movements."

Primitive reflex patterns that persist beyond their normal developmental window are frequently associated with sensory, movement, and (eventual) academic challenges. If we view retained primitive reflexes as untransformed remnants of the hereditary body, this makes perfect sense. For if the hereditary stream has not been overcome, the physical body is not yet really a home, and it will impair a child's ability to function in the world. It is increasingly recognized—even outside the sensory integration and physical/occupational therapy fields—that guided movement experiences help a child to work through many retained reflex patterns and that there is very often an associated improvement with academic challenges. The work of authors like Sally Goddard Blythe make clear the essential role of healthy movement experiences in the life of the young child.[39] There are predictable, even lawful ways that this process unfolds—which can be addressed in effective, albeit sometimes rather mechanical forms of intervention (such as occupational or physical therapy exercises).

A much broader lens for observing this process of movement integration stands at the heart of the Waldorf Extra Lesson work, as described by Audrey E. McAllen. Her work—with continued elaboration by Joep Eikenboom—provides wonderful insights into the archetypal activities that should unfold out of the organs of the astral body for every child.[40] In this way the Extra Lesson work addresses the human being in its universality and can be broadly applied to many different kinds of children. Out of these insights, pedagogical exercises using movement, drawing, and contrasting color have been developed, which support archetypal sensory experiences so that the "I" and the astral body can better settle into the etheric and physical bodies. In many Waldorf schools the Extra Lesson and its related developmental assessments have become a valuable lens for viewing motor and sensory health. They offer an important pedagogical framework for seeing where support can be given. They provide tools to help each child move through archetypal experiences to a more complete integration.

That overarching understanding of the pathway into the hereditary body is different, however, from a more individualized, constitutional understanding of movement. They can complement each other, but they are different. It is often helpful to evaluate a child in the context of overall developmental progress (a kind of pedagogical view, related to the Extra Lesson) and then look toward the individual constitution to better understand why a child may be struggling to find a healthy pathway into the body.

Steiner emphasized the importance of observing movement. He placed it into the context of too little movement and too much movement and into the polarity of what we can explore as either "feeble" or "maniacal" movement.

Steiner explained that limited movement of the limbs is an expression of incomplete transformation of the hereditary body, because it is too dense. This is very much the same picture that Steiner gave for the earthly child, though in this case relating specifically to movement. When a child's experience is dominated, held down by the physical body, the body cannot act as a flexible vessel for the child's intention. In a certain sense, the child has been lamed by the physical body; the child is held back. If we observe the child in this situation, movement is slow—if it comes at all—and often clumsy. In the setting of imitative activities, the child commonly has good attention but poor participation. The limbs appear heavy, as if the child has not yet woken into the limbs that day (which is true, because they are not properly connected with the astral body). When movements do begin, they are often a beat late. Children are not so much asleep as experiencing a kind of persistent gravity. Children are usually aware that the limbs are not doing things as they wish and will even express frustration at not having the limbs be able to accomplish what is desired:

> We can recognize this condition in children by noticing how they react if we say to them, "Take a few steps forward." They will be unable to do it. They do not rightly understand what they have to do. That is, they understand quite well what we say, but do not convey the meaning to their legs; it is as though the legs do not want to receive it.... When we find this—that children have difficulties when we ask them to do something that involves the use of the legs, that they hesitate to bring their legs into movement at all—this is an early sign for us that their physical body has become too hardened and is unwilling to receive thoughts.[41]

Physical forces dominate and are not lifted into fourfold activity. The "I" may decide to initiate an activity, but it is not conveyed. The astral body does not bring tone to the muscles, and the etheric body struggles to bring levity to the limbs—"This stimulation [of the astral body] is not passed on to the etheric body, least of all to the physical."[42]

When Steiner described this kind of imbalanced movement to the participants of the curative course, Education for Special Needs—the course of lectures given to establish an education to support children with special needs[43]—he used the German word *schwachsinning,* literally *schwach* ("weak") and *sinnig* ("sensed"). That term has traditionally been translated in English anthroposophic literature as "feebleminded," though the term has unhelpful negative connotations that are not true to Steiner's original description. Newer works have used the term *constitutional sensory weakness,* which may sound less judgmental but still does not fully convey the physiologic process. A more useful translation might be "a sensing activity that has feeble limbs."

For these discussions we will simply refer to this more earthly side of the polarity as "feeble movement" (in order to avoid the confusions and reactions that inevitably arise from referring to a child as "feebleminded," which seems like a harsh judgment of intellectual abilities, when what we are really referring to is a limb process). The weakness comes not out of a problem within the head system, but rather with an inability to convey that activity properly to the arms and legs. The head is feeble only because it is unable to overcome the physical density of the limbs. These are children who "like best to let their hands and legs [you can notice the same thing in the hands] hang anyway and flop onto things."[44] It may seem from the outside that there is no activity or interest, but the lack of movement really stems from the physical body's burden (in contrast to other reasons for not wanting to participate, such as distraction or refusal as a means for getting attention). "The urge to do nothing, even when all the conditions are present and ready, the urge not to let the thought go over into work and action, is connected with feeblemindedness."[45]

We can look for another confirmation that the children's challenge lies primarily in the limbs when, trying to connect to the limbs, they also experience frustration and melancholy. Melancholy has been described as a quality of the earthly constitution: "Even when [earthly] children do not seem to be melancholic, there is, nonetheless, a nuance of melancholy alongside the apparent temperament. This is caused by the child's earth nature."[46] We find a parallel picture for the feeble constitution where Steiner used much the same language: "In such conditions the body bears too heavily on the soul, [and] we will find that moods of depression and melancholy also occur."[47]

The imbalance for both the earthly constitution and for feeble movement lies in the density and relatively impenetrable quality of the hereditary body, and so we can now start to look for a kind of spectrum of expression for this process: we may see it in an unsculpted, malleable quality of the child's limbs and trunk (earthly) or in a feeble limb activity, characterized by slow, impeded movement, or as a pervasive heaviness and melancholy, brought by the dominant experience of the physical body (both constitutional descriptions).

On the opposite side of the polarity we see a very different kind of limb activity. We see lots of movement, but movement that is undirected and rarely guided by any conscious intention. In this situation the density of the physical body is easily overcome, so it is not hard to create movement (evidenced by the fact that there is a lot of movement), but that movement activity is not integrated with the head. The head prefers to stay within the realm of its own activity, because at some level it still has not created a connection to the body. Movement happens, but out of habit or happenstance. Such children "perpetually move their fingers, catching hold of everything and kicking out in all directions with their feet."[48] The fingers move in the space around these children in much the same way that our eyes (appropriately) might dart about a room, scanning without deep examination. Steiner named this kind of superficial, excessive movement "maniacal."[49]

The heavy melancholy seen with feeble movement is now absent. Instead, children with maniacal movement use the body casually; movements remain largely unconscious. We can liken this to the astral body of very young children as described earlier, whereby a baby's kicking sends signals to the astral body, but they do not make any lasting impression. The astral body's connection to the limbs stays very young. It has not really connected with the limbs as organs.

There is a definite sanguine character to this kind of movement, but it is not necessarily joyful. A more classically sanguine temperament may flit from one thing to another because everything is so interesting, like wanting to make sure to meet all of the guests at a party in order not to miss a single one. In contrast, the maniacal child touches everything—sometimes in an invasive way—but does not really engage with any of the objects. Interaction stays a bit abstract, dispassionate. One object is treated just the same as another. Instead of all of the guests being fascinating, none of the guests is really worth talking to for any length of time. The many encounters hold minimal interest.

That kind of superficial interaction is very common and even consciously cultivated in many parts of modern life. The endless stream of sensory impressions that compete for our attention exacerbates this kind of superficiality. It bombards us and thereby trains us to commit less of ourselves to any specific interaction. Why engage when there are so many impressions to choose from? Why commit energies to more deeply engage with an impression if we learn that it might well be fake (particularly when there are so many virtual realities that surround us with screens and speakers)?

As a matter of simple sensory survival we all have to become more numbed, more maniacal in our sensory habits. What if every image and sound seen during an hour-long television show came all the way into us and made a deep soul impression? That would be totally overwhelming. The developmental challenge is that when there is no safe space for integration, it becomes easy for the "I" and the astral body to stay too much in the head realm, so that the limbs are left on their own. We, as a society, stay very much in the head realm. Whenever we see excessive, superficial movement, we can understand that the "I" and astral body, coming from the spiritual world, are staying too peripheral to the physical body and most especially to the limbs. This quality of unformed movement bears some relationship to the unformed head of the cosmic child, who stays too much in the spiritual stream and does not penetrate the body properly.

Appreciating these gestures is important, because the more we can connect a particular behavior to the spiritual process that stands behind it, the more tools we have for meeting and supporting the child. The earthly/cosmic and the feeble/maniacal polarities have traditionally not been linked in this way, but when we come to understand them as part of larger developmental gestures, they seem very much to be related therapeutic lenses. These two constitutional polarities are not necessarily synonymous, however. It is not a given that we will see unformed limbs in all children with feeble movement or rounded head and facial features with maniacal movement. Things appear slightly different in every single child.

This diversity of manifestations should not be interpreted as a suggestion to create some kind of a checklist, which now has to be completely met so that a child can be considered a particular constitution. That is not the intention at all. Such links are really only an invitation, so that if we are working a child who exhibit slow movement and then, out of deeper interest, we take off the child's shoes so that we can touch the feet, we can be pleasantly surprised by the soft and formless feet. Such consistencies can lend us more confidence that we are observing a true constitutional picture.

Chapter 6

Therapeutic Indications

Exploring the therapeutic indications for the feeble and maniacal polarity help make the realities of the process of integration come even more alive. The main therapeutic task is to help weave the four members together. We know that the "I" and astral body come through the spiritual stream and the physical body through the hereditary, but their meeting can really only happen with the mediation of the etheric body. We can therefore look for ways to strengthen the mediating activity of the etheric body as a way to balance and support either extreme of the polarity. Indeed, Steiner's therapeutic indications for this polarity live in this middle realm.

Before we come to Steiner's specific indications, it is important to understand that there are four differentiated, but related activities within the etheric body, which Steiner described as four "ethers." While they are all part of the general etheric activity, they correspond to and support the activities of the physical, etheric, astral, and "I." These four ethers constantly pour into one another in dynamic interaction—they are true mediators. Through them the physical body is lifted and lightened, and the "I" and astral are able to bring form and direction to the body's activities. We will try to understand this interaction by tracing their activity from two directions: first from physical substance up to the higher members and then from the spiritual members on high down to an earthly orientation.

We can begin by tracing the pathway of a mineral, dead substance, as it comes into a living being. This is a lifting activity. It provides the foundation for further refinements of substance that allow what is physical to move to the state of a plant, then to an animal, and finally to that of a human being.[50]

In the plant (which as an organism contains a physical and an etheric body), mineral substance that is normally subject to the laws of gravity is shifted to a state of levity. Through this lifting, what is normally "lifeless" substance becomes "living substance."[51] Gravitational forces acting out of the center of the earth, which continually pull down toward that center, are met and countered by lifting etheric forces that act from the periphery. This interaction between lifeless and living substance is dynamic and does not go only one way. There is also a continuous release out of the plant's living substance back toward a mineral state. What rejoins the mineral state is inherently different from its original form—an example of this would be the bark of a tree. Bark is hard, a mineralized shell released from the cambium of the tree. It is no longer living in a dynamic growth state, but it has certainly changed from the mineral world (the soil of the earth) from whence it began. This process of lifting and releasing is continuously happening because of the presence of etheric forces. This lifting activity is made possible by what Steiner described as the life ether, which in a plant sustains the ongoing engagement and enlivening of mineral substance through the activity of the roots. In the human being, that same kind of lifting and enlivening activity takes place through the process of absorption, from an inner space—the lumen of the intestine—into the flowing activity of the surrounding lymphatic system.[52] The life ether is active wherever there is a continuous lifting and release of substance between the lifeless and the living state. It can be thought of as a circle of activity (see page 49, bottom of fig. 1).

In an animal (which has a physical, an etheric, and an astral body), that same activity of the life ether lifts substance from the mineral realm into a living, plantlike activity, but then etheric activity continues further. What was made into living substance goes on through further refinement to become "sentient substance."[53] What was previously living and dynamic now provides the foundation for capacities related to sensing the environment. In an animal there is therefore a bidirectional streaming: some enlivened substance is released back toward the mineral realm, but another portion is held so that it can be lifted higher through the activity of the chemical ether. The chemical ether finds its greatest physiologic expression in the forming and dissolving of chemical and molecular bonds, a shaping of what is enlivened but as yet unformed substance. Substance that is now lifted up toward sensing activity builds a relationship to the astral body. This kind of sentient substance is made possible by the activity of the light ether.

From sentient substance there is also a continual release back toward living substance and then eventually a further release back to mineral substance. Steiner stated that the end product of this twofold release in an animal is its manure. Where for the plant organism there is only a single ring of activity, in the animal there exists a twofold streaming mediated by the activities of the life ether, the chemical ether, and the light ether (see fig. 1).

Each human being—in addition to physical, etheric, and astral bodies—also has an "I," so that a threefold process of separation and excretion takes place. Substance that in an animal has been raised to a sensing capacity now undergoes an addition level of refinement: "Substance, which then becomes the bearer of the self-conscious spirit, is separated out of the sentient substance."[54] What was simply sensing (in the realm of the light ether) now becomes self-sensing. The awareness of oneself as a distinct, independent being comes about in the realm of the warmth ether. The warmth ether is most immediately connected to spiritual forces and makes possible the integration of parts into a whole. It is the warmth ether that transforms substance into human substance. Even here the process is still dynamic. From the warmth ether's self-conscious activity there is a continual excretion of our animal nature and from sentient substance down to living substance and back down to the mineral realm.

This lifting activity also works in the realm of action and behavior. Here the beginning substance at the bottom of the process is instinct, something we receive as an innate gift but which really exists outside our own individuality. What can be outwardly observed as the physical, mineral body corresponds to instinct in the realm of our will. Like the hereditary body that we receive and then have to work to make our own, "When speaking of instinct, either in animals or in its weaker human form, we will always regard it as something stamped upon the being from without."[55]

As our life ether takes hold of and enlivens the physical body, so do etheric forces permeate our instinct, and like the activity of the chemical ether "instinct becomes impulse...more inward in its nature."[56] We have lifted what was outside and are now able to incorporate it into the inner realm. We move from the realm of the life ether to that of the chemical ether.

The astral body, or the sentient body, works to continue the refinement: "It takes hold of impulse, and then not only is this made more inward, but instinct and impulse are both lifted into consciousness, and in this way desire arises."[57] Desire can be characterized as an inward sensing process that arises out of the further refinement of what was initially an impulse. This is the realm of the light ether, giving form to activity, but that form is not static. Desire lives in a dynamic state, for when "speaking of desire you speak of something which is created afresh by the soul every time. A desire is not necessarily something belonging to the character; it need not be attached to the soul, but it comes and goes."[58] This coming and going is the lifting of substance from the living state to the sentient state, from the chemical ether to the light ether.

When we move one level higher, to the activity of the warmth ether, desire becomes "motive" or "wish," and "wish" is ultimately described by Steiner as "something that can be faintly heard beneath the impulse of will, but which is still of the nature of will.... We perceive this wishing particularly clearly when we carry out something which arises out of a motive in our will, and then we think it over and say to ourselves; what you did then you could do much better."[59] Sensed desire, lifted to self-conscious motive, becomes a seed for better activity in the future, a wish. For the result of our self-conscious activity is not just to judge our behavior in the past but also to create a refined secretion directed

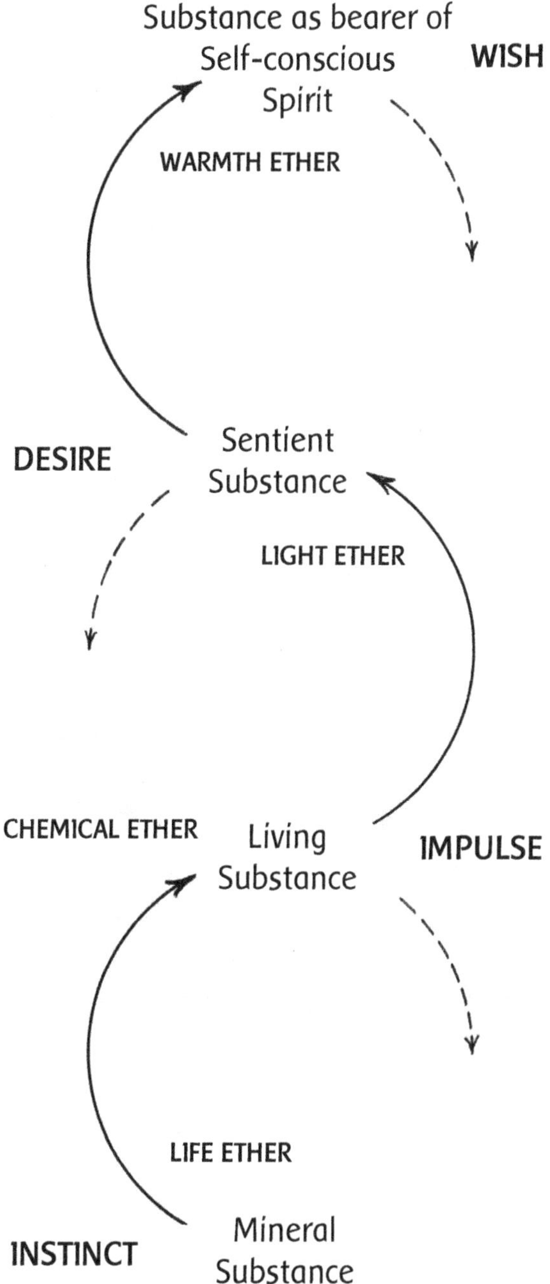

Figure 1: The upward streaming pathway of substance through the ethers, from lifeless substance to self-conscious substance

toward the future—one that says that a person will do it much better next time. The activity of the warmth ether stimulates us to continually improve and refine ourselves through future development.[60] That kind of intention can be considered the purest refinement of our hereditary body, in which our heritage of the past is fully claimed and now totally individualized for our work in the future.

The activities modulated by these four ethers—from lifeless substance to living substance to sentient substance to self-conscious substance and from instinct to impulse to desire to wish—make possible our life as human beings. The four ethers allow the spiritual stream and the hereditary stream to meet. If this ascending, lifting activity is weakened, we must support it therapeutically, and one of the places we can potently guide this interweaving is with the movement of eurythmy therapy. Through spiritualized limb movement we can encourage deeper integration. Steiner's therapeutic indications for movement, for the feeble and maniacal constitutions, are indeed eurythmy exercises, which relate closely to the activity of the four ethers.

Steiner began with the picture of lifeless, unpenetrated substance and the need to loosen and enliven it: "In the case of feebleminded children, what we have to do is bring mobility into their metabolic–limb system; this will also stimulate their whole spiritual nature. Let such children do eurythmy movements for R, L, S, and I ["ee"], and you will see its good effect."[61] This therapeutic sequence shows us exactly what feeble children need to overcome their unwieldy physical body. The differentiated qualities of the eurythmy sounds of this sequence take us through the ascending activity of the ethers.

Note that the following descriptions are not intended to teach the eurythmy gestures—that is really best done with a trained therapeutic eurythmist. Still, working to understand the archetypes behind the movements can give us wonderful insight into the needs of the child with feeble movement. Exploring the progression can also help us to develop imaginations for other kinds of medical or pedagogical activity that can lend a similar kind of developmental support.

The sequence begins with "R," a eurythmy gesture that is robust and invigorating: "The R expresses a rolling, a revolving; it the imitation of anything which gives the impression of turning, rolling, revolving."[62] The movement is done with the arms in large circles, going from above to the front, to below and then back. This movement is done in the vertical, or sagittal, plane. In the curative course Steiner alternatively described the eurythmy "R" as "a 'turning'; something is turning around, is revolving. There at once you have mobility."[63] In doing an "R" gesture, one can experience real energy and intensity. The energy and mobility it requires are integral to the gesture—initially, perhaps, even more important than the actual form. We can summarize by saying that the very first step for a child with feeble movement should be activity with invigorating movement and mobility, a deep in-breath, a stirring right down into the substance of the body.

The second eurythmy sound in the sequence is "L," which is also circular but more gentle and flowing. Movement is directed laterally, then inwardly, with an emphasis on creating a lifting, levity gesture from below to above, then circling round again. The hands, in parallel, rise up in the middle, slightly forward, move out expanding, and come down with the arms extended and slightly back, slowing at the bottom as they gather to then again rise up in front. There is just enough form to guide the movement but not enough to ever stop its progression. In Steiner's words:

> Think what formative forces the tongue is developing when L is spoken! L is the sound that signifies yielding or compliance, adapting oneself to fall in with something. And that is what the boy's organism needs; to be made pliant and supple, so that it shall be ready to adapt itself.[64]

Also:

> [There is] something creative, or formative, in the sound, and sculptors are very much tempted when working on the figures they are creating to make a movement of the tongue similar to the movement that the tongue makes when forming the sound

> L.... It was said in the old mysteries that *L* is the creative, formative element in all things and beings—the force that overcomes matter in the creation of form.[65]

> *L* was seen in the mysteries as a sound having special magical qualities, for when we give form to something it follows that we have power over it.[66]

This second step of the sequence helps children make their physical body yielding and compliant, so that it can then be given proper form.

The eurythmy movement for *S*, the third sound in the sequence, also has curving movements, but now with much greater form and even some fire. It is formed with the arms, but with intensity and faster movement, a crisscross weaving across the midline in front of the body. The *S* starts and stops in form, with swift movement in between. According to Steiner:

> The feeling lying behind the curved and sinuous line of S is really extraordinarily complicated, but primarily it may be said to consist of a powerful peace-bringing element, bringing calm and peace into that which is in a state of unrest, and this force carries with it the feeling of certainty, the feeling of being able to penetrate into the hidden nature of something and in so doing to bring about a state of calmness and rest.... S—a bringing of calm into that which is agitated, and the certainty that the means employed will have the desired effect.[67]

From revolving and mobility to yielding compliance, the child now takes a step toward calmness and penetration. It is essential, however, that the first two steps have taken place first, because for the child with a too dense hereditary body there can be no sense of rest and calmness unless the body is first brought into invigorating movement and mobility. The order of the sequence is important.

The sequence finishes with the eurythmy gesture "I" [referring to the German sound for the vowel, pronounced "ee"].[68] "I[ee]" helps a child come into uprightness. It is not a static uprightness, for the gesture arises out of a two-streamed stretching, pushing down against the earth with the feet and simultaneously up toward the heavens with the head, with one hand gesturing down and the other up. Where the "feeble" child initially was held captive by the gravity of the physical body, now there has been an overcoming, and the child's experience of the physical body becomes one of capacity, not just a burden: "Behind the sound *I* ['ee'] there is always a vindication of oneself, an assertion of oneself."[69] From revolving to yielding, from calmness to self-assertion, children experience how the inherited physical body can become a fitting garment for their true individuality. This sequence is immensely satisfying for feeble children, who inwardly long to find this kind of pathway for transformation.

We find some very practical applications for understanding the progression of this eurythmy sequence, for the child with feeble movement often runs into difficulties in two different ways. A first challenge comes if we expect a feeble child to be capable immediately, without a warm-up. (Remember Steiner's characterization of the situation where all the conditions are right for something to happen, but the child does nothing.) This brings frustration (even exasperation), but it happens because the feeble child's physical body resists. It is unwieldy, like a piece of wax that is cold and hard. No matter how much such children may wish to participate, they simply cannot do it at the drop of a hat. We need to identify these children, because it is unfair and may even add to their inherent melancholy if we expect them to move immediately, capably, and quickly into a new activity. They always first need to stir and loosen themselves to mobilize and penetrate their limbs.

Another challenge arises for children with feeble movement when they desperately work to create that stirring, revolving movement from the beginning of the eurythmy sequence (the *R* and *L*), but doing it at the wrong time. Then the adults around may throw up their hands and say, "When I need these children to move, they never move, and when I need them to be still or complete a task, they barrel around the classroom!" This sentiment may be true, but it fails to recognize that feeble children are not trying to be naughty; they are simply trying to stir their spiritual self into their physical. This longing for gross motor movement can evolve into a very challenging and also heartbreaking cycle if such children are never given an opportunity to do repetitive, big, stirring movements. If the activities offered to children are always too formed or too quiet and delicate, those with feeble movement then have to create a different, perhaps socially inconvenient pathway to lay claim to the physical body. Careful observation can help us appreciate whether such inopportune movement is naughty or whether it is a way of creating their own therapy. If big, exaggerated movements repeatedly arise from a therapeutic longing, then we need to create socially healthy activities for that sequence to unfold. We need to learn to think of big, stirring movements as being the developmental task of feeble children. It is very encouraging for children when that movement task can be supported within the context of their daily life. Practical work, especially when it contributes to the greater good, can become a wonderful outlet for the need to do repetitive limb work.

If we return for a moment to the indications for the early child, we are reminded that in addition to eurythmy exercises, Steiner also encouraged music and painting as very important spiritualized activities to lift and lighten the physical body. All three involve movement—of the limbs for eurythmy and painting, and of the lips, tongue, and vocal cords for singing—and all three are refined through repetition and practice. Eurythmy, music, and painting are also important, established elements in the Waldorf curriculum. It is not that great a leap to consider how the qualities of the four eurythmy gestures can be translated into many different kinds of activities: stirring gross motor movement, participating and responding, ensouling with story or imagination, and triumphing over the physical realm. A child with feeble movement patterns needs to regularly experience stirring gross motor activities, such as jumping, running, skipping, lifting, and rolling. These movements need to be carried on for a long enough time that the child is really able to fully penetrate into the movement and even be carried by it. This means that the child moves past being self-conscious about the movement and, it is hoped, even gets a little red in the face or begins to breathe harder. Stirring movements are already a part of many traditional children's activities:

- Traditional circle games often incorporate this stirring through fast movement, such as when someone is tagged and then has to run to try to catch the first child (as in the game Duck, Duck, Goose). These games are wonderful and even more satisfying for the child with feeble movement if the game can go on long enough for there to be repeated chances to run. Better yet, start with a lot of running and then progress into the chasing and the more careful tagging part of the game. The more children with feeble limbs can start with large, gross motor movement, the better they will then be able to participate in the game.
- Beanbag games, where something is tossed or passed over and over, also have this quality of repetitive gross motor movement. Again, for the feeble child, it is best if the game can be carried on long enough that it can first be experienced as pure movement; then, once the "molasses" has been stirred, the activity can become more formed and intentional.
- Jumping rope (what better way to overcome gravity?) is another wonderful opportunity. The more feeble children jump, the better they gets, but they may need multiple turns, as the first few will probably be unsuccessful. You will regularly see that these children improve as they loosen the physical body and better penetrate their limbs. After such a warm-up period, jumping can be supplemented gradually with rhymes and rhythms.
- For older grade school children, juggling is a wonderful, more advanced activity that brings the same qualities. What a triumph when children with feeble movement can juggle three balls successfully!

Out of such stirring movement the body becomes more flexible, and it is really only at this point that the child with feeble movement can begin to participate and respond in an activity. Group play now becomes more possible, as does imitative activity. There is more freedom to interact in a more responsive way. The child's experience of the body relates more closely to the "L"—yielding and compliant. We can observe that the child feels relieved. Earthly melancholy has lifted a bit, and the child is now better able to make use of the limbs. For some very earthly children, who are working to penetrate a quite dense physical body, much of their early childhood may be devoted to just getting to this step: "R" and "L," "R" and "L," "R" and "L."

The qualities of the additional eurythmy sounds, the "S" and the "I[ee]," can unfold in subtle but very satisfying ways when we involve children in movement that is practical and useful, in movement that is part of real work. Real work is different from just play or exercise because it is trying to accomplish something, and that accomplishment is important for the "S" and the "I[ee]" to really be experienced. Such work often involves repetitive gross motor activity, such as moving tables, carrying groceries, or maybe even rolling logs, but it does not stay there. A slightly tongue-in-cheek way to think about this need for gross motor movement is to consider what would happen if we were to develop a very modern but also quite materialistic approach to this problem. We would do a lot of research to determine what might be an appropriate substitute activity to replace "work." We would do many different kinds of analysis in order to identify the most essential parts, isolate them, and then create a machine that would involve a child in the most efficient kinds of stirring movement possible. That kind of machine might artificially replicate the beginning of the feeble sequence, but it would be creating gross motor movement just for the sake of gross motor movement. When we ask the child to help with tasks that are real and practical, we invite healthy form into the activity, and this is "S." Children do this naturally when their play becomes task-oriented, such as dragging logs or branches to one place and then slowing piling and placing the wood to make the walls of a house; or, rolling big balls of snow to make a snowman who becomes more and more refined in his form, eventually taking on a human likeness. Intention brings form into play, and working to do something well or correctly also develops moral health.

As recently as a hundred years ago people still lived very strongly with the morality and rightfulness of a specific trade. A child, grown old enough to be a youth, would be apprenticed to a master tradesperson. The child learned not only a method of earthly activity but also the rightful knowledge and lore that accompanied it. Different tradesmen—mason, smith, butcher, baker—carried out vigorous physical activity, but with the consciousness that it contributed in an important way to the health of the community. Such activity was also connected to spiritual pictures, with the trades related to archetypes of thought or interaction and protected by patron saints or spirits. In this way the physical work of the limbs was continuously lifted into the "major" mood of the morally healthy archetype and not allowed to fall into the minor strains of physicality performed only for its own sake. A young child is still living strongly with the memory of exactly those kinds of spiritual archetypes. It is reassuring and gratifying for a child to see those truths given earthly activity and to know that we do work not just for work's sake but because it is good.

The end of the therapeutic sequence, the "I[ee]," brings an experience of uprightness, of triumph over the weight of the physical realm. Now it is possible for an assertion of self and for the sense of satisfaction that comes through feeling capable in the body. After a lot of work and movement the child can now come to rest. In daily activity or play this experience comes when there is a moment dedicated to standing back and admiring what has been done—looking at the beauty of the bread that has been baked or the work that has gone into building a fort out of logs. In that moment the weight of the physical body is overcome and the body, as home, put into proper order. In the imaginative language of a fairy tale, this step often comes at the conclusion of a story, when the youth or maiden is crowned as a king or queen. That, too, is an expression of "I[ee]" (see fig. 2).

This therapeutic progression clearly finds its greatest potency by having a child do the exercises with a therapeutic eurythmist, but there are many instances when we are looking to find as many ways as possible to support a feeble child. Then it is both fair and appropriate to consider how the elements of this progression can be woven into the daily activities of a child. This can be brought in two simple but very helpful ways: we can turn to large, stirring movement to help engage and "lighten" the body, and then we can help the child find real work that helps contribute to the outside world.

We come now to the complementary pathway for a child with maniacal movement patterns. Here we again must work to facilitate integration through the weaving of the four ethers but this time in a descending motion, from the spiritual world down to the earthly. The therapeutic task for this sequence is to bring consciousness and intentionality all the way down into the limbs and the metabolism. Where the therapeutic gesture for the child with feeble movement begins down below and works its way up, the sequence for maniacal movement starts in the cosmos and comes down. The progression begins in the highest of the ethers, with cosmic warmth, which then, as it moves down, enlivens the activities of light ether, chemical ether, and life ether.

Rudolf Steiner described that pathway from the spiritual world down into the body as a kind of respiration with the cosmos, whereby "a human birth continuously occurs out of the macrocosm."[70] This birthing from the spiritual world begins with "an extraordinarily fine reception of warmth from the macrocosm—inhalation of warmth and exhalation of warmth."[71] Such inhalation of warmth is connected most closely with the head and nerve pathways, but "the warmth carries with it light, macrocosmic chemism, and macrocosmic life, or vitality. Light ether, chemical ether, and life ether from the macrocosm are carried by the inhalation of warmth into the human organism."[72] Each

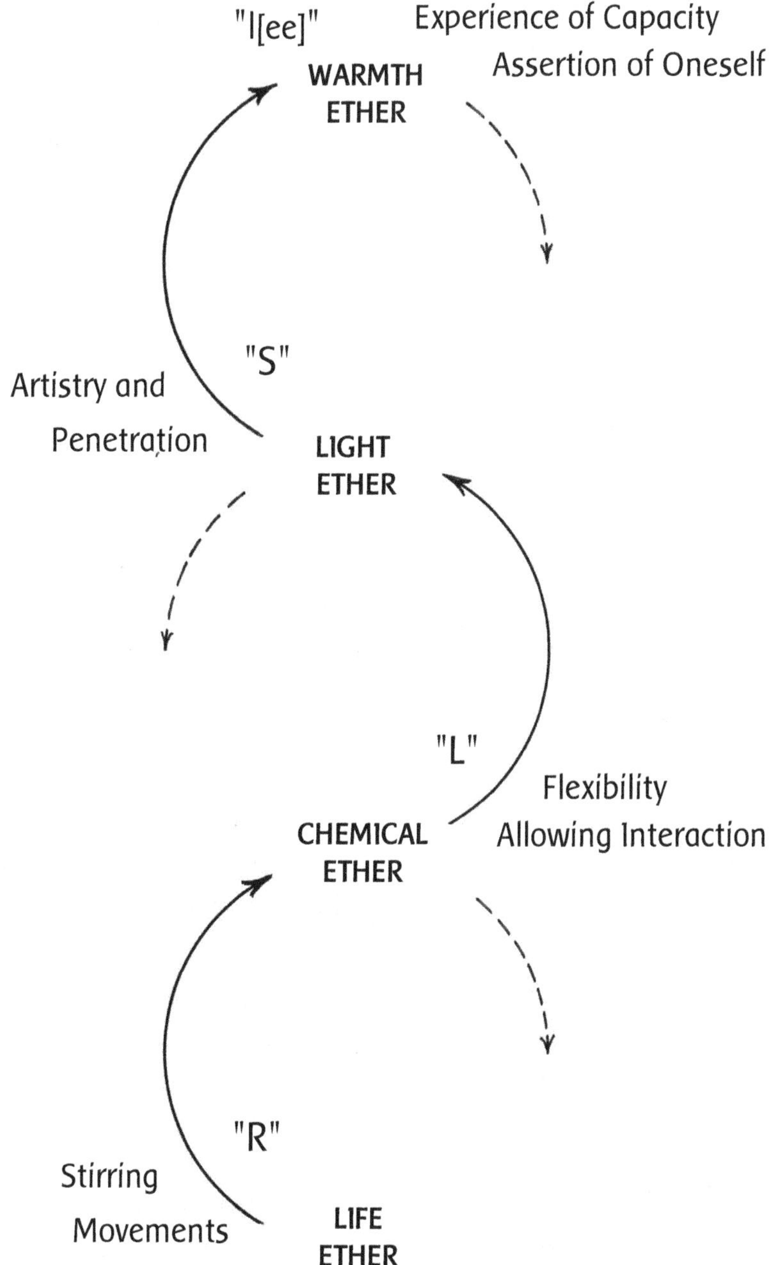

Figure 2: The upward-streaming pathway through the ethers, in relation to the eurythmy sequence "R, L, S, I"

ether unfolds its own activity, giving rise to our physiologic activity and the physical structures that serve it. Through this downward cascade of formative activity, thinking, feeling, and then willing develop.

We find anatomical expression of this downward cascade as well: out of the more global warmth ether comes light ether, which allows for thinking activity. Light ether stands behind all sensing activity and the form of our sense organs. According to Steiner, at the upper border of our respiratory activity, light ether comes to a stop, and the chemical ether becomes most active. The chemical ether unfolds its activity to the threshold where inhalation meets exhalation and then stops. Beyond respiration, in the place between exhalation and metabolism, we find the life ether. This cascade brings different formative activities, and out of the formative activities come the actual shapes of the organs. Those formative activities manifest physically in the formation of the nerve pathways, followed by the architecture of the arterial circulation, then the venous circulation, and finally the lymphatic system (see fig. 3).[73] This continuously birthed formative activity, breathed from the cosmos, provides the pathway for the spiritual stream to come into relation with the hereditary body.

When this cascade of formative activity is weakened or incomplete, movement loses its guidance and intention. This cascade is where we need to work therapeutically for children with maniacal tendencies. Excessive, unguided movement does not benefit in the same way from loosening the physical body, because these children are not so much being held back by the physical body as they do not come into a proper relationship with it. Rather, there needs to be a proper housing of the "I" and astral body within the physical and etheric, so that the limbs and their movements can be truly known and directed. This downwardly directed therapeutic pathway has its own eurythmy sequence, as given by Steiner: "On the other hand, when we have children with a tendency to mania, then, knowing how it is with their metabolic–limb system, we will have them do the movements for *M, N, B, P, A* [as in *father*], and *U* [as in *Ruth*]."[74]

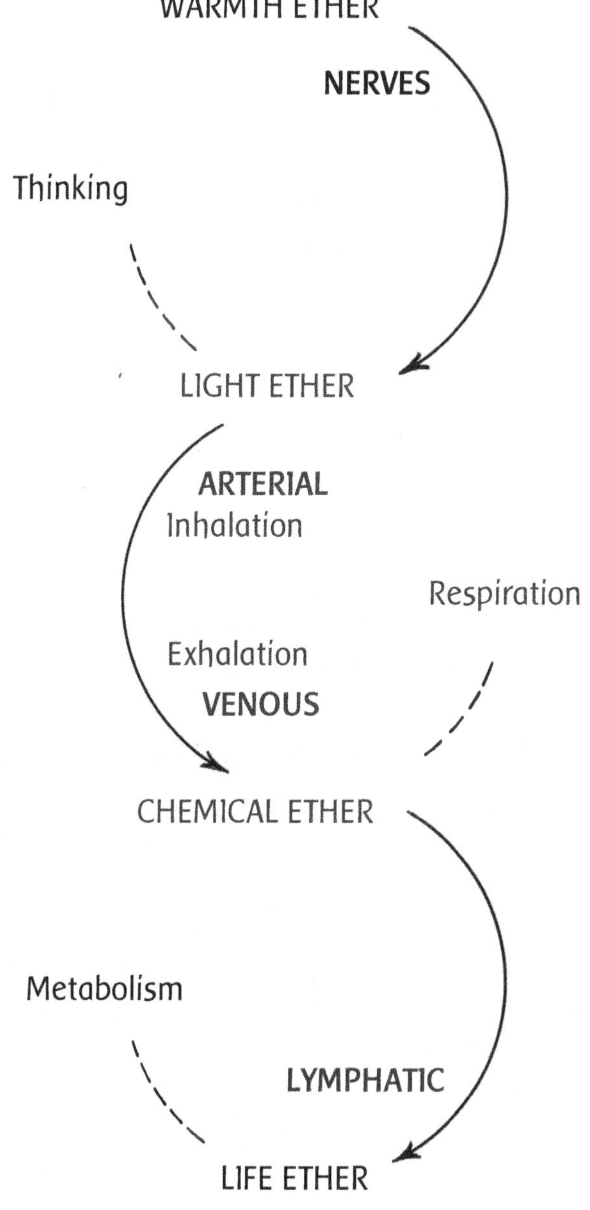

Figure 3: The descending pathway through the ethers, from the nerves to the lymphatic system.

The child with maniacal movement patterns shows excessive movement that almost seems to take on a life of its own. Instead of having trouble establishing movement and requiring repetition to fully come into the limbs, maniacal movement comes easily and then is quickly abandoned—which results not in the movement's stopping, but continuing and sometimes repeating without guidance. This brings about a certain rigidity within the etheric body, because when the etheric is not held by the higher members, it will echo on without adjustment or refinement. The etheric body faithfully holds an impression, like a ship that has been launched into the sea but has no one holding the rudder.

The first sound of the maniacal therapeutic eurythmy movement sequence is *M*. "M" warms and allows a stuck activity to be breathed out so that a fresh activity can start anew: "We have therefore to see that the out-breathing is stimulated as much as ever possible, and that the boy himself participates in it. This happens in *M*, the sound that belongs particularly to the out-breathing. When it is done in eurythmy, the whole limb system comes in to help."[75] The gentle, wavelike movement of the arms, front to back and back to front at the height of the heart, slows and integrates the speed of the head and the speed of the limbs. The child's activity up until now has been too much independent limb and too much independent head. Now the two are softened and brought together. The warmth of "M" helps to unite attention with activity: "In the way in which the sound is carried on the stream of the breath we feel that it conforms itself to everything and understands everything. *M* signifies that which is deeply felt and understood...imitation, combined with understanding."[76] The beginning of the maniacal eurythmy sequence supports exhalation and allows for new feeling and meaning.

Then comes *N*, which is related to the warmth and respiration of *M* but lives more in boundary. It anticipates (and in some ways mirrors) the maniacal tendency to too quickly abandon and dismiss:

> Understanding mingled with a feeling of repulsion, understanding tinged with irony.... Why make such a fuss over it? Of course, it is absolutely obvious—*N*.... To get into the right mood for the *N*-movement, we should imagine that we are dealing with someone who is quite stupid, someone who, in conversation, keeps placing great emphasis on very ordinary things. We want to make such individuals realize that they really are too stupid, that we can understand the whole matter very quickly and wish to get away from the whole thing as quickly as possible. That is the experience."[77]

Children with maniacal movement cannot sustain the "M" gesture alone—it does not take long before the child loses interest. If the "M" is continued, the movement soon becomes mechanical, which is exactly what happens when the limbs are abandoned by the higher members in the head. The "N"—reaching out and down slowly with one's arms to find a boundary, then suddenly lifting up and pulling back—allows children to inhale back into themselves (moving back toward a more limited engagement, a kind of dismissal); it matches the children's own natural inclination. Finding the right moment for that retreat within the "N" movement asks the child to better ensoul the limbs, because the "N" movement is complete only when there has first been a real penetration and meeting, before pulling back. Its therapeutic strength comes from the fact that it works to meet the children exactly where they are. "N provides the tendency to lead back into what belongs to the intellect."[78] After uniting head and limbs, "N" allows the child to consciously retreat back a little, but only after an awareness of deeper encounter.

The therapeutic sequence as a whole works very strongly with these kinds of paired activities and contrasts, between "M" and "N," "B" and "P," "A" and "U." Taken as single movements alone, the "M" and the "N" share a process of asking the child to foster thoughtful encounter and then to release. In "M" it is the release of the movement (say, forward) and then waiting to join the movement again as it comes back. For "N" it is the shift from slow approach to sudden rejection. There is a shifting alternation built into each individual movement, but as a pair they contrast with each other and build a larger polarity for the release moment, with the "M" as an outbreath and the release of the "N" as a retreat back in. "M" asks something very new of the child. "N" allows the child to do what is more natural. They work together to create a rhythmic feeling activity between exhalation and inhalation.

A similar activity comes through the pairing of "B" and "P." Now the activity relates more intimately to the body. This pairing directs the child to experience the body (not just the head) as home. Where the "M" supports a breathing out, "B," in a complementary way, helps the child to settle in. "B is always an enveloping, a kind of shelter. To put it somewhat crudely B might be said to be the house in which one lives."[79] The "B," with arms reaching out to a wide expanse and then settling in to find an embracing gesture, lets the child come in to find a boundary and hold it. "B" begins with movement, then defines a space within. The child is led to the experience of feeling "Here I am, housed within this space, housed within this body." We come from the outside in.

Steiner regularly linked "B" and "P," though we can experience their difference just through the sounds: the "B" sound is made more with the lips pressed together, the cheeks and the inner space of the mouth filled with air. Our awareness of the mouth is inward with "B." With "P" the lips are more pursed, pushing outward, and the air stream is directed out. Awareness is directed out. The eurythmy gesture for "P" marks a boundary, but instead of the arms turned in toward the body in an embrace (the inner space), the arms, raised up to the level of the brow, turn out. They come in to meet a boundary and then push out, and that boundary is carried all the way down through the body. The boundary is defined from the inside, looking out. Like the "N," the "P" brings acknowledgement of boundary, but now more related to the body. This second pairing helps the maniacal child find and better settle into the body as a home (*B*), then allows the child to consciously experience a boundary with the surrounding world, now from inside that home (*P*).

In *A* and *U*, we come to the third pairing of the sequence. *M* and *N* brought an exhalation and then an inhalation. *B* and *P* help children experience the body as a house, defined through its boundaries. With *A* and *U*, a much stronger formative activity arises, one that connects not just with breathing or with the body but with the earth and the cosmos. These two vowel gestures bring reverence and then solemnity. In the "A" gesture (*a* as in *father*), the arms are gently but fully extended into a V-shaped angle above the head:

> In *A* there lies a feeling of wonder, astonishment.... O human, you have derived your being from two different points of universal space. You must stretch out your arms to lay hold of the forces streaming in from these two directions, and in so doing you take into yourself what gave you birth. You must feel how these forces are streaming through your arms and coming together in your breast. This will give you a real experience of the sound "A."[80]

The radiating experience of the "A" connects us with the world, so that we can feel fully part of it. From this connection comes wonder, such a different experience from the usually superficial engagement of the maniacal child.

With *U*, children powerfully penetrate all the way down into the body, down into the limbs. For children who rarely fully engage with the body or direct movement consciously, *U* is powerful medicine: "*U*... [is] chosen to help children become aware of themselves in themselves."[81] Again, just as each of the pairings begins with quieter gesture (the exhalation of "M," the housing of "B, the wonder of "A"), so now the second gesture helps to the pull the children in. For *N* it was understanding with repulsion, and for *P* it was the boundary of the house. "Behind *U* is the feeling of becoming smaller, of being chilled and stiffened with cold. There is the feeling of drawing back into oneself, of holding fast to oneself."[82] The retreat is not simply away from the world, but pulling deeply back into oneself (see fig. 4).

This paired eurythmy sequence for maniacal movement is a real journey. The different elements are described in detail because as a sequence they help us to better understand what the maniacal child is looking for. Ultimately, the child whose fingers and hands are constantly striking out at the world, without guidance and without reverence, does long to find a richer connection to the surrounding world. By the very nature of their incarnation process, these children do not yet know how to make a meaningful meeting place. If their inclination for separate head and separate hands is left too long, then the world does indeed look to be a very boring place. There is little experience of meaningful connection. To counter this, the maniacal child needs help in learning how to look at the world with a long enough gaze to realize how interesting the world can be.

How can this be brought into wider application? Can we bring the underlying gesture of these movements into daily activity? As we have seen, for the child with feeble movement the starting place is stirring movement. For the child with maniacal movement the answer does not come through moving more but instead through breathing into an experience of less movement so that the activity of the limbs can be better ensouled. The important elements we can find in architecture of the eurythmy sequence are these:

- There is a breathing back and forth between the pairings, encouraging the child to breathe out and then pull back.
- The alternation repeats, so that with each "breath" the children are invited to become more and more deeply settled in themselves. Without this kind of alternating breathing (including the opportunity to pull back), maniacal children are not likely to stay engaged for very long.
- Also, the first steps of the pairings are all quieting, creating the space for a different kind of activity to begin. They act as an invitation for something new.

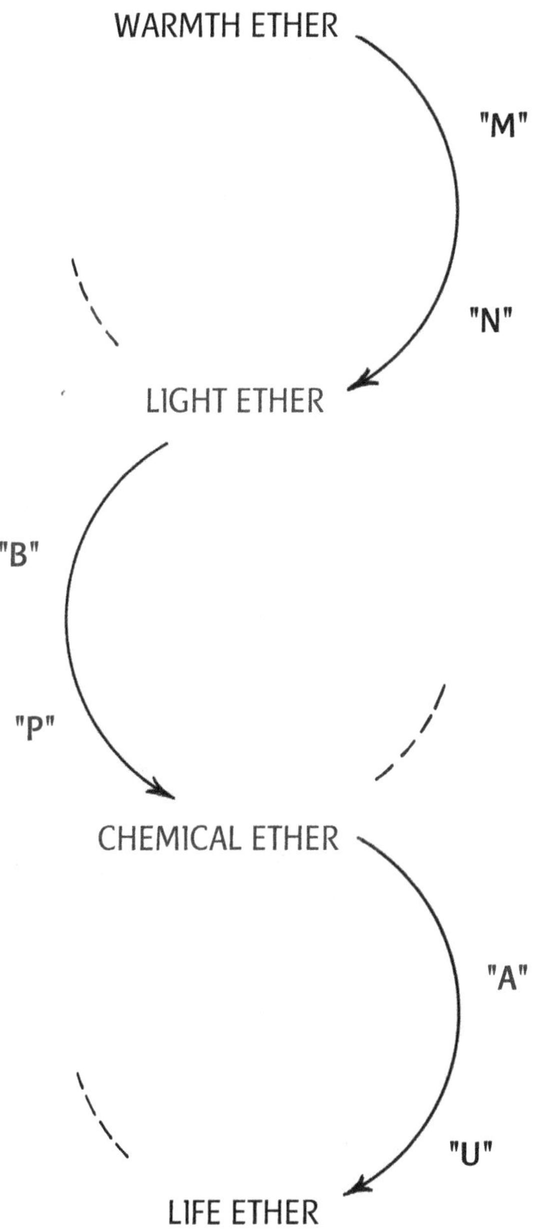

Figure 4: The descending pathway through the ethers, in relation to the eurythmy sequence "M, N, B, P, A, U"

- The gestures become more and more powerful and settle more and more deeply into the body. The breathing of *M* and boundary of *N* deepen all the way down to the wonder of *A* and sense of self in *U*.

We can find further clues for broadening this maniacal sequence by incorporating Steiner's indications for the cosmic child, who stays too easily in a contemplative gesture. The movements of the eurythmy sequence have complementary pedagogical techniques. Steiner reminded us how for the cosmic child the experience of boundary can be evoked through "moods, feelings, tensions, curiosity that are again relaxed, satisfied, and so on."[83] We can create a complementary activity to the paired gestures of eurythmy limb movement through creating an alternation of mood and imagination. Strong, shifting feeling awakens awareness within the child and makes it possible to connect more with the outside world. There arises an enhanced relationship between world and self that is accomplished through feeling. We do this naturally when we slow down enough to really observe, which is usually most easily done when we consider the natural world. The child with cosmic or maniacal tendencies needs to be invited to find that connection. In general, imaginations invite that kind of deeper consideration.

Some examples, which could come at the start of a circle time in the classroom to gather everyone's attention or as a pause on a walk are these:

- Begin with a quiet observation of the natural world, such as listening for the rain, feeling the wind on our faces or the warmth of the sun on our backs (an experience similar to the eurythmy "M"). It often works better if we are calling forth a sensory experience that is not strictly visual. The eyes are connected very strongly to the head pole, where other senses (touch, warmth, and hearing, for example) relate more to the body as a whole.

- Then use an imagination that allows us to pull back a little into ourselves, like a raindrop that falls on our cheeks or the wind that pulls off our caps (*N*, retreating back into ourselves a little).
- Children do just this kind of breathing into the world whenever they carefully notice the world and then collect some treasure to bring home (like picking raspberries). Create stories or imaginations which first breathe out into the world and then come back into themselves.
- Fostering a slower, considered approach is an essential element for quieting the maniacal tendency. Quick observation—which is what much of the technical world is rapidly training us to do—really only allows us to categorize, a very superficial engagement ("That is a flower"). Moving beyond that fast impression to instead notice the varied beauty of the natural world, such as how a flower grows over days or weeks, or seeing the variations of color or form in the clouds overhead creates a more loving relationship. We look again and again to see what is new and different. Almost like comparing two pictures in which some of the objects have been changed, this kind of activity invites us to really look and penetrate. If we only glance, we will never notice that there is anything different. We must help the child find a deeper gaze.
- When that deeper gaze can be directed toward a living being, it is even better, because then the child recognizes (perhaps initially only subtly) that the physical world does house spiritual activity—we just have to look more reverentially to see it.

If we take this one step further and consider the natural world in relationship to our own selves, it helps us come into an even richer relationship. That relating between self and the natural world underlies many important elements in the Waldorf curriculum: "Get the children used to seeing the human being as the confluence of all world phenomenon.... It is really impossible to regard something in relation to the human being without feelings."[84] That bridging to the natural world has important consequences for our social and moral perceptions as well.

Because the polarity of integration is really a process, a movement (not an isolated fact or static diagnosis), it is important that we do not forget that these are therapeutic sequences. This means that whether we are working with feeble limbs or maniacal movement, there really is a beginning, a middle, and an end. We cannot effectively start in the middle—we will not get far asking a child with feeble movement to jump right into the sharpened awareness of *S* or, alternately, expect a child with maniacal tendencies to immediately find "reverence" (like the *A*). We cannot artificially jump from the beginning to the end. Experience confirms that the first element needs to be nurtured for a long time and will always serve as a healthy starting point. Out of that foundation further steps will evolve.

We too often expect a child to have the maturity to jump right into an interaction without due preparation. So we need to nurture movement through real work and feeling through warm imagination. When the feeble child joyfully finds a connection to the limbs through the stirring of *R* or the maniacal child experiences the first glimmers of warmth and reverence through the exhalation of *M*, then a child will very often move on to evolve the next step out of herself. For, as with so many development patterns, when one stage is really ripened and full, it will flow very naturally over into the next step.

Chapter 7

Grimm's Fairy Tale "Iron John"

A Picture of the Inherited Body and Its Redemption

Fairy tales can provide very helpful guides for understanding the spiritual processes that stand behind our human physiology. They describe quests, struggles, transformations, and resolutions. These are indeed also the elements of a healing process.

The challenge in working with a fairy tale is that we may be tempted to take its elements too literally; then the process of transformation that stands behind the plotline can get lost, for the facts of a tale are but symbols for greater truths. The characters and events of a fairy tale very often relate to larger spiritual processes, so it is important that we not get too caught up in the nouns and instead focus more attention on the gestures and verbs of the story. We can experience this firsthand in the German fairy tale "Iron John" (also known as "Iron Hans" or "Einsenhans"), which puts into pictorial language the process of the weaving together of the spiritual and hereditary streams.

The narrative of "Iron John" takes us through the challenges, pathways for healing, and ultimate resolution of the integration process. It begins by contrasting two different places, a palace and a forest, and the threshold that exists between those two worlds:

> There was once on a time a King who had a great forest near his palace, full of all kinds of wild animals. One day he sent out a huntsman to shoot him a roe, but he did not come back. "Perhaps some accident has befallen him," said the King, and the next day he sent out two more huntsmen who were to search for him, but they, too, stayed away. Then on the third day, he sent for all his huntsmen, and said, "Scour the whole forest through,

> and do not give up until ye have found all three." But of these also, none came home again, and of the pack of hounds that they had taken with them, none were seen more. From that time forth, no one would any longer venture into the forest, and it lay there in deep stillness and solitude, and nothing was seen of it, but sometimes an eagle or a hawk flying over it. This lasted for many years, when a strange huntsman announced himself to the King as seeking a situation, and offered to go into the dangerous forest. The King, however, would not give his consent, and said, "It is not safe in there; I fear it would fare with thee no better than with the others, and thou wouldst never come out again." The huntsman replied, "Lord, I will venture it at my own risk, of fear I know nothing."
>
> The huntsman therefore betook himself with his dog to the forest. It was not long before the dog fell in with some game on the way, and wanted to pursue it; but hardly had the dog run two steps when it stood before a deep pool, could go no farther, and a naked arm stretched itself out of the water, seized it, and drew it under. When the huntsman saw that, he went back and fetched three men to come with buckets and bale out the water. When they could see to the bottom there lay a wild man whose body was brown like rusty iron, and whose hair hung over his face down to his knees. They bound him with cords, and led him away to the castle. There was great astonishment over the wild man; the King, however, had him put in an iron cage in his courtyard, and forbade the door to be opened on pain of death, and the Queen herself was to take the key into her keeping. And from this time forth every one could again go into the forest with safety.[85]

This introduction to the wild man in the woods really presents the birth story of every young child. It begins like many other fairy tales in the realm of the "King," who in this story is the child's father, but who in a larger sense represents our spiritual heritage. The beautiful palace where the King lives can be understood as our "home" before birth, when we are still in the spiritual world. The great forest, in contrast, is a completely different realm, and when someone enters the forest, he is never to be seen again in the King's palace. The wild forest stands as a picture for the physical world. The King's palace and the wild forest are quite separate from each other, for a birth into the physical world is simultaneously a death out of the spiritual world, and the soul through birth effectively disappears from the awareness of the spiritual world. In the story, all those who ventured into the forest and come into contact with Iron John disappear.

Iron John can be considered a picture of the physical body, the hereditary stream. The King, in fact, decrees that any person should open the door of the iron cage—to encounter Iron John—"on pain of death," a death out of the spiritual world. With our physical birth we engage with the hereditary body and come into a relationship with Iron John. Iron John himself is wild and frightening, "brown like rusty iron." He does not belong in the King's palace. He must be bound and locked in an iron cage. His iron qualities are important, because they belong so strongly to the earth. As a therapeutic substance, Steiner described iron at some points as "the metal of incarnation" and as a substance that has special healing properties because it requires us to continually overcome its earthly foreign nature. Its outer world physical properties must continually be overcome within the body.[86] It has a healing effect precisely because it is constantly stimulating us to engage with it and master it, which is exactly the developmental task of the young child in meeting and transforming the hereditary body.

The story then tells of the King's eight-year-old son, a boy who plays with a golden ball in the castle courtyard. Through this activity of his limbs (tossing and catching), the boy comes into contact with the wild man. The golden ball inadvertently bounces into the iron cage, and the wild man declares that he will not give it back unless he is freed. He needs to return to his own realm in the forest. The boy resists but eventually fetches the key from beneath the Queen's pillow, returns, and opens the cage. With this deed he becomes very afraid, aware of the fateful consequences of what he has just done, and consequently asks to go with the wild man into the forest. Iron John takes him, and so the boy leaves the realm of his father, the King, and goes to live in the wild wood.

We all begin in the palace of the King. That realm is quite distinct from the wild forest, but at the "midnight hour"—a time described by Steiner as the moment at which we decide to incarnate again into an earthly body—our whole orientation shifts toward the physical world (the wild forest), with planning and preparation for the hereditary body we will meet. We all are then working to meet Iron John. It is through the mother, the Queen, that we make that connection. The key underneath the Queen's pillow can perhaps be thought of as a picture of pregnancy and the birthing process. In the act of unlocking the iron cage the boy in the story pinches his finger, a pain related to the meeting with a hereditary body that does not fit very well. This meeting is a destiny moment, one in which a child's connection with the spiritual world loosens so that he can come and meet the needed experiences of his earthly life. The fairy tale is not complete just by encountering Iron John; we must work with him, and he gives us tasks. This is true for the body as well. After he has slept a night in the forest:

> The next morning the man took him to a well, and said, "Behold, the gold well is as bright and clear as crystal, thou shalt sit beside it, and take care that nothing falls into it, or it will be polluted. I will come every evening to see if thou hast obeyed my order." The boy placed himself by the margin of the well, and often saw a golden fish or a golden snake show itself therein, and took care that nothing fell in.[87]

This gazing—quietly and reverently, as Iron John instructs—requires full engagement with the world. For children who tend toward quick, superficial engagement and movement, this would be a very challenging task indeed. It would instead be easy to ignore the pool or to run wild circles around it, but that is not the task when working with Iron John. Now we come to the story's relationship to the polarities of movement. For the boy, like any children who "perpetually move their fingers, catching hold of everything, kicking out in all directions with his feet,"[88] struggles with the stillness of the task:

> As he was thus sitting, his finger hurt him so violently that he involuntarily put it in the water. He drew it quickly out again, but saw that it was quite gilded, and whatsoever pains he took to wash the gold off again, all was to no purpose. In the evening Iron John came back, looked at the boy, and said, "What has happened to the well?" "Nothing, nothing," he answered, and held his finger behind his back, that the man might not see it. But he said, "Thou hast dipped thy finger into the water, this time it may pass, but take care thou dost not again let anything go in."[89]

What does this mean, that the boy's finger is turned golden? On the one hand, it is certainly a marker of the boy's error, of his impulsivity, and Iron John recognizes this. At the same time it also stands as an expression of a healing, as the start of a purification process. What the boy has been doing unconsciously—perhaps for his whole life—is now suddenly made more wakeful. The boy is told to carefully watch the well, then suddenly pulls back when he realizes he has trespassed with his fingers. But the deed is already done. He thoughtfully engages and thereby looks more deeply into the well than he would have otherwise, then pulls back with startled consciousness. That kind of breathing alternation of going out and then pulling back in, echoes first the warmth and engagement of *M*, then the "understanding mingled with a feeling of repulsion"[90] that we find through *N*. The boy's therapeutic sequence has begun. He enters into a different relationship with the world around.

The process is not done. To transform, the boy must continue to work with his assigned task, to push further and deeper. His careful guarding of the well continues, though it is followed by another trespass:

> By daybreak the boy was already sitting by the well and watching it. His finger hurt him again and he passed it over his head, and then unhappily a hair fell down into the well. He took it quickly out, but it was already quite gilded. Iron John came, and already

> knew what had happened. "Thou hast let a hair fall into the well," said he. "I will allow thee to watch by it once more, but if this happens for the third time then the well is polluted, and thou canst no longer remain with me."[91]

Maniacal movement is an inclination that expresses itself most clearly in the limbs (a golden finger), but it is an imbalance that really must be healed from the head down. The gilding of the boy's hair is perhaps a marker of the beginning of a transformation of the head pole. With this second gilding, the boy's consciousness becomes more deeply seated within him, with a stronger awareness of his boundary, in much the same way that the *B* and *P* help a child to feel more properly housed in the body. His task continues:

> On the third day, the boy sat by the well, and did not stir his finger, however much it hurt him. But the time was long to him, and he looked at the reflection of his face on the surface of the water. And as he still bent down more and more while he was doing so, and trying to look straight into the eyes, his long hair fell down from his shoulders into the water. He raised himself up quickly, but the whole of the hair of his head was already golden and shone like the sun. You may imagine how terrified the poor boy was! He took his pocket-handkerchief and tied it round his head, in order that the man might not see it. When he came he already knew everything, and said, "Take the handkerchief off." Then the golden hair streamed forth, and let the boy excuse himself as he might, it was of no use. "Thou hast not stood the trial, and canst stay here no longer. Go forth into the world, there thou wilt learn what poverty is.[92]

That "poverty" brings him into a new set of tasks and a new set of healing experiences, but we can see how a therapeutic process has already been given to him. His third trespass into the well is no longer related to an unguided impulsivity. Now the transformation comes through watching and gazing—"trying to look straight into the eyes" in very much the gesture and the reverence of *A*. It is followed with an even stronger awareness of trespass, of self, and the responsibility for one's actions—"U.... helping the children to become aware of themselves in themselves"[93]—where the whole of the head is now gilded. Three times the boy gazes out, three times it is matched with startled awakenings of boundary. The boy's learning to gaze into the golden well gives us a beautiful imagination for how the maniacal child can be guided into deeper and richer engagement with the world.

After the boy's experiences in the forest, where he came into a kind of communion with the beauty and sanctity of the natural world while gazing into the golden well, he is now forced to leave the woods and go to the city to do "work." Through this second set of tasks he is taught to rouse his limbs into meaningful activity, though he does not yet know how:

> Then the King's son left the forest, and walked by beaten and unbeaten paths ever onward until at length he reached a great city. There he looked for work, but could find none, and he had learned nothing by which he could help himself. At length he went to the palace, and asked if they would take him in. The people about court did not at all know what use they could make of him, but they liked him, and told him to stay.[94]

In this second part of the story we find a different set of tasks and trials, which are much more connected to the heaviness of feeble movement. The boy goes to the city and longs to find his place in it but does not yet know how to make use of the physical body—"he had learned nothing by which he could help himself." This feebleness finds its therapeutic balance by spiritualizing, by leaving the wild woods and returning to a "palace." We can consider the boy's journey to the city a movement back toward the spiritual world, the realm from which he originally came. Even at his return the "court did not at all know what use they could make of him" because he has not yet overcome the density of the hereditary body. The physical body must be transformed, which he will achieve through work and service:

> At length the cook took him into his service, and said he might carry wood and water, and rake the cinders together.... The cook...exchanged him for the gardener's boy. And now the boy had to plant and water the garden, hoe and dig, and bear the wind and bad weather.[95]

The boy's new tasks bring opportunity for stirring and mobilizing the physical body: first in the cook's service, carrying wood and water, and then hoeing and digging for the gardener. These are all very much *R* activities. As he works, the boy becomes more capable, and as a result his tasks change. In the story the boy soon meets the King's daughter (who lives within the realm of her father's "palace"). In her presence he finds evermore capacity and flexibility, and he is even teased and taunted a little by the princess, as she begins to see that he is no common boy. The teasing conversation expresses movement—evidence of the boy's increasing capacity for interaction and exchange—like the eurythmy "L."

The boy moves beyond simple tasks and soon begins to find his own strength and initiative. His actions now extend beyond just the simple acts of a youth as he comes to the King's rescue as a mysterious knight. This happens when the King's lands are threatened and the boy decides he will fight in the battle, out of his own free will. The other youths he works with scorn the thought of his joining the fight and disdainfully leave him at home with a lamed horse. The steed (like his own feeble body) at first can only limp into activity, "hobblety jig, hobblety jig." But by working with Iron John the lameness is overcome:

> Not long afterward, the country was overrun by war. The King gathered together his people, and did not know whether or not he could offer any opposition to the enemy, who was superior in strength and had a mighty army. Then said the gardener's boy, "I am grown up, and will go to the wars also, only give me a horse."
>
> The others laughed, and said, "Seek one for thyself when we are gone, we will leave one behind us in the stable for thee."

> When they had gone forth, he went into the stable, and got the horse out; it was lame of one foot, and limped hobblety jig, hobblety jig; nevertheless he mounted it, and rode away to the dark forest. When he came to the outskirts, he called "Iron John," three times so loudly that it echoed through the trees.
>
> Thereupon the wild man appeared immediately, and said, "What dost thou desire?"
>
> "I want a strong steed, for I am going to the wars."
>
> "That thou shalt have, and still more than thou askest for."
>
> Then the wild man went back into the forest, and it was not long before a stable boy came out of it, who led a horse that snorted with its nostrils, and could hardly be restrained, and behind them followed a great troop of soldiers entirely equipped in iron, and their swords flashed in the sun. The youth made over his three-legged horse to the stable boy, mounted the other, and rode at the head of the soldiers. When he got near the battle-field a great part of the King's men had already fallen, and little was wanting to make the rest give way. Then the youth galloped thither with his iron soldiers, broke like a hurricane over the enemy, and beat down all who opposed him.[96]

The boy has found the possibility for flexibility and capacity by claiming the physical body and making it his own. The gleaming swords, snorting steed and storming forces of his troop must surely relate to the qualities of the eurythmy "S"—"a powerful peace-bringing element, bringing calm and peace into that which is in a state of unrest."[97]

We come again to a threefold repetition within the boy's valiant deeds. With Iron John's assistance he is given a worthy, swift steed. He rides to the King's festival and there is able to catch a golden apple, thrown into the air by the King's daughter. He repeats this feat three times: first in red armor on a red steed, then as a white knight on a white steed, and finally as a black knight on a black steed. Each time the boy nimbly catches a "golden" apple. Just as earlier in the story the boy's finger, then a single hair, and then his whole head were made golden at the side of the well, so now the limbs (as an expression of the hereditary stream) are able to perform valiant deeds and win golden apples. The boy takes them home with him, a picture of the redemption of his heavy limbs.

Through these deeds of work and service the youth comes closer and closer to the King's daughter. She recognizes that he is not only a "gardener's boy." At the end of the story they wed, their union an integration of the physical body (the boy's journey with Iron John) and the spiritual stream (the King's daughter). Through the wedding the boy is also reunited with his own father and mother (a king and queen). As a last step of transformation at the end of the story the wild man Iron John is himself also redeemed:

> And as they were sitting at the marriage-feast, the music suddenly stopped, the doors opened, and a stately King came in with a great retinue. He went up to the youth, embraced him and said, "I am Iron John, and was by enchantment a wild man, but thou hast set me free; all the treasures which I possess, shall be thy property."[98]

This is perhaps the last step of the sequence, the eurythmy "I[ee]": with "the sound 'I[ee]' there is always a vindication of oneself, as assertion of oneself."[99] The minor tones and melancholy of the physical body have been released. Iron John—as the earthly body—has found the possibility to be a king again while still possessing all the treasures and capacities of the physical realm.

This fairy tale "Iron John" gives us such beautiful imaginations for the integration process. It can enrich our own inner picturing as we approach a child, asking: "Is this a child who needs to learn to sit and gaze into a golden well? What can I do to help this child find an experience of reverence? Or is this a child who does not know what to do in the world and rides only a hobblety jig, hobblety jig horse? How then can I help this child find worthiness and capacity through work that serves a moral purpose?" It is said that fairy tales are whispers from the angels—whispers that can show us paths to better physical and spiritual development.

Chapter 8

Seeing Morality as an Expression of the Earthly–Cosmic Polarity

There is an additional lens we can explore for the meeting of the spiritual and hereditary streams, for this integration process manifests in yet another way. Moral sensing also arises out of this fourfold interweaving of the physical, etheric, astral, and "I."

This means that there is no absolute or single way to work with a constitutional picture. It also means that when we identify an imbalance, there are multiple potential therapeutic pathways available—for example, for feebleminded movement it is not only the activity of *R, L, S,* and *I* ["ee"] that is important but also how a child is supported through inflammatory illnesses and encouraged to participate in "spiritualized" activities like music and painting. When we gain the right constitutional understanding, it is possible to support and stimulate developmental growth on multiple levels.

The fact that there are varied, related expressions of the integration process also means that when we are unsure about where a child lies on a particular polarity (say between feeble and maniacal movement), we can look to other spheres of life in order to gain additional information. For when a constitutional leaning is true, it presents a consistent pattern (i.e., if there is a strong inclination toward feeble movement, then there will frequently be a feeble capacity for moral sensing as well).

The working of the "I" into the astral body, into the etheric, and into the physical body also makes possible our reaching out to morally perceive another human being. When this fourfold weaving is incomplete, we will see imbalanced moral perception. For just as we learn how to walk, step by step, so too must we build our morality step by step, experience after experience:

> We invariably bring into the world a faulty will system; consequently we never, under any circumstances descend to earth to become physical human beings, bringing with us our morality. We have to acquire morality, little by little.... Ethics and morality have to be acquired anew in each single earthly life.[100]

Moreover,

> You must realize that everything that has to do with morality, everything of which it can be said that our conception of it must needs include moral impulses, comes to expression within earth existence alone."[101]

It may seem a shocking thought—that we do not automatically develop into moral human beings. According to this spiritual law, morality cannot be preached; it must be built up as a living capacity. Preaching, as a set of rules, speaks to the head, whereas true moral sensing must develop through experience and interaction in the realm of the limbs.

Our ability to morally sense the other has come into societal consciousness in new ways as more children today are struggling to find this capacity. Rates of autism spectrum disorder diagnosis have increased significantly in recent decades, which means that the fourfold process of integration has become more and more challenging for the children who are incarnating. We can gain more understanding about how this relates to the earthly and spiritual streams by looking at one type of autism spectrum disorder: Asperger's syndrome.

Asperger's syndrome can be subtler than many other types of autistic disorders because a child with Asperger's syndrome is usually intellectually and developmentally mature—in some aspects even precocious—but unable to fully sense the social nuance of a situation. We can build a therapeutic understanding of Asperger's syndrome by connecting it to the cosmic and maniacal side of the integration polarity. The child's spiritual stream is held back. The "I" and astral body do not penetrate all the way down. They have not yet found a way to gaze into the golden well.

The following characteristics are part of the formal diagnostic criteria for Asperger's syndrome:

- marked impairments in the use of multiple nonverbal behaviors, such as eye-to-eye gaze, facial expression, body posture, and gestures to regulate social interaction
- failure to develop peer relationships appropriate to developmental level
- a lack of spontaneous seeking to share enjoyment, interest, or achievements with other people (e.g., by a lack of showing, bringing, or pointing out objects of interest to other people)
- lack of social or emotional reciprocity.[102]

Included in these diagnostic criteria we find, too, a description of the link between limited moral interaction and patterns of limited, superficial social engagement. These social hindrances are often accompanied by "restricted, repetitive, and stereotyped patterns of behavior, interests, and activities,"[103] such as:

- "[an] encompassing preoccupation with one or more stereotyped and restricted patterns of interest that is abnormal either in intensity or focus.
- apparently inflexible adherence to specific, nonfunctional routines or rituals.
- persistent preoccupation with parts of objects.
- stereotyped and repetitive motor mannerisms (e.g., hand or finger flapping or twisting, or complex whole-body movements)."[104]

The last of these diagnostic criteria shows that there is an observed relationship exists between moral sensing and movement. These last mannerisms—stereotyped and repetitive motor movements—are really unguided, unpenetrated, maniacal movements. When Steiner characterized the maniacal pole in the curative course, he indicated how superficial or mechanical patterns of limb activity will also be seen in behaviors of a more spiritual or mental nature.[105] He gave the example of children who have gained the skill for doing something with their hands:

> Let us say, they learn to draw a face in profile. Now, they simply cannot stop; whenever they see others, they immediately want to draw their profiles; it becomes quite mechanical. This is a very bad sign in children. Nothing will persuade them out of it. When such children are about to draw a profile, I can talk to them as much as I like; I could even offer a sweet—they go on just the same; the profile must be drawn! This is connected with the maniacal quality that develops when intellect runs to excess.[106]

Steiner also described how this tendency toward mechanical repetition can already be present in very young children:

> If we notice little children growing very happy and animated because of something they have learned—I mean, the way one learns things before the change of teeth—when we notice, for instance, that a child who is learning to speak takes inordinate pleasure in some recently learned sound, then we must be prepared for the possibility that things may go wrong with that child!...Egoism in the tender age of early childhood—they will perhaps click their tongue with satisfaction.[107]

The concern, of course, is not that the child has acquired a new skill but that there is an "egotism" around the skill—a heightened awareness around one's own activity—with a kind of rigidity. That excessive, inwardly directed attention may foreshadow an inability, or unwillingness, to look outward.

These stereotyped patterns result from a superficial penetration of the hereditary body. That kind of incomplete penetration often creates a mechanical or superficial gesture in the realm of social interactions, as well. The child's consideration of another human being takes place just enough to notice that a person is present as an object but not long enough to truly recognize the individuality within the "object." Because of this superficial meeting, there can be an almost moral equivalency between a chair and another human being. Such children meet only the surface of the world because they cannot, or will not, engage with it in a deeper way.

That kind of quick, surveying activity is not entirely wrong; it just needs to stay in the right realm. It properly belongs to the physiology of the senses. In the head pole the "I" and astral body act more directly with the outside world (not diving into the etheric and physical). That kind of independent activity of the higher members stands behind all the sense organs.[108] Steiner characterized the nerve–sense pole in this way:

> Human beings develop their human qualities mainly in two directions: toward the pole of thought and ideation and the formation of mental pictures, and toward the pole of will. Now as for the mental process, the thought process—that is ill if it is not a thief, and a persistent one, too! The brain–mental organization, the whole life of ideas, has to be a downright thief and has to apply no moral considerations whatsoever in connection with what it must and should receive. It must have the intention and habit of acquiring everything for itself.[109]

Our senses do not wish to really engage; we are simply observing and collecting impressions. If I look at a delicate flower with my eyes, I leave it in the same condition as it was before our interaction. In contrast, if I meet it with my will (such as with my fingers or my feet), the flower will not be the same after I have touched it, picked it, or stepped on it.

In a museum it is appropriate that we only look and listen. We look at everything. We are indeed a kind of thief for the impressions we meet, but the theft stays in the realm of the senses. Naturally, we are not allowed to just take a painting off the wall and bring it home with us. Then we would be "acquiring" everything for ourselves:

> But this aptitude for thieving must not, for heaven's sake, slip down into the will organization! The will has to be modest and restrained. It has to be sensitive, and have a feeling for 'mine and thine'—a feeling which develops only gradually in contact with life in the outside world.[110]

When we are in a healthy balance we are able to shift so that we can move from the thief—surveying a broad range of items and impressions—down to the more modest will interaction, which acts as the foundation of our morality.

Suppose we are going through two different kinds of museums: one with multiple wings and a massive, world-famous collection of art and one that holds only three works. In visiting one of those massive institutions (like the Metropolitan Museum or the Louvre), it is very easy, if not at a certain point essential, to fall into a superficial sensory activity. There is simply not enough time or energy to be able to relate to every work of art in a meaningful way. If we have a guidebook that lists all of the most famous works, we could quickly move from room to room and see all of them in an afternoon, but we are unlikely to have been moved by or really even remember very much about any particular painting. We may have "seen" it, and it now belongs in our collection of sensory impressions, but without much meaning.

If we become members of the museum and make repeated visits, then our relationship to the paintings would change. We could perhaps spend an entire afternoon looking at a single work of art (perhaps even repeated days for the same work of art). Our interactions would be much narrower but so much deeper, and what we carried as a living experience of those interactions would be richer. It is those slower, deeper impressions that we carry around with us as the treasures of our happy memories.

By living in a world where so many things are continuously competing for our attention (noise, screens, bustle) we are pushed to interact with the world in an increasingly superficial manner. This is not only because we are always rushed for time but also because the whole world is filled with so many things and we own so many things and feel pushed to acquire so many things. For a child whose own natural inclination is to relate to the world in a cosmic/maniacal manner, today's world only too easily encourages and reinforces that form of interaction. The less we use our limbs, the more our modes of interacting with the world become dominated by the activity of our heads and sensing—quick, abbreviated, transient. It is socially appropriate that our world has developed the possibility for texting and tweeting as almost constant, evermore abbreviated interaction. We are all becoming more and more maniacal and consequently more "autistic" in our interactions as human beings as well. We have less and less opportunity to gaze deeply into the golden well. It makes perfect sense that as our physiology becomes more one-sided toward a nerve–sense activity that Asperger's syndrome has emerged as a modern social experience. We are now forced to ask—socially, pedagogically, and medically—how do we consciously learn to build our morality?

In this vein, Steiner described a condition in which the activity of our head so dominates our overall activity that it moves beyond the nerve–sense pole and comes all the way down into the limbs. He called it "kleptomania." It is not a coincidence that it shares the term *mania* with the maniacal movement described earlier. It is a related expression of a superficially engaged "I" and astral body, but one that shows itself now in the realm of morality instead of movement.

Kleptomania can be defined as "a persistent neurotic impulse to steal especially without economic motive."[111] This indicates a pattern of activity that does not come out of a deep inner motivation. Usually a person steals out of need or vengeance or selfishness, but kleptomania is an activity that happens without significant inner longing. What should happen in the head, where objects are briefly examined and taken in, carries over into the limbs. All kinds of things are superficially examined and then frequently taken with the fingers. This is very close to Steiner's description of maniacal children, who "perpetually move their fingers, catching hold of everything." All kinds of objects are taken with kleptomania—pencils, notes, tissues, and wrappers, items important and mundane:

> If the astral infiltration of our brain (if I may so express it), which is, as we said, entirely justified in seeking to acquire everything for itself—if this astral infiltration makes its way down into the metabolic–limb organization or into the rhythmic system, then the urge to seize hold of everything for oneself begins to manifest in the will. The urge may at first show oneself in a comparatively harmless manner. You may notice a child beginning to take whatever is within reach, gradually piling up a little store or collection. Naturally one tries to check such a habit whenever it begins to show itself, and so it does not assume large proportions. We must accustom ourselves however to detect the tendency.[112]

All kinds of things are taken because there is insufficient interaction to appreciate the value or significance of the object. Steiner alternately described the process in a slightly different way:

> The head does not recognize property rights, it recognizes only an absolute ownership of everything that comes into its realm. The other pole recognizes morality. When, however, the function of the head enters the will, kleptomania results. This illness results because the aspect that belongs in the head exists in the will. Stealing is quite different from a tendency to kleptomania.[113]

Property rights grow out of a healthy sense of self and other. The self is emphasized in nerve activity, the other through the limbs. Children with kleptomaniac tendencies need to be guided toward a healthy limb activity (like the maniacal child), so that they develop a capacity to modulate properly between the self and other.

Steiner gave therapeutic indications for kleptomania, which we can summarize as treatments to help a child build balanced interaction by properly incarnating into the feet. This begins (as with the indications for the cosmic child), with strong feeling:

> You will then have to approach children with this understanding in your soul, and to proceed to educate them morally and ethically, doing it as effectively as you can and with the utmost inner vitality—never in a lackadaisical way! Working in this way with inner vitality, you will make up stories in which the kind of thing the children do is carried to absurdity. You will tell them a story about stealing, and you will go on doing this again and again. In this way you will actually intervene in the children's karma, you will be working right into their karma.... Qualities that are in their right place in the sphere of ideas have, you see, sunk down, in such children; they have gone right into their toes, into their fingertips. Naturally, we must know this if we want to educate them. Under some circumstances it will even be good to introduce in the stories gestures that come naturally to kleptomaniacs themselves.[114]

Additionally:

> It will therefore be good for teachers to awaken in children a feeling for the good—the meaning of *good*—by bringing it about that children look up to their teachers and take them as their pattern and example. That is why in our Waldorf school education we take particular care that authority should make itself felt at this age of life.... The teachers will then speak of things that are "good," always in such a way that it arouses the children's interest and enjoyment, and speak of things that are "bad" in a way to arouses their antipathy. For this to achieve the desired result, it is, of course, essential that there is first a natural acceptance of the teacher's authority. If this is necessary in the case of so-called normal children, it is in the very highest degree necessary in the case of children such as we are considering.... It is most important that, by virtue of the authority we have with the children, we would find it possible to speak with them quite plainly and unreservedly in this way, showing them how objectionable such a habit is. However, this must not be done too early. It has to be brought home to the children's intellect; by attempting this too early, we can easily kill everything. We must go to work with our stories in the first place, and then

> gradually lead to this appeal to the intellect.... Such stories always work, but we must be patient.[115]

Other indications for kleptomania include therapeutic eurythmy exercises, using vowels that work right down into the legs. (Notice that the therapeutic eurythmy sequence for the maniacal constitution finishes with vowels: "A" and "U.") Eurythmy vowel exercises guide the child's descent with penetrating activity:

> Very good results can also be obtained from the use of curative eurythmy, but it must be carried out with tremendous energy. A boy must be asked to make all the movements that belong to the vowels with his legs, for what we have to do is expel the intellectual element from the will, while at the same time impelling the will into the striving, or taking pains, that lives in the vowel sounds.[116]

Steiner also described methods for bringing consciousness to the limbs by using tight elastic socks (tight enough to draw special awareness to the feet)[117] and even having such children hold their own feet:

> It is also good to punish the children by having them sit for a quarter of an hour and hold their feet or toes with their hands. From the perspective of strengthening the will, that is something that you can do against kleptomania.[118]

Then comes a recommendation for combining foot holding and memory exercises. The relation of memory and the limbs is explored in more depth in part 4 as another physiologic process where sensory activity moves out of the head to come into relation with the limbs:

> It is better if both things are done together—that is, to remember backward while holding onto the feet. We may not make an error here. The exercises should be done for a quarter of a year.[119]

These are all therapeutic tools for helping children to bring their "I" and astral body down into the realm of the limbs. We are given a whole range of characteristic behaviors and qualities linked with a repertoire of healing experiences. To briefly summarize:

- When we find unformed, sculptable features in the head, we know we can work to evoke strong feeling.
- When we see maniacal movement, we can look to the alternating, settling sequence of "*M, N, B, P, A, U.*
- When we see repetitive patterns or superficial social and moral engagement, we can seek to help the child penetrate deeper into the limb realm, by bringing eurythmy vowels that go right into the legs, using tight elastic socks, foot holding, and backward memory exercises.

As we might predict, moral sensing can also be a challenge for the earthly child. For the pole opposite to kleptomania Steiner gave the name (now perhaps not so surprisingly) feebleminded (German: *schwachsinning*). We have explored how a child with feeble movement has difficulty bringing the limbs into movement because the hereditary body is too dense; with feeble moral sensing the child has a related kind of challenge in understanding and holding on to moral insights. These children have a hard time learning moral rules. As an example, children might do something—for example, hitting, pushing, or yelling—and feel regret when it goes badly, but they are likely to do the exact same thing again the next day. Being able to grasp morally and incorporate an understanding of what is an allowable interaction often eludes feeble children. Steiner characterized this physiology of morality during a faculty meeting in which some of the older students at the first Waldorf school were discussed. They had been caught stealing. Steiner described the inability of one of the boys to raise his consciousness to a higher moral law and also how the boy was dominated by a very strong hereditary stream:

> [He is] someone who is never quite here. He does not go around like other people, but more like a sleepwalker.... There is, therefore, a clear case of feeblemindedness inherited from both

> father and mother, which inhibits him from comprehending what is allowable or not. He cannot grasp it, it always slips away from him. It is like trying to grasp a piece of glass that has been covered in oil.... If a human being is to develop moral impulses, the etheric body must be able to grasp the physical body, but that is not the case with him. He is incapable of saying this is good so I may do it, and that is not, and so forth.... Just think for a moment how strong the hereditary influence is in him. It is really very strong.... Feebleminded people are lacking in their capacity to retain judgments. They simply cannot grasp the judgment. That has nothing to do with logic. It is a purely psychological phenomenon.[120]

This dominance of the hereditary body limits the child's capacity to learn to judge what is permissible in social situations. The condition shows up as the need to be told over and over again how to do something or, more likely, how not to do something (how not to hit another child, how not to yell in the classroom, how not to grab at a hot pot), with the child acting as though he has never heard that instruction before. On a certain level the child knows that he should understand and remember what is being told. The child is not trying to be dismissive or naughty. He simply cannot grasp the judgment; it is like trying to grasp an oiled piece of glass.

Children with feeble moral sensing are earnest about wanting to do the right thing. Their remorse, when things do not go well, relates to the melancholy that comes from a dominant earthly body. These children are generally aware of the behavior, aware of their incapacity, but they cannot do anything about it without finding a better way to take hold of the physical body. (This is quite different from children with a kleptomaniacal tendency, who will generally meet a correction not with remorse but intellectual rationalization. If an apology comes at all, it is usually mechanical. If we tell such children not to hit other children and then become distraught when they kick someone, they might argue, pointing out that we never said anything about kicking.)

The therapeutic process is the same for both kinds of feebleness—to work to mobilize and loosen the physical body so that it can become a proper vehicle for the activity and impulses of the higher members. This is done through gross motor, repetitive, intentional work.

While the feeble–maniacal polarity describes movement and the feeble–kleptomania polarity relates to moral sensing, the same fundamental spiritual-scientific observation underlies both processes. A child may not necessarily exhibit an imbalance in both realms, but if we find one expression, it often proves useful to look for the other as well. When we find echoes of the same process in both movement and moral sensing, it should strengthen our confidence that we are working with the proper constitutional lens.

Chapter 9

Putting the Pieces Together

Looking at Movement to Understand the Child Who Is "Lazy" or "Isn't Interested in Participating" in the Classroom

After looking at several different expressions of the process of the meeting of the spiritual and hereditary streams, we now return to movement. The initiation and guidance of movement are really the core expression of the polarity of integration. Whenever there is a question or concern about how a child moves, we should return to this polarity of the will. When young children are asked to move their bodies, we can see very quickly how the fourfold weaving of the "I," astral body, etheric body, and physical body is taking place. Observing imitative movement is particularly informative because it asks the child not only to be mobile and responsive in movement (a challenge for those children who incline toward feeble movement) but also to be attentive enough to follow along through a whole series of gestures, songs, or games (which is challenging for those who are on the maniacal pole). Observing movement always gives insight into whether there is a dominant spiritual or hereditary stream.

For the child with feeble movement, the body cannot move well without first being warmed and loosened—this really should be understood as a kind of spiritual law for the feeble child. It leads to some obvious challenges. From the outside it can seem as if the child is just too lazy (because the child does not move when asked) or is not interested in participating (because the child does not move). The lack of movement may have nothing to do with lack of initiative or of interest. The child may deeply wish to be cooperative but cannot because the body is not yet compliant. This is especially true if a movement sequence is too complex (continuously changing, without repetition) or if it moves too quickly. There is then simply no time or space for children with feeble movement to find a way in. By the time they start to penetrate down to their feet and toes, the group activity has already moved on to something completely different. This can be compounded by the temptation (from the teacher's side) to feel that such children are not participating because they are bored or not paying attention, and thus the sequence is made even more varied or animated. This will not entice the feebleminded children into movement. They may long to participate, but they are simply not capable that quickly.

When we see challenges in initiating movement (perhaps reminding us of small children trying to push their arms through the sleeves of a bulky winter coat with their mittens already on—pushing, pushing, pushing), we should look to see how far the children have penetrated into their limbs. How much of the limbs has been claimed? Is movement initiated repeatedly from the upper arms and from the elbows? Are the wrists used skillfully, or are they rigid or floppy? Are the children really sensing with their palms? Do they use their hands as if they were wearing mittens? For feeble children, the penetration and skillful use of their limbs often gets better in the course of an activity (with more stirring), but the start is usually awkward.

We can similarly consider how these children interact with other. When the feeble process is strong, the children's play will often be a beat behind. They very much want to enter the play, but it takes a little time to find their role in the game, and then they often want to continue in that role or activity even after the other children's imagination has moved on. The feeble children wholeheartedly participate, but it just takes a little time.

Feeble children love to play the same thing over and over. This strengthens their experience of capacity and comfort. The story of the play does not necessarily start off where it ended the previous day but has to be built up again. Repetition is needed.

Similarly, with manners, the child may need to be reminded what to do every day. This will get better with time, but the basic expectation may have to be set anew each day. The child in time does become more and more capable and able to act independently, so that eventually a prompt or gentle reminder may suffice instead of complete instruction.

We can lovingly support the feeble children by providing sufficient time and repetition for them to work all the way down into their physical body. Integration is aided by big body movements, such as running, jumping, crawling, or marching (*R*). The movement does not need to be precise. It should be simple enough that there is very little possibility for doing it incorrectly. It also needs to be big enough that the children can really experience the movement as stirring, revolving, and mobilizing.

Movement needs to be repeated for a long enough time that these children really find their way into participation. Whether this can be accomplished with four or seven or fifteen repetitions can really be determined only by watching the children. A rough rule of thumb is that, at about the time most adults are starting to get bored with the activity, the children with feeble movement are just really starting to find their way into it. Do not worry too much that the activity will become boring. Small children (who all, appropriately at some level, still have feeble movement) love this kind of repetition.

The activity should not be rushed but can deliberately get a little faster once there has been some warm-up time. The passing of beanbags could be one such activity. Exercises in body geography are helpful, though the goal for the feeble child is to emphasize different parts of the body in order to get the child to mobilize and flexibly penetrate the different parts (much as in the gesture of the eurythmy *L*).

Consistency serves as an anchor. It is not uncommon to see a feeble child fall out of the group movement and stop participating but know that at the end of a game or verse there will be a jump or a falling down. The child then waits, waits, waits for that moment to arrive and joyfully joins back into the movement at that moment. That predictable anchor moment brings reassurance and invitation to rejoin. It is like the chorus of a song when everyone can sing along.

Once the child has found a way in, the activity can move more into the realm of archetype and the experience of being a capacity within the body. This can now involve more specialized movement or activity (*S*). An example is to invoke the honor and worthiness of the trades, be it as a carpenter, a baker, a shopkeeper, or a knight. Once the body has been stirred and made accessible, more specialized tasks or stories can be brought in. The body is elevated to proper activity that strives to contribute to the outside world. Real work that involves limb movement usually brings all of these qualities (such as sweeping, chopping, grinding). These kinds of activities are by their very nature repetitive, though not in an abstract or artificial way. Like the boy in "Iron John," the child finds ways to use the body in the service of the "King" (as a cook, gardener, and warrior). It is particularly nice to finish an activity with some recognition of accomplishment (the eurythmy *I* ["ee"], for example). This echoes the ending of fairy tales, which tell us that they all lived "happily" or in "peace" (see fig. 5).

This experience can really only come after the other steps have been worked through—first stirring, then mobilizing, and then coming into specialized movement or tasks. Such an *I* moment can perhaps be felt best in transitions. It is very easy to fall into the habit of needing to prod or rush the feeble child into the next activity. For this reason it is lovely to allow a little breath of time to see what has been done, to reflect back on it a bit. This could be as simple as a word of appreciation: "That is a lovely fort." Or an acknowledgment of what has been accomplished: "Wow, we have peeled a lot of vegetables!" That little space helps decrease resistance when it is time to move on to the next activity. (Otherwise the child may be inwardly feeling, "I am just now finally feeling good in what I am doing, and now you want to me stop and start all over again with something completely new!") Breath is very important. Otherwise, if all things are fast-paced, the feeble child

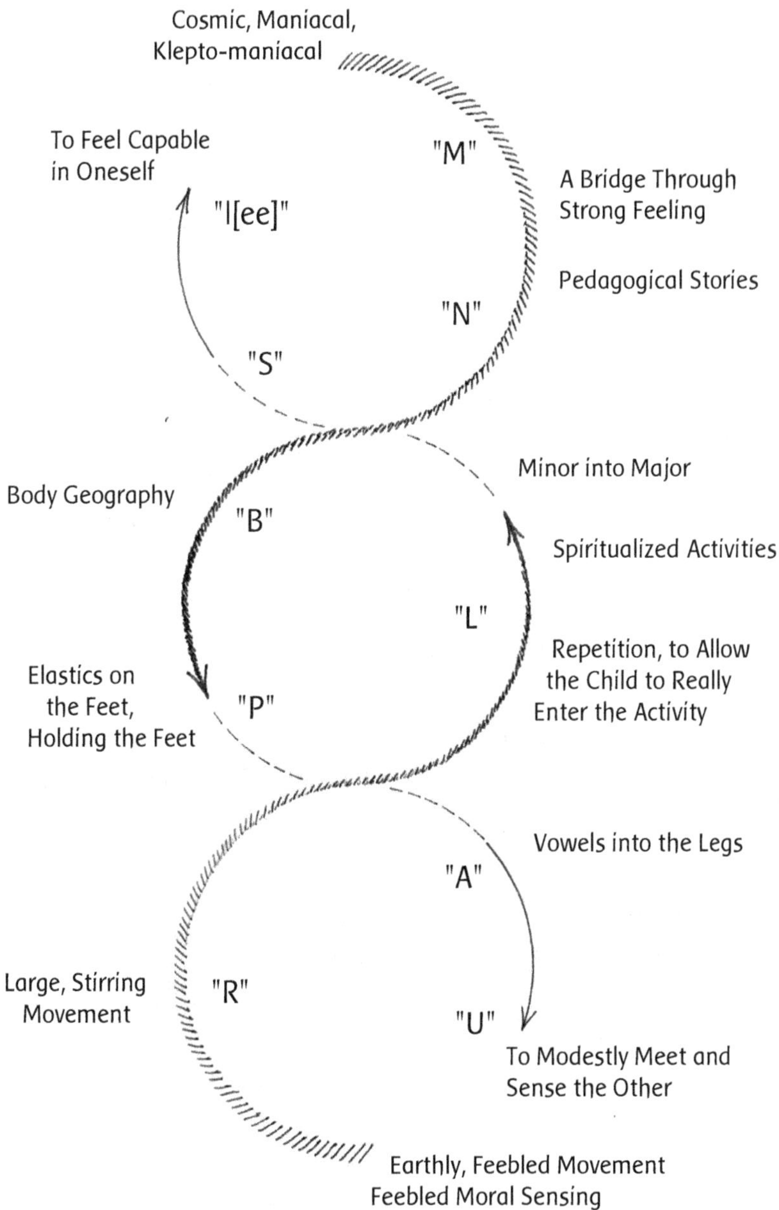

Figure 5: The upward and descending pathways combined, summarizing the therapeutic gestures for both the feeble and maniacal constitutions

may spend the whole time always being a beat behind and never really feeling himself fully capable in the world.

A child with maniacal movement obviously has polar movement patterns, but this can create similar frustrations or concerns: a) the child is too lazy (now not because the child is not able to move, but because the child does not engage, especially if it is an imitative activity—like following the gesture in a song or circle activity), or b) it looks as if the child is not interested in participating (because the child is not doing what is being asked). These are, in broad brush strokes, the same "symptoms" as were described for the feeble pole, but they clearly require a different kind of guidance.

With respect to movement, maniacal children actually move a lot, but it is not related to the overall group activity, or these children initially start an imitative movement but then fall out of it quickly. They often switch into restless movement. The form of a child's gesture may be correct, as one with maniacal patterns may be quite capable with the limbs, but it is hard the child to sustain the gesture, which quickly falls away. Alternatively, the head and the hands may be doing the movement properly, but there is little connection between them—with poor tone and no radiation into a movement; the child moves as if guided by marionette strings, without continuous connection.

There are several considerations in terms of social behavior. The child may have trouble settling into an activity. This may be an important aspect of the child who orbits around the room, perhaps preferentially talking with the adults (which is different from a true hesitancy to engage, which is described in more detail in discussing the hysteric constitution in part 3).

Such children may join the play but with little consideration of what the others are doing. This is not the same as the example of those who collide with others or knock things over because they are moving and cannot stop, which is more likely in feeble movement. Rather, this pattern is related more to a rather superficial regard for what is already happening—e.g., wanting to play with a particular toy and not really being concerned about whether someone else is already playing with it or how it will affect that other child if the toy is taken away.

This form of social interaction can also show itself through statements that include a lot of facts but little true conversation or exchange. When another child gets upset, there is an explanation—perhaps quite logical—but little expression of sadness or apology. There is not much experience of boundary or violation of boundary.

The way to help a child with maniacal movements and interactions comes through being invited and guided into deeper engagement, in several ways. A bridge from the dominant head process to the neglected limbs can be built through the feeling life. Making things faster or more clever usually does not invite better participation from these children. Instead, creating a living picture, an imagination, does inspire more engagement, especially when it is brought with rich enthusiasm.

Slowing a child down enough to notice what has changed helps to create this feeling space. The child's inclination is to almost immediately move on to something else. As an imagination builds, the child's attention may flit back and forth several times.

A further step comes by building a connection between the imaginative picture and then collectively looking for its physical manifestation. This might come through something like a story about the changing of the seasons and then looking for the changing colors of the leaves in fall or finding the first buds on a tree in spring.

Caring for a plant or an animal over time also helps to build this feeling bridge. Such activity asks the child to look more deeply: Does the plant need water? Is the soil dry, or is it flooded? Does an animal need more water? How do I learn to gently hold a rabbit so that it feels safe and calm?

Observation that has practical application is also a good method. In speaking about a kleptomaniacal child, Steiner said:

> This boy should be taught some practical job. He should learn how boots are made. "He could make boots for the whole family." He could also learn gardening. And he should be encouraged to solve all manner of small practical problems.[121]

Body geography also works with the maniacal child by building a bridge between an imagination and the child's own (physical, hereditary) body. Bringing in body geography helps to ground an imagination so that it does not remain too superficial (and sometimes helps avoid having the child debate and discuss what is being brought, rather than really entering it). Working back and forth between a story and the body creates a sort of natural breathing alternation, much like the therapeutic eurythmy sequence for the maniacal child.

After warming and inviting the child into observation (*M* and *N*), experiences of body geography encourage the child to enter more into the realm of *B* and *P*. Here is a description by Steiner of body geography and imagination:

> A pictorial approach is always likely to work on children, especially when the picture is connected with their own corporeality rather than with something outside their periphery. An example of such an approach was when I asked a boy to grasp his left lower arm with his right hand and gave him other tasks. Anyone unfamiliar with the methods of the Spiritual Science will hardly be able to appreciate the difference between impressions made on a child by such an inwardly perceived picture and by outside pictures that are more remote and abstract because they lie beyond the child's periphery.... Only the pictorial element—that is, only what awakens feelings through a pictorial quality—can enter the soul life.[122]

Attention and interaction with others, in reciprocal interaction, is also helpful. Meeting others is enriched and deepened when it is part of a larger picturing or imagination, for if the exercise gets too mechanical, it loses its therapeutic potential. Some examples could include these:

- Beanbag exercises that involve passing in a group. These bring the activity of opening and observing in order to receive the beanbag from another child (more like the first gesture of the eurythmy pairings "M," "B," and "A"), which then shifts to the need to connect with one's own activity—like meeting the beat or passing with enough precision to get the beanbag into the next child's hand (a kind of "N," "P," "U"). These movements ask the child to feel himself in active relationship with the environment.
- Similarly, games or dances with partners, where we must not only move ourselves but also do so in relationship with those around us. Trying to get the children to greet one another with feeling and acknowledgment (such as with a low bow and a smile) is one example. The maniacal child can very easily slip into a mechanical pattern (perfunctory bow, not even necessarily directed at the partner or noticing that there is a new partner). The most therapeutic element in this case is seeing that each partner is really an individual human being.

The more we observe children and practice these kinds of activities, the more we begin to appreciate that many different kinds of normal classroom activities can provide a therapeutic experience when we can help the children enter into them in the right way. Then it is not so concerning to hear that body geography and beanbag exercises can be helpful for both sides of the polarity. Repetition and consistency are healthy for all young children. We can differentiate their benefits by recognizing that (a) the child with feeble movement needs repetition to mobilize into the limbs, as each repetition allows the child to work a little bit further down toward the fingers and toes, and (b) children with maniacal movement benefit from repetition because it allows an imagination or inquiry to be revisited and deepened, thereby building greater interest for the world. In this way it is possible to do the

Table 3: Summary table for earthly and cosmic, feeble, and maniacal constitutions

Between Heaven and Earth: The Polarity of Integration relating to the development of the metabolism and limbs and to patterns of *will*	
We can see expressions of it in the sculptural quality of the body as described through the earthly/cosmic polarity that arises through the meeting of the spiritual and hereditary streams.[1]	
Earthly The weight of the hereditary body cannot be escaped; melancholy; the limbs and chest are not sculpted (the tissue is plastic).	**Cosmic** The spirit stays too dominant but disconnected; the head is unsculpted (the features are plastic, not well defined).
We can see expressions of it in Movement as described through the feeble and maniacal polarity.[2] (*Education for Special Needs,* June 30, 1924)	
Feeble Movement (related to the earthly pole) Hesitates to bring the legs into movement; the urge to do nothing, even when all the conditions are ready.	**Maniacal Movement** (related to the cosmic pole) Never waits for a command; perpetually moving fingers, catching hold, kicking out; repetitive, mechanical movements.
We can see expressions of it in Morality as described through the feeble and kleptomaniacal polarity.[3]	
Feeble Moral Sensing Cannot grasp a moral principle, even when repeatedly told—like trying to grab a piece of glass covered with oil.	**Kleptomaniacal Moral Sensing** Head forces come into the limbs, the limbs then act like a thief; no real sense of personal boundary or property, dispassionate.

Therapeutic Realm Balancing activities for this polarity of integration are *activities.*	
For the Earthly Child	**For the Cosmic Child**
The need for spiritualized activity (music, eurythmy, painting), passing from the minor to the major mood.	The need to evoke strong feelings in order to build a bridge for more connection to the world.
Feeble Eurythmy "R-L-S-I" Stirring movements that are repeated long enough so that the child can really enter in; movements that get them a little out of breath and contribute to a feeling of capacity (e.g., real work).	**Maniacal** Eurythmy "M-N, B-P, A-U" The alternation of opening to the outside world, and then pulling back to consciousness of one's self. **Kleptomaniacal** Building memories and imagination of the past; having them hold their feet; eurythmy vowels down into the legs; pedagogical stories developed with real enthusiasm.
Fairy-tale picture The cook, the gardener, the knight Activities of the world, in service to the king (spiritualized activity)	Fairy-tale picture Gazing into the well Reverent attention as a path to loving interaction

Both poles (as with all small children) benefit from repetition so that they can better enter into the activity: one to gradually mobilize the body to a state where it is really accessible to join and the other to build enough interest so that there is a willingness to join in.

* June 13, 1921 in *Education for Adolescents.*
† June 30, 1924 in *Education for Special Needs.*
‡ July 15, 1924 in *Faculty Meetings with Teachers,* vol 2.

same activity, but with a different emphasis consciously included for each type of child—one day might be focused on those who need the mobilizing movement and the next on deepening the intention and engagement for those who stay too superficial. The main elements for both sides of the polarity are summarized in table 3.

Very often one can resist the temptation to create a whole new set of exercises to prescribe for a particular constitutional problem. Instead, we should work to see how these elements are already present in many of our everyday experiences and classroom activities. Then we are better able to understand what we already do. The Waldorf curriculum, as given by Steiner, was created with these incarnation pathways and hindrances in mind.

Chapter 10

The Process of Integration in Later Life

as a Path of Self-development

> As a consequence of an unspiritual, scientific outlook we see only the human exterior. Therefore it is essential that, in order to arrive at a real spirit-filled social organism, we must recognize that divine activity is at work in our neighbor. We shall not arrive at this realization unless we actually do something about it. One thing we can do is to strive to deepen our own soul life.[123]

The integration our earthly and spiritual streams plays out most dramatically in the first seven years of life, but it does not end there. It is a process that continues throughout our biography. We are continually challenged to overcome gravity and the weight of the physical body while also being challenged to push beyond superficial engagement with the outside world. One of these two poles generally dominates during the early years of life, but as an adult it is possible to experience both poles of an imbalance—sometimes simultaneously. This is because we are really only in a healthy balance when we are able to connect to both poles and hold both of them at once. We are naturally blessed with times when things do find a contented equipoise, but they are usually followed by periods of flux and disorientation. This means that we are asked to repeatedly trace the pathway of integration anew. Falling out of balance—in one direction or the other—is a common and very human experience.

As an example, most everyone experiences the inertia of the physical body and the struggle to lift it into movement in early spring. This is a very common complaint, that things feel intractable at that time of year. Winter is starting to lift in the world outside, but there is a lingering experience of darkness and heaviness inside. This is the season of Lent in the Christian tradition, when there is a dying process that precedes a cycle of renewal (though this annual experience, which is universal, is felt far beyond any specific religious practice or teaching). It is a time for feeling stuck, depressed, and often caught by the past. It is healed not through abandonment but by a penetration of the obstacle and finding a way to lift it to a more dynamic activity. The consistency of this seasonal soul experience can enhance our understanding of resurrection as a quest to renew the physical body. Resurrection is a spiritual archetype, one that we are always participating in (thanks to the activities of the life and chemical ethers, through the lifting activity of "R-L-S-I").

Another traditional, but perhaps less esoteric expression of this process is spring cleaning. Spring cleaning usually entails more than just dusting and sweeping. It is digging through the collections of earthly objects we possess and deciding what is still useful and what should be given away. And it can feel so good! When we finally start the process and gain momentum, we can accomplish things that we has been wanting to do for weeks, months, or even years. The experience is not so much one of loss but rather of liberation and health when what is no longer needed can be given or thrown away.

Sometimes the inventory of what we need to work through is not physical at all. We may feel that we are stuck in "molasses." Everything feels more difficult and takes more effort. This could happen when we have been ill (when our etheric is depleted) or when we really have a pathologic depression (which is usually related to a liver imbalance, the organ of the will), but it also comes about when we are on the cusp of needing to make a change. It is an expression of the feebleness that arises when what we have brought with us from the past does not fit anymore. We cannot penetrate it because we are outgrowing it and it does not belong to us anymore. A melancholy sets in, which is the harbinger of an emerging developmental step, like the feeling of body aches and irritability that comes at the beginning of a flu. This feeling often marks a biographical shift. An exaggerated experience of density stimulates the impetus for change.

It is very common to see these kinds of shifts emerge on a seven-year biographical rhythm. The major integration process of the hereditary and spiritual streams has come to some completion by the end of the first seven years and the eruption of the first adult teeth, but we find echoes of this process at the end of every seven-year cycle.

A first repetition of this process (at the end of the next cycle of seven years) comes with the entry into adolescence. It is a striking example of biographical shift. It definitely is an earthly time, with tremendous physical growth that often outpaces broader developmental maturation, so that the body does not feel like a good fit anymore. The penetrating spirit cannot quite keep up; heaviness and awkwardness set in. This is generally more physically pronounced in boys than girls, as boys are particularly influenced by the state of the physical body—Steiner described how in a male incarnation the physical body and the "I" play a more prominent role, while in female incarnations it is the etheric and the astral bodies that predominate.[124] During early adolescence girls may, in contrast, experience the heaviness more as emotional sadness or social isolation. Adolescent boys often seek remedy through strong physical sensations of touch and gravity, which help them to really feel themselves in their bodies (like a child with feeble movement). Sports activities, rough or extreme play, and even physical violence can all be understood as different variations of a stirring activity during this window. For girls, stirring may come through a shifting of social connections or through a longing to learn practical tasks. The beginning of the menstrual cycle is also a physiological pathway for breathing between an intensive connection to physical substance (through the buildup of the uterine lining) and then a release of tissue that is no longer needed.

Adolescence brings with it a longing to individualize the body, to claim it as "mine"—something along the lines of saying "The way my body looks and feels does not really reflect who I am as an individual."

Then the development of a personal style—through clothing, makeup, haircut—helps to make the body a more accurate reflection of the spirit inside.

For some individuals the integration process never quite feels complete, and then the body does not feel like home, regardless of how it looks from the outside (beautiful or not). When this experience is strong, many people seek ways to alter their experience of the body. They shift the ways in which the "I" and astral body connect with the etheric and physical bodies through experimentation with alcohol and drugs and through extreme activities ("I have never felt so alive!"). A broad range of adolescent behaviors can be understood as attempts to overcome the density of the physical body—like fighting, piercing, stimulant drugs, and aggressive sexuality—stirring, stirring, stirring!

On a fundamental level the contentedness of our adult biography is influenced by how well we are able to make the hereditary body our own during early childhood. It underlies the way in which we can unfold our will. Steiner spoke to this relationship and what happens if our spiritual kernel, our "I," is unable to free itself from the experience of the physical body:

> We must try to avoid everything that permits the "I" to be too strongly absorbed by the organism or to become too dependent on it. You will understand how serious this is when I tell you that the cause of criminality and brutality in people lies in the fact that their "I" was allowed to be absorbed too strongly during their years of growing up.[125]

What starts as a longing for stirring limb experiences in the young child can become a powerful desire to forcefully shift the dominant physical body when the earthly experience extends beyond its proper developmental window. This can be one root cause of destructive behaviors in teenagers or young adults and can be considered whenever strongly stimulating activities or substances are sought.

A different, but perhaps equally common way to work with the experience of dominant physicality is not to push through it to loosen it, but instead to abandon it. This comes out of a desire to try to lift away from the experience of the body altogether, a kind of mini-death. Many kinds of sedatives and opioid drugs lift us out of the body. Anorexic eating is also a pathway to reduced experience of the physical body. Suicidal depression—so often arising out of an experience of being stuck with no possible way out, of being trapped—shows us what might be the darkest side of an unmitigated hereditary stream. The possibility to bring ourselves out of those dark places arises out of our capacity to make ourselves anew, to find a new home in our earthly life.

A healing path for the adolescent or teenager stuck in this earthly phase can be created in much the same way that we would strive to meet a younger earthly child: by working to lift the earthly realm back into the spiritual. Specific pedagogical activities (related to the indications given for the earthly child) were given by Steiner for balancing the way the "I" integrates with the other members. Those indications come in a series of lectures known as Balance in Teaching and presents a kind of natural evolution of the earthly/cosmic polarity but now adapted to meet the experience of the older child and young adult. It addresses how the child's "I"-organization orients itself in relation to the physical body, with this polarity traditionally referred to as "too much" or "not enough" integration (see next page, table 4).

The opposite condition comes when there has been "not enough" penetration, a failure "to induce a rightful fusion of the 'I' with the rest of the organization."[126] Then "the 'I' remains too far outside, with the result that such children become dreamers or visionaries, or they will be generally useless in the world, living in the grip of fantasies. That is the other extreme—the mistake of not letting the 'I' sink deeply enough into the organism."[127]

This superficial side of the polarity results, not surprisingly, in a lack of meaningful engagement. When a child's cosmic constitution

Table 4: The polarity of too much and not enough "I" integration

For too much "I" integration	For not enough "I" integration
Characteristics and indications "When...we notice that children are becoming too materialistic, that the 'I' tends to become too dependent on the body, we need only have them draw on paper those geometrical forms that are otherwise grasped more by thought. The moment we let the children draw geometrical forms, we create the counterpoise to an excessive absorption of the 'I.'" "A certain heaviness in their singing, then we must try to guide them to practice more spontaneous listening rather than musical memory."	Characteristics and indications "If we see the children becoming too dreamy through the stories of history, then, when the right moment arrives, we must permeate the subject with ideas, with the great interrelationships in history." "If children tend to become too dreamy and romantic through lessons in geography, this can be counteracted by having them grasp concepts such as differences in altitude above sea level or by leavening the geography instruction with other kinds of thinking, related more closely to geometry; that will bring the 'I' back into their organism."
Supportive activities "There are whole subjects that help us when we want to protect the 'I' from being sucked into the organism too strongly. These are above all geography, history, and everything where the emphasis is on the picture element and on drawing."	*Supportive activities* "Everything in teaching that necessitates forming mental images of number and of space, such as geometry and arithmetic, helps the 'I' settle itself well into the organism as the child forms such images and works on them. Equally, everything in speech of a musical nature, rhythm, recitation, and the like help in this. Music, especially the training of memory for music, will be especially beneficial for somewhat fanciful children."

(Sept. 22, 1920, *Balance in Teaching*)

is not overcome (for we can see that the "not enough" constitution may arise as an extension of the cosmic constitution earlier in life), the older child never finds a real anchor for being interested in the world: "Concentrating merely on contemplation leads the children to a stunted, prosaic adult life, with a tendency to boredom. They will have a superficial view of life, will not feel inclined to observe accurately, will not pay attention to events around them... [and will] become benumbed, confused adults."[128] The danger that comes from not having the "I" and the astral body fully penetrated in the etheric and physical is boredom and the desire to be constantly entertained.

As has already been discussed, such prolonged superficiality is strongly encouraged by many aspects of our modern, electronic life. With so many virtual opportunities to be quickly and transiently engaged, we are all constantly being influenced to migrate toward a "not enough" connection.

We have more information sources today than ever before, but our engagement with them is so superficial that we are very often less well informed. The format for the information we receive has consequently changed, to give us just the essential character of an event or an interaction: in a sound bite, a headline, or a tweet. Such brevity is very different from older, traditional forms of communication that strove to capture the very essence of an experience, like the carefully crafted distillation process of a haiku. There is no time to gaze into the golden well. We are standing at a point where our society is rampantly entertained, increasingly bored, and in danger of being profoundly spiritually undernourished, all at the same time.

This is of particular concern because it stunts our experience as human beings. It blunts our feeling bridge to the world and weakens our capacity to really meet the other person as a true human being. In adult life, stirring movement and strong feeling remain important experiences, but the process of integration becomes, on many levels, a path of self-development. As a final consideration, we look at how a series of meditative activities, described by Steiner as the six "subsidiary" or "basic" exercises, can help us to consciously support and renew the interweaving of our earthly and spiritual aspects.

Chapter 11

The Six Basic Exercises

These exercises stand as a foundation for almost any kind of meditative work. The German word given by Steiner to these exercises, *Nebenübungen,* can also be translated as "near" or "next to" exercises, in that they should be done as a kind of preparation or companion to any other kind of spiritual striving. They help us to be healthily incarnated in the body, by working through a process of conscious integration.

The first five exercises are control of thinking, control of actions, equanimity, understanding every being, and complete openness. The sixth of the six exercises is the integration of all five exercises, thereby working toward inner harmony. Each exercise is practiced for a month, so that the whole course is experienced over the course of half a year. In working through the sequence, it is a common experience to find that dedicated daily activity with one exercise naturally evolves into the next exercise of the sequence. It is truly a developmental pathway. The order and course of the meditative exercises are therefore not artificial or arbitrary. They guide the individual consciously through a path of self-control and self-awareness, related to the process of integration, making deeper moral sensing possible.

The first, control of thinking, is also commonly referred to as the pencil or paper clip exercise, for it asks us to center our thought activities on a simple practical object:

> To begin with, we must master our thoughts, particularly our train of thought. This is called "control of thoughts." Just consider the way thoughts whirl about in our souls, how they flit like will-o'-the-wisps; one impression rises here, another there, and each changes our thinking. It is not true that we govern our

> thoughts; rather, our thoughts govern us completely. We must reach a point where we can, at a certain time of the day, become so absorbed in a thought that no other thought can enter and disturb our soul. In this way, we hold the reins of thought life for a while.[129]

Focusing on a simple man-made object (Steiner's specific recommendation) reduces the number of associations we bring to an object and also creates the possibility for tracing the origin and the manufacturing process for the object. Although such a man-made object is of the outer world, the process of holding it in thought is a completely inward one. For a few moments of the day we bring the content of the outer world in and raise it into a consciously directed process.

What is this activity from an anthroposophic perspective—in other words, what does it require of our spiritual activity? This first exercise asks us to bring will into our thoughts. We are bringing the activity of the limbs (the will) into the realm of the head (our thinking). To make an object really alive in our thinking, to form an image and hold it as thought content, we have to completely enliven it. Through a will activity we are lifting and spiritualizing our earthly thoughts.

The therapeutic indication for the earthly child is, as we have seen, "spiritualized activity," to lift the melancholy experience of the physical body from one of density and heaviness to a reconnection with the child's spiritual heritage. We have seen how there can be echoes of this heaviness again in adult life. This control of thinking supports us in renewing the conditions of our earthly life. It brings the possibility for more conscious flexibility. Then we are overcoming not the heritage of our earthly, hereditary stream, but rather of deadened, materialistic thought: "In respect of our world of thought we are entirely dependent upon the experiences brought to us by our birth, by our destiny. But through the will, which rays out from the depths of the soul, we carry into what thus comes to us from the outer world, something that is inherently our own."[130] Parallel to the way that we seek stirring, physical activity to loosen the physical body, we can also spiritualize ourselves through stirring up our will, all the way into our thinking:

> How, in reality, do we become inwardly more and more spiritual?...We become more spiritual through the inner, will-permeated work we carry out in our thoughts...and the greater the strength and intensity of this inner radiation of will into the sphere of thinking, the more spiritual we become.... Freedom dawns when we enable the will to become a mightier and mightier force in our thinking.[131]

Practicing control of thinking also helps us to recognize the physical body: "Through concentrated thinking—through our concentration exercises—we become gradually conscious of our physical body as something outside [of us]. We feel it as something that is there and that belongs to us to a certain extent."[132] This recognition is liberating, for it is precisely through this differentiation that we are freed enough to realize that conditions of our physical incarnation influence us but are not of us. We gain enough distance and perspective to appreciate that the melancholy of the hereditary body is sometimes necessarily with us but that it does not have to define us.

> Esotericists must learn to pull back with their soul-spiritual nature and free themselves from the physical. Then they will learn to observe their physical body. It helps for this if we gather our thoughts together, as much as possible, to a point, concentrate on this point, immerse ourselves in it, and dwell within it for a time. Through such concentration, a strengthening of the force of thinking takes place, and through this we can gradually succeed in observing our physical body.[133]

Recognizing the physical body allows us the possibility to continue to evolve beyond it, a true process of spiritualizing.

The second basic exercise, control of actions, brings a polar movement. Now instead of bringing will up into our thinking, we are asked to bring thought and intention down into our deeds. This pathway, of thought into will, helps to overcome the superficiality of the cosmic, maniacal, and kleptomaniacal experience and brings us right down into the details of what we are doing:

> Here it is necessary, occasionally at least, to act in ways that are not precipitated by anything external. Whatever is initiated by our place in life, our profession, or our situation does not lead more deeply into higher life. Higher life depends on such intimate matters as one's resolve to do something that springs completely from one's own initiative—even if it is something absolutely insignificant. No other actions contribute anything to the higher life.[134]

While such deeds could be viewed as insignificant, the process of carrying out a small act at exactly the same time of day is a huge challenge. The vast majority of our lives are spent in habitual patterns and reaction. It is rare to be completely present in what we are doing. If we return to the imagery of "Iron John," there are few moments during the day when we are truly gazing into the golden well. To become so interested in how we interact with the world that we wait and wait for that right moment to come in order to do the right deed at the same time every day is a powerful practice: "Consider how little arises as the result of your own initiative. Consequently, you must spend a little time performing acts derived only from you."[135]

It is a common experience with this second exercise—be it taking off and putting on a ring at noon or putting on your left shoe first in the morning instead of your right—to remember, only after the fact, that we should have done it, sometimes minutes, hours, even days later. We may have been firmly committed and really interested in carrying out the deed, but the time slipped by unnoticed. This happens because we are not connected with our "time" body, which is the etheric body. Our astral body and our "I" may have been carrying the intention, but their connection to time and to the etheric remained too superficial. When we instead carefully watch what we are doing so that we notice the time leading up to a particular moment, we strengthen our connection to the etheric body. Then, when we carry out the task, using our limbs, we connect all the way down to the realm of the physical body. A penetration, from the heavens down, is completed.

It might be possible to accomplish this second exercise out of rigid duty or obsessive preoccupation. Perhaps for this very reason it is given as the second exercise, after we have first worked for a month on attaining freedom. For when we chose to do something every day, at the same time, out of a place of freedom, it refines our activity in the world. Whereas will into thought creates freedom, thought into will brings about love:

> But by what means do our actions evolve to greater perfection? How do we achieve greater perfection in our actions? We achieve this by developing in ourselves the force which can only be designated by the words: devotion to the outer world.—The more our devotion to the outer world grows and intensifies, the more does this outer world stir us to action. But it is just through unfolding devotion to the outer world that we succeed in permeating our actions with thoughts. What, in reality, is devotion to the outer world? Devotion to the outer world, which permeates our actions with thoughts, is nothing else than love.[136]

The second exercise, with careful waiting (protecting the well to make sure nothing should fall in) brings us to a place of loving connection with the world.

The first exercise helps us to continually overcome the density and rigidity of taking on the physical body. The second helps to overcome the superficiality that limits our engagement with the world. The earth lifts up to the heavens, and the heavens pour down to the earth. Out of this twofold movement comes the possibility for the third of the basic exercises: equanimity.

> People fluctuate back and forth between joy and sorrow. One moment they are beside themselves with joy, the next

> unbearably sad. Thus we allow ourselves to be rocked on the waves of life, on joy or sorrow. We must reach equanimity and steadiness. Neither the greatest sorrow nor the greatest joy must disturb one's composure. One must become steadfast and even-tempered.[137]

Such composure comes when we have been freed from previous patterns. We strive to not always react to things in a particular way. A healthy point of balance in the middle (which holds true for all of the polarities) does not exist as a static state. It comes from being able to consciously hold both extremes at the same time—both joy and sorrow. It means full integration, no longer captured in either the earthly or the cosmic polarity.

Once we have strengthened our process of integration and are better balanced and healthy in ourselves, we are then in a place where we can truly begin to meet the outside world. If the process of integration is imbalanced, we have seen how it limits our moral interaction. In a way, the younger child (of either the earthly/feeble or cosmic/maniacal inclinations) cannot fully meet the other because the child has not yet come into himself. Integration of self needs to happen first. A person might decide at certain points in personal development that "I just need to be more loving to the world" or might say, "The fourth exercise seems like the best; I'll just skip to that one!" But the fourth and fifth exercises are really only possible when a foundation for loving the world has been laid down through practice of the first three. Within the sequence of the six basic exercises it is only at this point that we can rightfully begin a moral encounter.

The fourth exercise moves us out into the world to practice "freedom from prejudice."[138] We could also call it the practice of positive engagement with the world. Prejudices are the reasons we find to stop looking at the world, because we think we already know it too well. The fourth exercise challenges us to not get stuck in the experiences we carry out of the past (a kind of inheritance) and to move beyond superficial observation. We are instructed to look at everything we encounter carefully, so that in it we can find the good:

> Try to approach what is wonderful in every phenomenon of outer reality. You will see that everything contains an aspect that can be affirmed. Do as Christ did when he admired the beautiful teeth of the dead dog. Practicing this will lead you to a great ability to tolerate anything, and you will gain an understanding of everything and of every being.[139]

We find the good—that which can be "affirmed"—by looking through the physical to see the spiritual inherent within it. This should form our practice for the fourth month.

The fifth month's exercise comes as the culmination of the sequence. By first integrating ourselves and then looking to find the spiritual essence that stands behind or within the physical world, we can then shift to a gesture of openness toward all that we encounter:

> The fifth quality is complete openness toward everything new that meets us. Most people judge new things according [to] the old things they already know. If someone comes and tells them something new, they immediately respond with an opposite opinion. But we must not confront a new communication immediately with our own opinion. We must instead always remain alert for the possibility of learning something new. We can learn, even from a small child. Even if you were the wisest person, you should be willing to hold back your own judgment and listen to others. We must develop this ability to listen, because it enables us to encounter matters with the greatest possible openness. In esotericism, this is called "faith." It is the power not to oppose, which weakens the impression made by the new.[140]

This fifth step brings us into true communion with the world around us, with the future, with the wisdom of the spiritual world. These fourth and fifth exercises challenge us to overcome the inheritance of what we carry with us and make it new—to push through our prejudices and find the good, to hold back our judgments and listen. Then, in the sixth exercise, we are asked to bring them all together.[141]

These six basic exercises could also be considered a therapeutic tool for the polarities we have been considering. For the stirring we engender in ourselves by working through these meditative activities will also flow over into the children we strive to help. An example of this would be our intentional engagement in the first exercise (*control of thought,* will into thought) to improve the ways we guide children with an earthly or feeble constitution, for such liberation of thinking frees us from the gravity of the physical body.

Alternatively, by taking up the second exercise (*control of deeds*, thinking into will), we learn how to improve the way we model intentional, fully guided activity as we work to support very cosmic or maniacal children. Certainly practicing the whole sequence allows us to model stronger and richer moral capacities in the world and refines our ability to sense the spiritual in the world (learning to see the good and to be open to what is new). It will encourage and reassure the children we work with, as they continuously look to know how to engage with the earthly, physical world.

PART TWO

THE POLARITY OF DIFFERENTIATION: BETWEEN BLOOD AND NERVE

Chapter 12

Sensing into an Experience of Self through the Foundational Senses

We have explored the developmental mandate of the first seven years as the penetration and individualization of the hereditary body. This can be accomplished only through the full fourfold interweaving of the "I" with the astral body, which then mutually enter the etheric, and all three take hold of the physical body. When this interpenetration successfully unfolds—through the warmth and activity of inflammation, through movement, or through moral encounter with the world—then the child will have a healthy experience of will. As the child nears the end of the first seven years and has successfully worked through this integration process, we see aspects of developmental ripeness emerge. We can even define some of the qualities we would expect to be present when this integration process is successful.

Starting with movement, we expect that the child will move capably and fluidly (stuck in neither a strongly feeble nor a maniacal movement pattern). Also, we expect that the child will be able to engage with the world with the beginnings of true moral perception. Engagement and movement—those are both activities, both dynamic qualities, that are appropriate for the will. It is very difficult to capture the healthy qualities of the metabolic–limb pole in static characteristics. Some of the sculptural aspects of the polarity described in the last section can be seen in a photograph (the formable quality of the head relative to the limbs), but most of the characteristics of the polarity of integration cannot be captured in a static image. We really need to see the child in activity.

For this reason, observing the will pole requires a different kind of perception. As an example, we do not learn to swim by looking at someone swimming while we are sitting on the side of the pool. To learn to swim, we have to dive into the water and get wet, we have to be in the process. Observation of the will similarly requires that we find ways to appreciate the child's experience of the body from the "inside." Practicing imitation, even mimicry, can be a very helpful therapeutic technique. In time we can learn to feel the experience a child has of the limbs without needing to move our own limbs in imitation. We live into their experience through imagination. It involves a kind of empathy—feeling with the child. It is not a static measure, not writing down measurements or taking a photograph. We feel into the child.

Steiner did speak about photographs in relation to the limbs and about the activity of the bones and muscles—but in a completely novel way, which helps to clarify the kind of observation needed. In a series of education lectures given to support the founding of the first Waldorf school, Steiner discussed the movement of a joint, in which two bones (or "laths" or "poles") are connected in a straight line, then bent (contracted) to form an angle:

> It is a thoroughly machine-like movement. You also carry out mechanical movements of this kind when you bend your knee and when you walk. For in walking the whole mechanism of your body is brought into continuous movement, and forces are continuously at work. They are pre-eminently forces of leverage, for forces are actually at work. Imagine to yourself that by some kind of photographic trick you could arrange that, when a man was walking, all the forces and nothing of the man, should be photographed; I mean the forces which he applies to raise his knee, to put it down again, to bring the other leg in front. Nothing of the man would be photographed except the forces. If in the photograph you could see these forces developing, it would be a photograph of a shadow, and even in walking itself you would see a whole series of shadows.... You live continually in forces. It is not in the least true that we live with our "I" in our visible body. We live with our "I" in forces.[142]

These shadows, these forces, are the activity of the will pole. Even though we have organs of movement (muscles, tendons, ligaments, and bones), to see the physiology of will, we need to understand that it is the activities, not the architecture, of the organs that are of primary importance in the metabolic–limb system.

Children learn to feel into the will pole through these forces, but not passively—as we do when we look at something from the outside. Children learn to feel into their own body by engendering these forces. Consequently, they will be unable to feel the activity of their limbs adequately if they have not moved them sufficiently. It is the full interpenetration of the four members that makes it possible to move the limbs and also that same interpenetration that allows one to feel into the body. We can extend our answer to the question "What does a successful integration look like?" by recognizing that there is a relationship between healthy movement and the capacity to feel into the forces of our own body, into the photographic shadows. We usually think of sensing as an outwardly directed activity, but our sensing activity needs to extend not only into the world of external objects but also into our inner world of forces.

There are specific, identifiable steps along this inward pathway into the body. Steiner carefully described them as sense capacities, though to do so adequately, he needed to expand beyond the commonly identified five senses.[143]

Steiner placed in the middle of our sensing world the capacity for vision, which lies in a neutral kind of position with regard to our inner and outer worlds. We encounter visual impressions all day long, most of them resulting in only a superficial kind of cognition. The majority of them do not make a deep impression or effect a significant change in us. Vision is the sense through which we most commonly encounter an object or person. "The sense of sight transmits to us the surface of external corporeality which confronts us in color, brightness, or darkness."[144] Our eyes may brush past an object, or what we see may stimulate us to look more deeply and really engage with it. The process of gazing more deeply, really looking carefully at something in the outer world takes us out of ourselves. We forget ourselves a little bit in order to really connect with what is seen outside. That visual engagement and inquiry begin an outwardly directed sensing pathway. In contrast, to begin a more contemplative activity, to become more in tune with our inner world, we often close our eyes. That frees our sensing activity to move more inward. For this reason, we can consider vision as a kind of neutral, "middle" sense.

What do we meet when we take a step further into ourselves? Steiner suggested that we come to the sense of taste. Through our sense of taste, an outer object begins to exercise an inner effect as it meets a person's secretions. We come into more intimate relation with something through tasting it than by just seeing it. A very delicious or a very unpleasant taste certainly pulls our attention into ourselves. The pathway of inward sensing then really begins with taste.

If we trace the pathway a step further, we come to smell. Even just considering the anatomy of the sense organs, we can see that the mucous membranes of the nose are more inward. (For example, we cannot casually lick or sip with our sense of smell the way we can with our sense of taste.) The olfactory nerve links directly back to the brain so that smells have a more immediate effect than taste and result in "quite an important change in our inner being."[145] Smells have an almost visceral effect and commonly bring strong emotional associations. It is hard to be completely objective and noncommittal when it comes to smell. It provokes an inward reaction in us, good or bad. So the inwardly directed sensing pathway goes from vision to taste to smell.

Going another step inward, Steiner placed the sense of touch. We are all, of course, very familiar with the sense of touch, and this placement of touch as a sensory activity more inward than smell can feel quite unexpected. We are used to thinking of touch as a way that we reach out to understand the qualities of the objects around us, and that is certainly true. But that information about outer objects actually comes as a secondary experience, because it really only arises from an extrapolation of the changes we experience within our own body:

> When you touch objects, you actually perceive only yourself. You touch an object and if it is hard it presses forcibly on you; if it is soft its pressure is only slight. You perceive nothing of the object, however; you sense only the effect upon yourself, the change in yourself. A hard object pushes your organs far back into you. You perceive this resistance as a change in your own organism when you perceive by the means of touch.[146]

This understanding is therapeutically very useful, for it helps orient the sense of touch as a core human experience. We know that children's physical and emotional development can be interrupted if they do not receive regular healthy touch as an infant. Viewed in this way, touch is not just an outwardly directed meeting but indeed an essential step on the inward pathway for knowing how we are, in our bodies. We experience calm and nurturing reassurance through the experience of deep touch, whether through a massage or a hug or, as an adult, through sexual intimacy. When we look to the larger realm of sensory integration disorders that are so prevalent today, it is clear that children who experience disturbances within the sense of touch not only experience challenges in relating to the outside environment (being at one moment hypersensitive and at the next moment almost numbed) but also often struggle with accompanying challenges of self-regulation. In truth, we should reverse the order of that sentence, because the inability to really sense oneself comes first, and through that inability to feel "the effect upon yourself, the change in yourself" comes the disturbance with the outside world.[147] That marks an archetypal developmental progression—that in order to properly meet and sense the outside world, we must be able to first sense into ourselves. For this reason it is very helpful, when there are outwardly observable behavioral or learning problems, for us to look to this inward sensory pathway to see where disturbances might lie. To accurately sense the outside world, we have to first not be distracted by the ways we cannot properly sense ourselves.

The inward pathway: from vision to taste to smell to touch—these are all members of the traditionally acknowledged five senses (with only hearing left out). The next inward sense is not part of those five but is still well known, its organ centered in the inner ear. It is our sense of balance (which can also be described as our vestibular sense). In coming to the sense of balance, we have crossed a certain threshold, because our vestibular sense is not stimulated by anything from the outside (which was indeed the case with vision, taste, smell, and touch). It is a sense devoted to our own position and orientation. We know that we are shifting our position (when spinning, bending, or riding on an elevator) because of very small crystals (*otoliths*), suspended in fluid (the *otolymph*) of our inner ear. It is only in rare circumstances—like with an earthquake—that our sense of balance informs us about the activity of the outside world; its activity is to tell us how we are changing our position in relation to gravity and to the outside world:

> Then, if we press still further into our interior, we come upon a sense which is no longer mentioned, as least not often. It is a sense by which we differentiate between our standing up or lying down, and through which we perceive when we are standing on our own two feet, that we are in a state of balance. This experience of equilibrium is transmitted by the sense of balance. There, we penetrate completely into our interior; we perceive the relationship of our own inner being to the world outside, within which we experience ourselves in a state of equilibrium. We perceive this, however, entirely within our inner being.[148]

In this description Steiner expanded the sense of balance beyond the strictly physical vestibular sensing of where we are in space to include the experience of "ourselves in a state of equilibrium." This is worth noting. This means we feel ourselves in direct relation to the world through touch and then in relative relation through balance.

There is an aspect of the sense of balance that allows us to find a comfortable place where we are no longer required to be actively engaged with the environment (as we are with the sense of touch) but also are not entirely cut off from it (as when we are asleep). That equilibrium allows us to enter into quietly observant activity, open to noticing the world but not dependent on it. That middle space also belongs to the sense of balance.

A further step, one that is even more inward, is the sense of movement. It is today commonly identified with the proprioceptive sense, which means the ability to consciously sense the changing movement of our bodies (particularly the position of the limbs in space). The specific nerve endings within the muscles and joints that make this sensing possible had probably not been clearly identified anatomically in the 1920s, but Steiner recognized it as a distinct sensing pathway. The sensory organs for taste and smell are easily identified. Those for touch are highly localized but spread throughout the skin. The vestibular organ in the inner ear is more hidden; we cannot see it from the outside, but it can still be found. The nerve endings for the sense of movement, however, are quite diffuse, and the sensory experience that arises from them is much more general. As Steiner put it:

> If we penetrate still further into ourselves we find a sense that inwardly reveals to us whether we are at rest or in movement. We don't only observe whether we are remaining still or moving simply by virtue of the external objects moving past us; through the extension or retraction of our muscles and through the configuration of our body insofar as the latter changes when we move about, we can inwardly perceive to what extent we are in motion, and so forth. This happens through the sense of movement.[149]

We see a progression whereby sensory activity has become larger and more of a whole-body experience, while the sensory organs become increasingly less defined. We are moving away from structure and more toward an awareness of forces.

Gross motor and fine motor development depend on our senses of touch, of balance, and of movement. They manifest in the way we move our bodies and interact with objects (like holding a fork or learning to ride a bicycle). An important additional aspect of the sense of movement is not just knowing where our limbs are in space (without having to look to see) but also modulating our movement. Think of a twelve- or thirteen-month-old child who is just learning to toddle and how walking essentially has two speeds: either standing/balancing or moving forward. Walking activity at that age is basically on or off. In time, the process of walking becomes much more refined, more nuanced, with many speeds and variations. An older child, however, who is still struggling to develop this sense of movement and has as yet still immature sensing will commonly exhibit movement that is too strong (and therefore often excessive, even hurtful) or so weak as to be ineffectual. Movement, even in this older child, still tends to be strongly "on" or mostly "off."

We can relate this modulation of movement back to the polarity of feeble and maniacal movement. In feeble movement there is not enough movement in general; then, when the limbs are loosened into movement, the activity is big and coarse. There is little nuance. For these children the sense of movement is clearly still a little numb.

A certain kind of movement numbness is also present for the maniacal constitution. For in these children there is a lot of movement, but it is not adjusted or adapted to the surrounding environment. Here there is actually also very little modulation—like a dim light that is left on all the time, regardless of whether there is dark night or bright sunshine. Movement is not guided, because it is not fully sensed; it carries on, on its own. The superficiality of the maniacal movement extends not only outwardly but also inwardly. If we try to imagine a "hand" of consciousness reaching in—from vision, to taste, to smell, to touch, to balance, to movement—that hand does not extend very far. In fact, for children who strongly exhibit either feeble or maniacal movement, there are very commonly numb areas in the senses of touch, balance, or movement. These body-oriented senses, which are so closely related to the will, remain underdeveloped.

The last, most inward sense in this progression is what Steiner called the sense of life. It is considered to be the fourth of the "lower senses," which include the sense of touch, balance, movement, and life.[150] The life sense is completely directed toward our inner world, to our sense of self. As Steiner put it:

> When do we enter the most into ourselves? When, within the general feeling of life, we perceive what we always have as our consciousness in the waking condition; when we perceive that we are; when we experience ourselves inwardly; when we sense that we are we. All this is mediated by the life sense.[151]

Steiner further ascribed the life sense to our sense of wellbeing, something we do not usually appreciate unless it has been disturbed. For it is really only when our inner world is disturbed—through hunger, through illness, through fatigue—that our life sense comes up into consciousness.

What is the sense organ for the life sense? It is even more dispersed than the nerve endings in the joints, skin, and muscles, because the life sense is connected to all of the normally sleeping functions of the body that lie below the level of consciousness. We could perhaps best say that the organ of the life sense is the autonomic nervous system. The processes of sleep, digestion, excretion, and reproduction all live within this realm.

The life sense stands as the most inward part of our sensing life, but it is a sensing that is easily drowned out by other sensory impressions or demands. Disturbances in the preceding senses (touch, balance, or movement) can influence and interrupt our ability to come to the sense of life. In fact, many sensory-seeking behaviors are attempts to self-stimulate ourselves in order to get further along that inward pathway. These are familiar behaviors; we all call on these instinctive activities to help us feel more collected—like crossing our legs or wringing our hands when feeling anxious or bouncing a leg, tapping a foot, or rocking or swiveling on a chair when we are bored. These stimulate the lower senses and help us to feel more centered and calm within ourselves. They help connect us to a more settled orientation with our body, which is particularly helpful when outer conditions require some vigilance and we are not able to let go of them fully enough to connect all the way in to the life sense.

These kind of self-stimulating behaviors shift and become disruptive to regular activity when one or more of the lower senses is particularly imbalanced. This happens when there has not been enough metabolic/will activity to be able to feel all the way down into the body. For the health of the lower senses develops in relation to experience. When one of the lower senses is still unformed and therefore immature, there arises an excessive need to stimulate that sense. This drive for stimulation is a two-edged sword; it leads to greater development and refinement of the sense (children seek out the sensory experiences they need), but that overwhelming drive can also blunt or block the development of a connection to the life sense. Excessive sensory demands (like continually avoiding any balance stimulation or repeatedly seeking out unusually strong touch stimuli) can become blockages on the inward path. Whatever senses lie further inward from the needy sense activity may also stay immature. They may not fully come to expression, because they are drowned out by competing (earlier) sensory needs. Let us look in more detail at how some of these competing sensory blockages can present themselves.

An Incompletely Developed Sense of Touch

The sense of touch can be imbalanced in two different directions: we may retreat from the world because we experience the change in ourselves too powerfully (hyperesthesia), resulting in avoidance of tags, belts, tight socks, scratchy fabrics, crunchy food textures, and so on, or we may seek to exaggerate our touch encounters so that we can truly experience ourselves in that meeting, because we otherwise do not really feel them (hypoesthesia) and therefore seek very strong touch—squeezing, crashing, hitting—to enliven an experience that is at baseline too numbed. It is very possible for children to also swing back and forth between the two extremes, alternating hyper- and hyposensitivity. That swinging shows that the modulation in the middle has not yet been developed, but deep, steady, and nonthreatening touch can be very calming and orienting for both extremes. Through the sense of touch we begin to permeate ourselves inwardly.[152] The work of Temple Grandin explores that relationship in depth, describing the therapeutic power of strong touch in autism.[153] Other authors have also explored the importance of the four lower senses in the life of the young child in great detail.[154] We can make the following general observations:

- It is essential that children be allowed and encouraged to move their bodies and explore the environment in dynamic ways. Our modern lifestyle tends to be very full with busy schedules but too often lacks significant activity of the four lower senses. Encouraging children to explore the environment (which is really an essential path of feeling into themselves) through lifting, rolling, crawling, wrestling, and hugging fosters natural explorations of touch.
- Children who have problems with tight clothing and itchy fabrics or who are very selective about food textures or, alternatively, who are continually falling, crashing, and squeezing and prefer for their clothing to be tight (like a cinched belt) are experiencing an imbalanced sense of touch.
- Bringing a child intentional, safe, steady touch sensations, through things like burrito rolls, playing with heavy beanbags, dry skin brushing, and large joint compression add a therapeutic potency to the experience of touch.

Both under-sensitive and overly sensitive touch reactions benefit from these kinds of experiences. The sense of touch grows stronger and matures through that experience. The way in which we bring touch to the child may, however, necessarily be quite different:

- Children who are still a little bit numbed in their touch experience continually find ways to push the physical boundary of the body hard enough so that it matches the sensing boundary of their astral body (which does not extend out far enough). Their need for strong touch is great, so finding socially healthy opportunities for strong encounter is essential. Repeatedly telling a child with numbed touch to stop engaging in those strong sensory encounters may actually delay/deny the development of that sense. In fact, when a child is repeatedly doing the same behavior and not listening to requests to stop, touching the child (touching the head, holding and gently squeezing the hands, rubbing the shoulders or back) while speaking may bring about better attention. Through touch one is meeting the child in the realm of the sense that is calling for so much of the child's attention. Similarly, meeting the child who seeks strong touch encounters with firm touch at the beginning of the transition (arriving into the classroom in the morning, getting ready to shift activities, or putting on a coat) grounds the child by helping to put the longing for touch at rest, which allows the child to better pay attention to outside activity.
- Children who avoid touch will also benefit from deep, steady touch, but they need to have the space and safety to initiate the encounter. As an example, children who are overly sensitive to touch will, with time, very happily come and snuggle into a teacher's lap if the lap is consistently offered and available. Bringing strong touch directly to the child is too frightening—for the astral sensing activity of the limbs of these children may extend well beyond the physical boundary of the skin. As with numbed touch, repeated opportunity to feel firm touch helps to sculpt the physical and sensing activities into a more cooperative relationship. If a touch encounter needs to happen, such as

> putting arms through the sleeves of a coat, presenting the coat and then allowing the child to choose which arm to put in first may ease the touch encounter. Asking children if they are ready to put on the coat usually only heightens their touch sensitivity. Clear, consistent expectation that the touch encounter will happen is another form of firm, steady touch, just in the social realm. Consistency is another way for a teacher or parent to bring healthy experience of boundary. In contrast, erratic or unpredictable expectations and reactions have a disruptive influence on how a child "touches" the world. (We explore this dynamic more fully in the third section of the book, focusing on the epileptic and hysteric polarity.)

An Incompletely Developed Sense of Balance

Balance tells us about our relative position to the outside world and also makes it possible for us to find our own inner equilibrium. Equilibrium may sound static, but it is not. It comes from being able to constantly adjust, to be able to sense our own activity and outside activity without being captured by either one. Our sense of balance allows us to release from the environment without totally losing hold of it. Like all of the senses, balance should have a kind of transparency so that we are sensing through it, without our consciousness being diverted to the sense organ itself. When the sense of balance is undersensitive, it is common to see a child exaggerate change in position in order to better feel the relative inner change (lots of spinning, falling, hanging, leaning, rocking). Here again is a pattern of exaggerated self-stimulation, though the activity tends to be more self-contained than with an undersensitive sense of touch (in which the outer world must be encountered in order to feel oneself).

If our vestibular sensing is too active (overly sensitive), connection to the outside world retreats, and our attention becomes directed very strongly to our own change. Anyone who has suffered from an episode of vertigo can relate to this (perhaps from an inner ear inflammation or too much time spent on a rocking boat). We feel unwell—dizzy, nauseated, and off balance, even to the point of vomiting. The experience of vertigo in this situation is not limited to a strictly mechanical incapacity that makes us wobble; we truly experience that we have lost our equilibrium for our whole sense of self, and we feel off. Then we retreat from any stimulation to our balance sense. This gives us a picture for the kind of protective self-possession that comes when the lower senses are markedly underdeveloped but overly sensitive.

Our sense of balance is not static; we can adjust it. With gentle repetition we learn to modulate our own sensing response—as, for example, when after the first few swings on a swing we are not so affected by it. We downregulate our vestibular sensing. Conversely, if the sense is too numb and then, when walking on a balance beam, we stop paying attention to the noise and activity around us in order to better sense the change in our body position, we upregulate our vestibular sensing. That is the kind of equilibrium we are all trying to unfold: to learn to balance dynamically, to keep the teeter-totter in the air without one side or the other clunking abruptly to the ground. It is a balancing that influences many areas of life.

We can summarize as follows:

- Patterns of repeated rocking, bouncing, chair tipping, or spinning can be understood as a child's attempt to exaggerate the shifting relationship of self and environment through the sense of balance (even adolescents who love to ride roller coasters!). If children with an immature, undersensitive vestibular sense do not stimulate their balance sensing strongly enough, they lose connection with themselves.
- Children who avoid fast movement, who shun swings, or who do not like to bend down to the ground or stand up too fast are frequently overwhelmed by their own overly sensitive balance sense. Great energies are then devoted to circumventing any quick shift in space, with a resultant emphasis on children's own experience—how can they

hold themselves steady? The process of protective self-awareness may drown out the external world and limit many forms of dynamic engagement.

- Helping a child to explore swings, balance beams, rising and falling, or jumping rope, all support the child's work to find physical equilibrium.
- Furthermore, any time children can be guided to adjust or modulate their activity in relation to the outer environment also works to strengthen the sense of balance. Such interactions have a threefold architecture to them: first acknowledging what a child needs or feels (such as being angry, being bored, desperately wanting to move), then giving a clear boundary as to what is possible or permissible in that situation ("But you may not scream in the classroom or hit another child"), and then helping the child find a middle pathway ("Why don't you sit down quietly for a few minutes until you are ready to play more gently"). Modeling that kind of modified interaction also helps a child strengthen the social aspect of the sense of balance. This threefold pattern is explored in more depth in the section on aggressive behaviors (see Chap. 25).
- The physical and social aspects of finding equilibrium overlap, so that a child who struggles to modulate social balancing (particularly the ones who want to do things too strongly, who seek strong physical balance stimulation) can be helped by providing regular opportunities for swinging, rocking, or balance-beam walking. Nurturing the physical organ of balance will help the child in unfolding the more social/spiritual aspects of equilibrium. Conversely, a child who too keenly senses changes in physical balance (and probably works hard to avoid them) can be helped through consistent expectations for engagement, often as part of a larger group activity. The safety of cohesive activity allows a child to better engage in digestible amounts of vestibular stimulation (and they may be more willing to do it if the whole class is doing it), which in time will work back upon the physical sensing capacity.

An Incompletely Developed Sense of Movement

As our sensing activity shifts yet more inward, there are, of course, many inner activities happening all of the time, of which we are only minimally aware. They are different from the limb and eye movements we carry out through the course of the day, which are to varying degrees intentional and conscious. The movements of breath (respiration) and blood (circulation) are different in that they are continuous and so intrinsic that we cannot live without them. We need to include these activities in the sense of movement as well. A very important quality of circulatory and respiratory movements is that they are also constantly modulated. It is a sign of health when our heart rate and respiratory rate rise and fall in relation to our activity.

Proprioception (the sensing ability to know where our body and limbs are in space from the inside, without needing to look at them from the outside) is part of the sense of movement too, but it is not strictly limited to geometric perception. It is not only the position of the bones, or laths (to return to Steiner's photographic analogy for the will system) but extends much more into the dynamic sensing of how our joints are moving and changing (the shadows of the forces). That sensing, that capacity for modulation helps us know when we need to move and when we need to be still, to know how much to engage. Outwardly this expresses itself through skills like catching a ball without looking or tying our shoelaces. In a way it is in our hands. We feel what we need to do, from the inside. It is very disconcerting when one does not have that connection and suddenly needs to look at one's movements from the outside—like the paralysis when a leg or arm falls asleep. For children who have not yet developed the sense of movement, in many ways their limbs are still mostly asleep, and they need to watch their bodies from the outside to see what they should be doing. This is particularly evident with imitative activities. These children will look to see where their arms or legs are in space, because they cannot feel it from the inside. Their proprioceptive sense is still so numbed that they need to return to a much more outward sense, vision (from movement past balance, touch, smell, and taste and back to vision) in order to connect to their activity. The movement then is characteristically quite halting, as the child cannot move fluidly; the activity must go back and forth between movement of the bone and muscles, then vision (and adjustment), then movement, then vision (and adjustment), and so on. The child cannot be in the activity, sense it, and simultaneously adjust it.

This is admittedly quite a complex skill, one that perhaps only the finest athletes, dancers, and musicians really perfect. Nonetheless, life is full of circumstances where we are asked to carry out an activity and simultaneously adjust or refine it—like pedaling a bicycle (a fairly rote motor activity) but then also speeding up or slowing down in relation to obstacles in the road or the increased resistance of going uphill. The sense of movement also builds through repetition and experience. Each time we do something, it becomes a little bit easier, more fluid, and we are able to move beyond the simple mechanics of the movement (which is more about pure proprioception and the building of muscle memory) and into modulation, which in time brings the possibility for a kind of movement mastery.

We should therefore think about an underdeveloped sense of movement not only in situations where there is generally poor awareness of the limbs in space but also when there are challenges in modulating movement activity. Here are some examples:

- Children with underdeveloped movement are guarded in their movements; they need to stop to look and check their movements against their neighbors ("Am I holding my hands the right way?"). They commonly move in spurts: movement—look to see if it is right—movement—check again—movement, and so on. Their activity lacks fluidity and continuity. (This pattern can also be seen in children who are very sensitive to the outside world and move fitfully out of fear of encounter—see part 3 and the descriptions of the hysteric constitution. These children are so busy directing their attention outward that they sacrifice their inner anchoring through the lower senses.) A very sensitive child often re-anchors happily and successfully into the lower senses when the environment is well known and safe, like a home environment versus a school setting, whereas a child with a truly undeveloped sense of movement may struggle with this in all settings.

- We should also consider the health of the sense of movement in children who have fluid movement but in whom the movement is either too strong (excessive) or too weak (inadequate). The movement is carried out, but there is no way to adjust it while doing it. The impulse for movement successfully comes down into the limbs, but the connection cannot be sustained, like pushing a canoe out into the river with no one to steer. The child cannot yet feel into the movement or modify the movement once it has started.
- Pushing (open a heavy door), lifting (a heavy versus a light object), dancing (especially with a partner), sawing or cutting (how hard or soft to push and pull), jumping rope (matching the speed of a jump rope), and weaving on a loom are all examples of ways for children to move and simultaneously adjust their forces of movement while they are active (not just apologizing or trying to compensate after the fact). These are all very healthy ways for a child to refine the sense of life and build on the health of the senses of touch and balance.

Chapter 13
The Pathway to the Life Sense

The sense organs that lie along this inwardly directed path—from vision, to taste, to smell, to touch, to balance, to movement—are all still connected to the world and therefore also accessible to outer observation. The final sense (the most inward), the sense of life, remains a bit more hidden.

Developmental milestones for both gross and fine motor skills give us specific measures for the maturation of the senses of touch, balance, and movement. They check to see whether an activity is present—for example can a child hop and get both feet off the ground? If a child cannot jump in that way by twenty-four months of age, we know that we need to look more closely at motor development and the senses of balance and movement. That kind of observation is fairly straightforward. Measures for the sense of life are less easily defined through such checkmark methods. In fact, it is debatable whether a life-sense category even exists in most developmental screening tools. What sort of methods allow us to know from the outside how children experience themselves inwardly—how a girl senses that she is "she"? Yet, at the same time, the health of the life sense influences nearly every realm of activity. To observe it, we need to free ourselves from outside measures and instead watch the pathway inward, to see how well a child is at home in the body.

It has already been mentioned that the life sense has a connection to our autonomic nervous system. As a starting place we can choose several largely unconscious, autonomic functions to consider. One is the imbalance we all experience as hunger. When we are hungry, we do not feel well. Something is not right. We might be tempted to use hunger as a shortcut, an approximation to say that hunger is the life sense. This is not quite accurate, because the life sense is related much more closely to an intrinsic knowledge of when we need to eat (before we get so hungry that it disturbs the rest of our activity) and to the knowledge of when we have had enough. We feel imbalance either way: eating so much that we feel unwell and the pleasure of food is gone or aching and distracted by our need for food. The life sense helps us know (from the inside) what we need to do. Thirst connects similarly with the life sense (asking when we need to drink water or when we have drunk enough water) as well as other bodily functions, like knowing when it is time to go to the bathroom, when it is time to sleep, and when it is time to wake up. These are all quiet signals that help us autoregulate and contribute to our sense of wellbeing.

In early life much of the life sense is related to the activity and proximity of a child's mother (or whoever acts as the primary caretaker). We can watch the progress of this pathway inward by watching a baby. Already immediately after birth, an infant is comforted by the taste of mother's milk. Breast feeding helps to make all the wrongs right and puts the whole child's physiology at ease. Suddenly the life sense is balanced; the child feels well, and the child's whole physiology calms. How did this happen so quickly? What prompted the child to connect so quickly to that inner sense of wellbeing?

Breast-feeding, as a sensory activity, is primarily rooted in the sense of taste. Of course, it also carries the experience of smell and touch, but the sweet taste of mother's milk is comforting and calming. We know this to be true because it acts as a balm even when it is given by the father or by a grandparent. So, in our very first days and weeks (even months) of life, our sense of taste helps connect us to the life sense.

As children grow a bit older, the possibility for soothing expands, and smell (in addition to taste) becomes a gateway to wellbeing. It is now possible to soothe and calm babies by simply handing them to their mother—with her familiar, distinctive smell—and baby feels better, even without needing to breast-feed. The taste of milk, which was given completely from the outside, can now more frequently be supplanted with smell, which, whereas it comes from the outside, is more of an inner experience. With this step, the sensory activity for calming moves further inward, and the child's capacity for self-soothing becomes a little more independent. We can almost think of it as the development of some soothing resilience, where children can find their place of wellbeing with a little less input from the outside.

As children continue to grow, another step comes as they learn to calm more through the gateway of touch, cradling, hugging, and snuggling. Taste and smell become less important for calming and soothing; at this point other familiar adults (a teacher, neighbor, or friend) can also help in calming the child. Why is this? It is because the sense of touch is again more inward. In fact, if we recall Steiner's description of the sense of touch, the child's experience is more one of feeling oneself, of saying, "Here I am." Receiving loving touch is helpful because it lends an experience of orientation, which is essential for self-soothing. By this point the child's capacity for being soothed has grown, so that the senses of taste, then smell, and now also touch can act as important gateways to an enhanced sense of wellbeing.

This process continues to expand and enlarge, though not necessarily with a silky smooth transition. At a certain point the child gets a little restless with these three sensory gateways (which often happens when the child is between six and nine months old), and now nursing or holding or swaddling is not enough—the child wants to be bounced. There needs to be more movement, and the child wants to participate in this movement. It can feel confusing for the parent, because what used to work beautifully does not seem to be enough anymore, and so there are desperate attempts to nurse more or to hold more or to bounce more and for longer periods of time. It can be exhausting, because it seems as if the child is demanding so much more sensory stimulus to reach the same point, and bewildering, because the child used to respond so well in the past. ("I used to just nurse, and my baby went right to sleep," or "Now I have to lie so that our shoulders are touching, because if I get up the baby will not go to sleep.") These can be times of high parental anxiety, but if we look at this progression, we can be reassured that when this kind of sensory restlessness emerges, it is a sign of another step on the child's pathway toward the life sense. We are charting our way from the sense of taste (of milk), to smell (of mother), to touch (of cradling), to now active touch (engagement) and the beginnings of balance (bouncing). This new restlessness represents a kind of developmental stretching, for what initially was given as a fully outer sensory experience (the taste of breast milk) is gradually supplanted by more active, independent capacities. When touch stops being a fully satiating experience, it is usually because the child needs to unfold a larger sensory experience that now includes active touch and balance.

It is striking that the timing for this transition generally comes during the same period that outer mobility sees tremendous development—with finding the strength to roll (four to five months), then to sit (six months), and then to crawl (nine months). This evolves into standing and walking (twelve to fifteen months). As a child becomes more skillful at exploring the outward, surrounding environment through gross motor strength and skills, there is a reciprocal progression inward, through the lower senses toward the life sense. This is appropriate, for as a child becomes more independent through exploration of the physical environment and the social environment, the child needs to feel more inwardly grounded and secure. Through these steps, the capacity for self-soothing becomes more innate. Children actively strive, step by step, to become more participatory in the process of their own soothing.

Another prominent developmental step also comes somewhere between six and nine months of age, and that is children's need for more regular eating and sleeping rhythms. Again, things have changed—just breast feeding a seven-month-old is not going to bring on sleep. At this point, regular nap times, predictable bedtimes, consistent snack and mealtimes become very important. Why do children need predictable rhythms? Rhythm allows us to begin to participate inwardly in our own physiologic processes. Take some very common examples: If a child learns that lunch comes at 12:00 p.m. every day, then soon that child's secretion of stomach acid and digestive enzymes will begin at 11:40 a.m. If bedtime is consistently 7 p.m., the child's nervous system starts shifting to a more anabolic, restorative activity at 6:30 or 6:45 p.m. The move toward consistent rhythms may be met initially with resistance, but it will quickly become a parent's best friend. Less has to be done from the outside, because through predictable rhythms the child's own inner participation increases (a kind of physiologic anticipation and preparation). It is no casual coincidence that this developmental shift comes at the time that a child really begins to outwardly explore the world through movement.

Many children, even before this six- to nine-month age span, are ready to more actively participate in their self-soothing through learning to have a transition time between nursing and falling asleep. When this space can be encouraged—so that there are a few minutes of wakeful activity between coming off the breast or bottle and then settling into sleep—dependence on the sense of taste changes. Sucking or nursing becomes more of a signal that it is time to calm, but it leaves room for children to practice taking up some of those self-soothing steps on their own. Where repetition and consistent life rhythms allow for greater anticipatory inner changes in getting ready for an event (like a nap or a meal), this space between nursing and sleeping encourages a child to carry on with the self-soothing, self-orienting process after receiving prompts and guidance from a parent. This transition space may again be initially met with some restlessness, as the child learns to grow into this space (though this is generally a fairly short-lived process). But offering the child space to practice self-soothing brings a lasting capacity that will help the child settle and stay asleep for longer periods of time. The child is then better able to fall back to sleep independently in the middle of the night. We can see that between six and nine months of age, as a child learns to sit and then crawl out into the world, there are continued openings for a more rhythmic, inner participation in activities and the beginnings of independent self-soothing.

In the next phase, between twelve and fifteen months, a child makes another big transition with outer exploration, learning to pull up to stand, to cruise (perhaps along the edge of a couch), and then to begin to walk. Gross motor movement has become more complex. Where rolling and crawling were primarily related to the sense of touch, standing and walking now also depend on the sense of balance and the beginnings of self-movement. The primary sense that makes standing and walking possible (balance) is one step further on the pathway through the lower senses. Balance has already been maturing, as between six and nine months a child enjoys the stimulation of bouncing or moving, but now through standing, balance has become independent. There is not yet much modulation (related to the sense of movement), for this early walking basically alternates between two speeds—stand and go. The sense of self-movement is just beginning.

Between twelve and fifteen months comes another window, where many children will happily wean from breast-feeding. In fact, at this age, some children express quite emphatically that they are done and have no more interest. Steiner indicated that it is appropriate for a child to stop breast-feeding when the child becomes independent in movement, and so this shift into more active movement and more independent ways of being helps explain why this is true. This kind of time line is not meant to be a hard and fast rule, for there are many different viewpoints and experiences relating to the manner and duration of breast-feeding. Even so, it is very helpful to know that such a window opens for many children and that it will not hurt their development to wean in the period between twelve and eighteen months, especially when one can see that a child is making joyful motor and social exploration of the world. Small children are by nature continually striving to develop more active capacities for self-calming and self-orientation; they blossom in relation to the maturation of touch, balance, and movement.

Let us look at how this finds expression in specific situations. We can all agree that as a child becomes more independent, a child also needs to learn to self-orient, for when we are less attended, there is less outside help available. This need for self-orientation (an aspect of self-soothing) comes up for small children whenever they are transitioning from one activity to another. A child who cannot self-orient becomes overwhelmed by the situation. How do children strengthen this capacity? They do so by falling asleep at bedtime. The same pathway we follow at night to withdraw our attention from the outside world helps us calm and orient in a busy or chaotic outer environment. We learn to recognize that "this is the process I know that helps me to feel well and able to find my peace," and that capacity flows over into other situations in which we need to calm ourselves—whether two hours later when we rouse at the end of a sleep cycle (and we have to put ourselves to sleep again) or when we feel lost or overwhelmed in a confusing situation. Children naturally go back to that calming process over and over, so that whatever a child experiences at bedtime the child will want to have repeated or re-created whenever she wakes in the night or whenever she feels insecure.

Children who fall asleep while nursing will frequently want to nurse back to sleep; children who need a parent to lie in the bed until they fall asleep will (completely understandably) get up to find a parent to fall asleep with. This is an interesting parenting paradox, because when it feels as if we are providing a wonderful, loving activity by giving a child a long, involved bedtime ritual (which we are), with lots of soothing interaction and reassurance, we simultaneously also need to be giving the child space to practice steps of self-soothing. When that space does not open, a child can become stuck, needing outside help well beyond the first years of life. As will be explored in the next section, the ability to successfully self-soothe as an independent skill should find a healthy and full development during the first seven years of life. At age six and a half to seven years, children become etherically independent from their mother, and this inner capacity for self-orienting and self-calming becomes pivotal.

We can summarize these points by recognizing that the inner pathway to the life sense can be supported in several ways. First, healthy movement underlies this whole process (which is really the process of integration explored in the previous section).

With regard to the process of calming and falling asleep, we can also lend support by gradually allowing a space between nursing and falling asleep (which greatly helps a child learn to settle into a rhythmic sleep pattern as they approach the six to nine month transition). Later, we need to be open to seeing when a child is ready to wean and to take a next developmental step, as part of a shift away from taste and nursing as routine elements in the soothing process (which often comes as the sense of balance strengthens and the child learns to walk freely, between twelve and fifteen months).

A third step we have not mentioned but that follows in the same progression is moving much of the bedtime ritual out of the bedroom and into a common space. The timing of this is less specific but can be considered by the time a child is really fully independent and mobile (running, hopping, leaping). This divided bedtime still allows an extended opportunity for reading a story, snuggling, or hearing stories about the day. It preserves the physical intimacy a young child needs for experiencing elements of smell and touch, but now it introduces a temporal threshold ("It is time for bed") and an accompanying geographic threshold (moving from the living room into the bedroom), which creates a space for the parent to actively calm and connect and then a different space for the child to independently chart the path to self-soothing. When these major parts of bedtime preparation are done (bath, story, cuddling, conversation), the completion of the process in the bedroom can become quite short (a verse, then a hug and kiss). If we think about parents providing a share of the soothing process, at birth it is probably about ninety-five percent. As a child learns to find the soothing space between nursing and sleeping and then to fall asleep without nursing, the parenting share drops, and the child's capacity grows. By the time a child reaches kindergarten age, the larger share of the soothing process can be taken on by the child. Then bedtime becomes more of a reminder, a marker that it is time to begin the transition to sleep than an attempt to provide sufficient stimulation to make the child go to sleep. This third step has the advantage that it simplifies the number of sensory experiences a child receives as part of the final calming process into sleep, so that when the child's sleep lightens in the middle of the night, there is less of a need for parental contact in order to go back to sleep (because the place to talk and cuddle is in the different space of the living room, not in the bed the child is lying it). The introduction of such a time and location transition has proved helpful in many situations in which the process of falling asleep and staying asleep in one's own bed has become problematic or even quite dysfunctional.

A related piece of this process involves close observation of how children, and for that matter adults, invoke sensory experiences in order to self-soothe. What do we do when we are anxious or in a socially nebulous situation? We stimulate our senses of touch, balance, and movement—we rub our brows, cross and uncross our legs, twirl our hair, bounce a foot, or clench our hands in fists. When the outside world is not predictable, we create inner security by invoking the lower senses, which helps us connect to the life sense as an inner anchor. Many people also engage in these same kinds of behaviors when they are getting ready to fall asleep, such as rubbing the face on a pillow (touch), rolling to the left two times and then to the right once (balance), or yawning, stretching, and moving around several times before settling in (movement). Those are all behaviors that help us release from the outer world and come more into our inner realm.

Children learn to do this, too. It is important that there is, again, the space for them to experiment with this self-orienting as part of their sensory maturation. Too often any kind of self-stimulating movement at nap time or bedtime is perceived as restlessness, and then there is the temptation to want to intervene. We decide we need to bring more reassurance and comfort from the outside (which we can do for the senses of taste, smell, and touch but less so for balance and movement and really not at all for the life sense), or we rush in to squelch the behavior because it is disruptive. There are naturally many instances where a child uses movement as a means to delay going to bed, but those movements are usually directed out—escape. The kinds of self-stimulating that relate to the inward pathway are usually about feeling oneself, about going inward. A child who moves, wiggles, rubs, or roles in the process of going to sleep may just need that space. If we continuously interfere in that movement process, we pull the child's attention back to the outside environment. Even an occasional escape route on the way to the bedroom may be an attempt to stimulate the lower senses. Watching children to see if they are truly distressed or just working to find connection to the life sense can be very informative.

Within these self-stimulating movements there can be behaviors that get stuck, where a sensory need is so strong that the child seems unable to move past it. Then that particular sensory pattern sticks out, like rubbing a hand on a pillow over and over, head rocking, bouncing, and the like. This usually means that a particular sense activity is still underdeveloped and that disproportionate sensory seeking is acting as a hindrance along the inward path. (The child cannot consistently move past it to get to the life sense.)

A certain subset of these self-stimulating behaviors get extra attention, things like thumb sucking or having a hand in the pants (genital stimulation) while lying down to fall asleep. Thumb sucking is primarily a touch stimulation, but one that is very early and connected to the sucking activity of a nursing baby. Touching of the genitals similarly stimulates very early, innate sensory pathways. Touch that demonstrates any kind of sexual knowledge or which is directed to another person should obviously prompt further observation and inquiry to see if there is a possibility of sexual abuse, but genital stimulation can be part of the inward path toward self-soothing. With these behaviors comes the challenge of appreciating that the self-stimulating represents a sensory need, but that is tempered with wanting to help the child shift to a more age-appropriate and/or socially appropriate activity.

One way of addressing this kind of behavior focuses on identifying the specific sensory aspect of the behavior (assessing whether it is taste, smell, touch, balance, or movement) and then trying to bring more regular practice and experience of that sense in a broader context. Several possible solutions can be tried:

- When the touch experience is self-stimulating (as with thumb sucking or genital touching), substituting other kinds of touch (back rubs, hugs, wrestling, deep touch, or joint compression) can help those younger touch patterns recede.
- If a child needs continuous touch experiences from the outside to fall asleep (i.e., from a parent), then healthy touch stimulation, with back rubs, hugs, wrestling, or compression can be incorporated earlier into the bedtime ritual, rather than introducing them right at the time the child is trying to fall asleep.
- For children who are big enough to have moved out of their crib, the process of touch seeking can be aided by having one side of the bed against a wall and adding a headboard and footboard so that there is a boundary on three sides of the bed that they can push up against. Heavier covers, such a down comforter or a couple of layers of blankets, may also feel good (assuming that the child is old enough and strong enough to move from under those covers when they need to). Children also often independently work to support their touch experience by doing things like filling the bed with stuffed animals so that there is almost no room left for sleeping. This facilitates a kind of "cocooning" that helps build

and maintain a proper sense of boundary. This decrease in the amount of physical space in bed, with more objects to encounter, can allow for more independent seeking of strong touch and boundary without a parent present.

- Greater daytime chances for building a healthy touch capacity through routine tasks and activities that involve the limbs can also help to balance bedtime needs.

For balance and movement needs that are so strong they inhibit the soothing process, there should naturally be greater opportunities for bouncing, balancing, and movement:

- These can even be incorporated as part of the bedtime ritual. Looking for these sensory patterns even gives insight into why young children often love to be dried off after a bath and then run around the house, just when it is time to settle down and go to bed, or why children suddenly decide it is time to wrestle when it is time to get into bed. Directly meeting and acknowledging these sensory needs can help shorten the overall transition into sleep (though such activities are usually best incorporated into the part of the bedtime ritual that is done in a common space outside the bedroom).
- Wrestling is not usually considered a part of most bedtime rituals, but it is worth mentioning, especially for boys (though many girls need it and enjoy it too). The emphasis lies not in winning or in hurting but in letting children really feel their own muscles, joints, and skin. Escaping a bear hug is a particularly popular exercise, as is hiding under a pile of cushions.
- If those activities seem only to rev up a child, daytime opportunities for building healthy balance and movement sensing can be increased instead.

A last variation fits into this discussion, and that is encouraging a child to shift to a sensing activity that lies a little further inward when a particular self-stimulating activity seems stuck. If we take thumb sucking as an example, we see that there is a certain progression for the sense of touch in relation to the mouth:

- Thumb sucking is foundationally a touch experience of the mouth related to nursing (from birth).
- The touch experience of the mouth then evolves, relating not just to sucking but also to chewing (usually beginning at around six months).
- Then a touch experience of the mouth arises that relates more specifically to speech (with the first formed words coming at about a year). Then comes a shift to fluent speech, singing, whistling, and so on.

We can therefore help older children who are thumb sucking explore more differentiated ways of experiencing the sense of touch in the mouth by bringing new or different textures of food by practicing verses or poems (even tongue twisters) or by learning to blow bubbles, leaning to sing, or, for older children, learning to play a flute or recorder. We thereby help children find ways to move their sensory experience farther out into the world—from the soft palate and tongue (sucking); to the hard palate, teeth, and tongue (chewing); to the tongue, teeth, and lips (speaking); to singing or playing an instrument—all of which moves sensory experience further forward in the mouth, bringing it into more and more conscious activity. By introducing sensory experiences that offer an older, more developed use of that same sense experience, children can be encouraged to move beyond the stuck pattern. We might ask: What is the natural refinement of that sensory experience? This can be done similarly for any sense that seems stuck.

A related variation looks at where the stuck sensory-seeking behavior is grounded (in which sense) and then strives to strengthen and stimulate the next sense along the inner pathway. Looking at thumb sucking again (or prolonged nursing), we can consider it a sensory activity that belongs to taste (particularly in children who always put things in their mouth or chew on their clothing, which is reminiscent of the crawling stage, when everything goes in the mouth).

The next sense along the inner pathway is smell. We could then consider introducing a lavender pillow at bedtime or something else that has a gentle, soothing smell. Very often young children treasure a much-beloved blanket or stuffed animal not just because of the feel or the associated emotions but because of the smell. Or, to move even a little further along the inward pathway (from taste to smell to touch), the bedtime ritual could include massage with a little bit of rose or chamomile body oil. Then we bring a soothing experience, helping children move away from a sensory experience that should have faded developmentally and instead helping them shift toward sensing that invites more participation.

These relationships between the lower senses are more helpful as developmental movements than as a rote system of developmental techniques. They speak to complementary gestures—motor movement out into the world and self-orienting movement toward the sense of wellbeing within. These parallel developmental capacities help us consider at what stages particular patterns find healthy expression and when those same developmental patterns stay too long and can even hold back development. Helping young children chart this inner pathway creates a healthy metabolic foundation for the learning and exploration that will come in the grade school years.

Chapter 14

Awaking into Thought and Sensory Activity

Through the Shifting Physiology of the Large-headed and Small-headed Polarity

Healthy metabolic–limb activity shows itself on many levels. Children who have entered the hereditary body and have successfully worked to make it their own experience joy in movement and seek movement. They also exhibit a level of comfort and contentment in the body, as they experiences a real capacity for more independent orienting and self-soothing. In addition to these measures of movement and self-awareness, there should also be good digestion.

When digestive capacity is good, eating is a pleasure. Foods can be properly transformed and their substance taken up into one's own body (a smaller, daily transformation of substance, reflecting the much larger bodily transformation of the hereditary body that is carried out over the first seven years). Appetite is also good, and if the parent asks about favorite foods or foods that are disliked, there may not be much response—because almost all foods are appreciated and the digestive process carries out its activity without much conscious consideration. It remains a properly unconscious activity. In addition, the child sleeps easily and deeply. These are all markers of healthy metabolic–limb activity in childhood.

There is often a dreamy kind of self-contained metabolic contentment in these children. They love stories and are frequently imaginative though not necessarily that accurately observant. Sometimes they strike one as being a little bit large in body and a little bit young in their awareness and interaction. They are frequently red-cheeked. On many levels they present a picture of healthy but dominant metabolic activity. When we see a two-, three-, or even five-year-old child with these qualities, they strike one as thriving and happy.

Toward the end of early childhood, particularly around the age of six and a half to seven, children start to change. They become more observant and more curious. They want to know how things work. The conversations one could have around them when they were younger now have to be edited, because the things one used to be able to talk about (between adults) are noticed and commented on, and there are more questions. Memory develops in new ways. Abstractions take on new importance—like letters, numbers, the meaning of street signs. On many different levels the child is waking up out of a dominant metabolic state into crisper observation and thinking.

The preceding description presents a kind of archetypal and in some ways idealized picture. Of course, many children do not follow that exact pathway. Some children will become wakeful much earlier—in fact it seems as if some children come out of the womb already asking questions and writing their names. Other children instead revel in this sleepy metabolic activity and hold on to it even into third or fourth grade. They contentedly allow the details of the school curriculum to go floating by. In light of this variation, one can look at every early-grade-school child and ask: Does this child seem relatively younger or older than the biographical age? Every child will naturally tend more toward slower, metabolically rich development or toward a more wakeful development that brings earlier awareness of the surrounding world. This discernment creates the foundation for understanding a second, broad developmental movement—the shift from dominant metabolism during the first seven years of life to the more wakeful activity of a grade school age.

When a child enters this transition at six and a half to seven years old, there is an accompanying shift from primarily substance-oriented, physically connected physiology (characteristic of the metabolic–limb pole) toward substance-free, body-free activity (a defining quality of the nerve–sense pole). The spiritual forces that stood behind the phenomenal growth and digestion of the first years of life now find other pathways for activity. In this way the engagement of the spiritual members becomes more differentiated.

Now let's consider how this shift from predominantly substance-oriented physiology to substance-free spiritual activity underlies a second essential developmental process in the life of a child. We saw in the first section how the four members of the human being interpenetrate: "I" into astral, into etheric, into physical. That is not the only way they can interact. If it were, we would be filled exclusively with activities of digestion, movement, and metabolism; but the "I"-being works into the body through multiple pathways. It can act more independently, diving directly into engagement with the physical body and

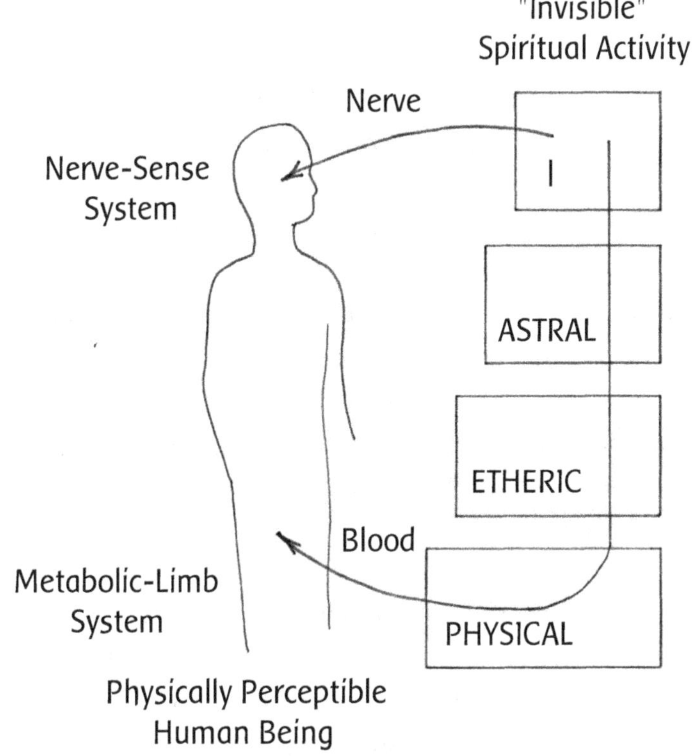

Figure 6: The spiritual activity of the four members for "blood" versus "nerve"

then releasing out again. In this pathway the "I"-being's activity is not mediated by the astral or etheric bodies (see fig. 6). This pathway of direct interaction into the physical, Steiner said, stands behind the activity of the nerves.[155] This nerve–sense pathway liberates us and allows us to be thinking beings, for this unmediated activity makes body-free activity possible. We can consider ideas, possibilities, and abstractions flexibly, without needing to physically recraft our bodies in the process. (That recrafting happens whenever the "I" dives down into the astral, etheric, and physical bodies through the blood/metabolic pathway. That fourfold pathway is constantly changing the physical body.) This nerve activity of the "I" is similar to a ray of light that passes through a clear window—the light needs the window to shine in or out of the house, but it does not change the window in the process. Our sense organs act similarly as windows for the "I."

There are very elaborate and elegantly structured nerve and sense organs in the head, which hold open a space for these substance-free activities. During their more formative, embryonic stage these sense organs start out as more vital organs (more connected to a fourfold metabolic interweaving), which is necessary for the substance of the organs to be shaped and transformed. They maintain some measure of flexibility even after the embryonic period, for the synaptic connections that create our neural networks are continually being refined. At a certain point, however, the organs of our nerve–sense pole do not significantly increase in size or shape. We do not grow new eyes or a new spinal cord at age seven. In fact, after the change of teeth, nerve and sense organs maintain a relatively constant physical form and function. They are very active with sensing activity, but they are no longer so connected to the metabolic transformation of substance—we do not completely reorganize the structure of our eyes or our ears every time we gaze or listen. When we are trying to solve a mechanical problem, however, we do consider many different permutations without needing to physically grasp the pieces and rearrange them for each new possibility. This thinking activity is possible because the activity of the higher members is liberated from an intimate connection with the substance of the physical body. This disconnection grows as the organs of the nerve–sense pole mature.

A physiologic polarity develops between nerve and metabolism. These physiologic activities exert opposing sculptural activities as well: on one side substance-oriented processes (of the will and metabolism) act in a loosening and energizing way, while substance-free processes (of the nerves and senses) exert a forming and devitalizing effect. From the head we gain form and organization. The head forces hold and dampen down metabolic growth forces. The head forces are the sculptors. Therefore, as a child matures and awakens into a crisper, more differentiated sensing experience of the world, there is a corresponding diversion of forces away from body-oriented physiology. That process continues throughout our biography, so that the tremendous etheric vitality of early life diminishes in consequence of wakeful, hardening forces, and the etheric predominance of early life gives way to astral (sensing) dominance at the end of life.

Steiner emphasized this shifting physiology and gave specific meditative indications for helping to observe it. He gave several variations, placing it among a series of foundational exercises that support general spiritual development[156] while emphasizing its role in medical meditative practice: "Now what you have to do, my dear friends, is strive with all your strength to attain imagination in your concept of the human being. In this connection, therefore, I would like to give you a few fundamental indications."[157] Steiner presented a twofold imagination to a group of young doctors and medical students gathered at Easter in Dornach, Switzerland, in 1924.

The meditation begins with picturing the form of the human being in the embryonic state and then transforming it into the picture of a child, making the two pictures as intense as possible—"as if your thinking were actually touching them."[158] The transformation is then carried further, into the form of an adult human being. Steiner indicated that in this process the shifting from embryo to child is the more difficult, while the connection between child and adult is not so very different:

> If you really carry this out, you will be aware of certain difficulties. You will feel: If I enlarge the head of the embryo to the size of a child's head, it becomes very big. I must compress it. I must also inwardly crystallize, as it were, all that in the embryo is still watery and fluid, being part of the fluid body so that it becomes the embryonic brain. Then you will have to stretch and give shape to the limbs in the embryonic state.... If you succeed in this, the imagination of the human etheric body will actually come to birth within you, and comparatively soon.[159]

Moving through this process does help us come into a relationship with etheric forces. We experience a process moving forward in time, similar to the growth and unfolding development of a plant's stem, leaves, and flower. This is a differentiated etheric process, because as the limbs grow longer and larger, the head becomes proportionately smaller. This etheric process is twofold—expanding (lengthening) and contracting (holding). It parallels the emancipation of etheric forces from predominantly self-contained, substance-oriented activity (limbs) to a more wakeful, forming activity (head). As the process continues the head must be compressed and crystallized and the limbs stretched and shaped. From this exercise we begin to see that it is natural and appropriate for a child to gradually move away from a metabolic-dominant condition (which maintains a certain roundness supported by outwardly directed metabolism) to one in which limb growth becomes more emphasized (as formative activity pushes inward giving shape and a more linear orientation). It is a spatial metamorphosis that moves forward through time. That is the first exercise.

Steiner gave a second movement, a second part of this exercise, which is to reverse the progression starting with old age:

> You can try to picture an old, sclerotic man—old men are, to a certain extent, sclerotic—feeling that you are touching him and

> in this act of spiritual touching you get the impression that he is really hollow.... Now let the picture of old age pass backward. When you let the picture of the embryonic structure pass over into the structure of childhood, you carried out a spatial metamorphosis—what happens now is that with old age you have the impression of a being who has been hollowed out, who sucks all the time, and this hollow being seems to be filled with force and energy when you let the picture pass back into the age of maturity.... And then the picture of the prime of life must be carried back to that of youth.... When we succeed in doing this, we get the impression of the etheric body being animated, beginning to ring and sound. This gives us an impression of the astral nature of the human being.[160]

Through this reverse sequence we see a progression of the activity of the astral body. Beginning with the sclerotic body of the old man, we start with what has become a predominantly substance-free activity of the astral forces. They have sculpted to such a degree that the body is now hollow and largely devitalized. As we move backward into earlier stages of life, the body becomes "filled with force and energy" and "animated." As we go backward in time, the astral body becomes more connected to the etheric and physical bodies. The centripetal, sculpting activity from the head, which dominates later life, shifts back into astral activity that is centrifugal, enlivening, metabolic energy in youth. The astral forces are the same; only the pathway that they use (the head in later life, the limbs and metabolism in youth) and their relationship to the other bodies differ—predominantly independent of the etheric and physical with age and diving into and through the etheric and physical in youth.

The entire meditation, as given by Steiner:

> Carry the human being's earliest time
> [—the embryonic life—]
> On into childhood,
> And carry childhood on
> Into the days of youth.

There will appear to you, condensed,
Human ether being
Behind the body's structure.—
[—physical body in its structure.]...

Carry old age's density
Back into the prime of life,
And the prime of life
Back into the life of youth.
There will ring forth in sounds of worlds
The working of the human soul
[—astral body—]
Out of the ether life.

We can characterize these shifting imaginations as follows (though for these meditative movements to come truly alive they must be practiced rhythmically and repetitively):

> As we envision a child moving forward through life, we see a transformation of the etheric body's activity. Through maturation the head becomes smaller and compressed and the limbs larger and longer, and we see a shift from body-oriented, metabolic activities to liberated body-free etheric forces available for thinking.
>
> When we move backward from old age to the prime of life and then to youth, we see the hollowness of an old man gradually filled and enlivened, so that it begins to ring and sound. In this (backward) transformation the astral body moves from an outward sculpting activity to an inwardly enlivening one.

Through these time imaginations we come to better understand the shifting relationship of the astral and etheric bodies. As we next explore, Steiner's introduction of a large-headed and small-headed constitutional polarity lives very much in that interaction, in the shifting spiritual activity between an embryo and an old man. As human beings we necessarily live in both activities, though at different stages of life they exhibit a particular prominence. We carry the seeds of our nerve–sense activity as an embryo, and we still carry ringing metabolism (though in smaller measure) into old age. The complete shift away from the capacity for metabolic transformation comes only at death.

This meditation was given to the young doctors, but it carries important insights for the course of overall child development and pedagogy. We saw earlier how in the meeting of the spiritual and hereditary streams, very often an imbalance expresses itself as a constitutional inclination (to either be held down by the earthly or to stay too peripheral in the spiritual). In a similar way, the activities of the astral and etheric bodies shift and evolve so that (ideally after the process of integration is complete) every child works to develop both substance-oriented and substance-free physiology. When that process unfolds in a healthy way, we see the archetypal milestones of an evermore skillful, wakeful activity that unfolds over the first seventeen or eighteen years of life. When the process is imbalanced, we can feel that the (etheric) shift of the first part of the meditation comes either too slowly or too fast. When it comes too slowly, there is a kind of sculptural stagnation, and the body (especially the head) is not compressed or crystallized. The limbs, hands, and feet stay relatively small. When the process is too fast, and wakefulness comes too early in life, the head becomes proportionately small, the limbs extended, and the activity of the astral body too "old." Where a child stands on this polarity (too late or too soon) influences patterns of learning, thinking, and physical maturation. This marks a second essential developmental process that can be carefully observed through a constitutional polarity.

Rudolf Steiner explored this process during two faculty meetings in 1923, in what has come to be described as the polarity of the large head and small head.[161] We can already see—through the experience of the meditation given in his course for young doctors (*Understanding Healing*)—how the proportion of head and limbs relates to a balance between forward and backward development.

The proportional size of the head does indeed prove to be a helpful measure of a child's shifting development away from metabolic growth toward substance-free thought capacities. It would be a mistake to believe, however, that a simple head measurement alone is an appropriate way to determine constitution. This physical measure really relates to a much larger dynamic between the metabolic–limb system and the nerve–sense system. Steiner began his discussion with the teachers (and Dr. Eugen Kolisko, who was present for the meetings[162]) by characterizing the threefold nature of the human being and its differing relation to physical substance:

> Of the three human systems, the metabolic–limb system depends most upon external material processes. When people understand the earthly processes playing out in physics and chemistry, they also understand which processes continue within the human being, at least to the extent that human beings have a metabolic–limb system. However, they learn nothing about the laws of the nerve–sense system.[163]

According to Steiner that system is freed, liberated, from interaction with the physical world:

> We have the nerve–sense system. We can properly understand that only if we are aware that there is a regularity in the nerve–sense-system that is not subject to the physical and chemical laws of earthly matter. We need to be aware that the human being rises above the laws of earthly matter through the nerve–sense system.... The nerve–sense system is thus capable of independently developing all activities related to the spirit-soul, because all material laws of the nerve–sense system are removed from earthly nature.[164]

The rhythmic system also is described, as it lies between and "naturally balances the two extremes." [165] This balancing is really a mediation between the head and limbs. The qualities of the rhythmic system are an expression of the relative strength between the metabolic–limb and nerve–sense systems, whether one dominates or is incomplete. The large-headed and small-headed polarity is a measure of these relative strengths, for we all incline one way or the other:

> These things form quite individually within every human being. This is particularly true of children. The activity of one system always predominates over the others, and we need to do what is necessary to create a balance. For that, we must have a capacity to really listen to how children express themselves, so that expression can become a revelation of what we need to do with the child in order to help it achieve a completely harmonious health.[166]

The large-headed and small-headed polarity finds its greatest expression around the change of teeth and into the early grades, though it can often be observed at a younger age and continues to express itself throughout adolescence.

If a child stays too much in the metabolic sphere and does not undergo the necessary refining and condensing processes that underlie healthy sense activity, then we can say the nerve–sense system has not yet been sufficiently sculpted. This is, in fact, the definition that Steiner gave for the large-headed constitution, a state in which "the nerve–sense system is not in order" and we can even see "the first traces of a tendency for mental [nerve–sense] dysfunction."[167]

What might this "dysfunction" look like? It means that the child's ability to be wakefully attentive to the outside world is compromised. The child tends to be "inattentive," "flighty," and "to turn away from what you present."[168] What the child needs is to develop the ability to be "better able to pay attention to the outside world"[169]—through the activity of the nerves. The nerves and senses allow us to relate to the outside world from a distance, abstractly; this is a very different activity from the intimate exchange and transformation that come through the metabolic–limb system. Nerve activity allows us to observe. Within metabolic activity there is little possibility for separation, as everything is combined in its interweaving, working to make everything into a whole (no longer separated into parts). This is true physiologically; it is also present in the soul life of the child: "When children show little tendency for differing imaginations, if they simply toss everything together in a fantasy, if they cannot properly differentiate, then the nerve–sense system is not in order."[170] When we look at this description in relation to the changing shape of the child, we can see that with a large-headed constitution children have stayed a little too embryonic, and maintain a developmental youth with respect to their biographical age.

The opposite is true for children with a small-headed constitution. Here the interweaving digestive activity is no longer dominant; in fact, the "limb-metabolic system is not sufficiently active throughout their being. Of course, such children feed their organic metabolism, but what the metabolism should be for the human organism does not sufficiently extend throughout their entire being."[171] On this pole it is the metabolic–limb system that is not in order and is too weak.

What is the result? The nerve–sense system dominates, so that such children become very aware of the surrounding world. This usually means that they are aware of more than they can digest organically. The sensory process is too strong and cannot be let go: "External observation of such children shows that they like to brood over things, but that they are also very strongly irritated by external impressions, that is, they react too strongly to external impressions."[172] This can take the form of distractibility on many levels, as attention is pulled in different directions at one time, toward sights, sounds, textures, and so forth. Where the child with a large-headed constitution remains too young and is therefore still inattentive, the child with a small-headed constitution is developmentally too old, too far along in the shifting of awareness toward the outside environment and is challenged by distraction.

This distraction is actually quite familiar to almost everyone today, for the energies we necessarily direct toward observing the outside world are overly stimulated and accentuated. Such sensing awareness is an undeniable sign of nerve–sense maturation, but it should not come too early. It is really an appropriate step only when it is built on the ability to fully work through what we take in. Metabolic activity and the transformation of the inherited body need to come first, then wakeful sensing. When this happens in a proper way, so that both the metabolic–limb system and then the nerve–sense system are well formed, a child will be open to the outside world, able to take impressions in, and also able to properly digest and transform those impressions. (In a parallel way we can see that an infant naturally becomes interested in solid food once the digestive organs needed to break down the food are mature, a change that is often heralded by the eruption of the first baby teeth.) For many children sensing activity becomes dominant too early, when there is still insufficient transformative capacity. The child cannot take what is given and digest it into a whole. Integration and combination remain difficult: "When children show too little capacity for synthetic imagining—that is, for constructive imagining where the child cannot properly picture things—if they are little barbarians artistically, which is common in today's children, it is a symptom that the metabolic–limb system is not in order."[173] Synthetic thinking, constructive imagining, and artistic ability (being able to draw or paint a part while holding an awareness for the composition as a whole) are all related to our ability to take ideas and impressions in and make them our own.

One further symptom described by Steiner is that "when there is a deficiency in synthetic thinking...children become pale. Children often become pale in school. We can handle that similarly to the condition of the astral body not being properly integrated into the metabolic–limb system."[174] The blood in the skin, which is an expression of the metabolic pole, is dominated by a nerve activity that constricts and forms the blood vessels, holding the blood back and making us pale. The pallor most children exhibit when they are anxious

Table 5: Basic characteristics of the large-headed and small-headed constitutions, per Steiner

Nerve–sense system not in order	Metabolic–limb system not in order
Large-headed constitution Large head with relatively small hands and feet The compressing and crystallizing of the head and accompanying growth and extension of the limbs are not yet complete. They still resemble the "embryonic" state.	Small-headed constitution Small head with relatively large hands and feet The compressing of the head pole has brought wakefulness but also devitalized the metabolism. The child already carries proportions closer to those of an adult.
Stays young too long	Grows old too soon
Too metabolic, cannot analyze	Too nerve–sense, weak constructive or synthetic imagining
Imaginative but inattentive, flighty	Brooding, irritated by external impressions
Red face, terribly annoyed by small remarks	Pale

(too aware), overly tired (awake too long), or weakened from illness (depleted metabolic forces) may be carried by the child with a small-headed constitution as a chronic state.

In contrast, when the metabolism dominates the whole physiology, we can see it coming all the way up into the head pole: "If that system develops too strongly so that you need to make only a small remark and the child immediately gets a red face and is terribly annoyed, treat that in exactly the same way as when the astral body and 'I' are not properly integrated into the nerve–sense system."[175] The astral body and "I" have not yet found a differentiated nerve activity, so the child finds it difficult to create distance from an impression. It is as though the child with a large-headed constitution cannot help but take the remark in and "swallow" it whole—thus the immediate redness as blood rushes to the head.

Steiner described this polarity on multiple levels. It is traditionally designated as the large-headed and small-headed polarity, but it is important not to get stuck on the size of the head (which would consider this polarity in only a superficial way). Looking at the relative size of the head and of the hands can be a helpful confirmation of a child's overall progress in this process, but the full picture of the polarity is best recognized with the designations of a nerve–sense system that is not in order or a metabolic–limb system that is not in order. Table 5 shows an overview of Steiner's characterizations.

It is key to understand and observe the polarity on multiple levels, because if there is a true constitutional leaning it will manifest in consistent, parallel ways. We can look at form (relative size of the head and hands), color (red or pale), sensing patterns (inattentive or irritated and brooding), and thought (cannot analyze or cannot synthesize). We can also hold the picture of imbalanced nerve or metabolic systems and see related constitutional signs revealed through patterns of illness, patterns of eating, and patterns of learning (thought).

Patterns of Illness

The relationship of nerve–sense and metabolic–limb activity stands at the heart of a threefold understanding of the human being. When these systems are out of balance, illness arises; most people show a consistent pattern of more regularly getting sick in one region or the other. Very often the medical history of children gives us a clue as to their constitutional leaning, particularly if they show a predominant pattern of head and neck inflammations or functional complaints of the digestive system.

For a still large-headed constitution, there is very commonly a pattern of repeated inflammations of the head pole: big tonsils and lymph nodes, ear infections, sore throats, sinus congestion (though usually not an allergic sinusitis). These share common qualities: tissue that is too large, too congested—we could even say, too "young." These inflammations in the head pole are an imbalance, but they are also a tool for the higher members, working through inflammation to further form and refine the head and its sensory organs. These kinds of acute illnesses are frequently accompanied by strong fevers with redness and swelling, all qualities connected to the dominant metabolic activity. The illness process may build quite strongly for these children without much consciousness or complaint, like a child who seems well during the day and then suddenly develops a high fever and even ruptures an eardrum, all within a few hours. This is an expression of strong inflammation without much awareness of what is happening, because the child's consciousness naturally leans more toward that (sleeping) metabolic side. For a child with a large-headed constitution, these acute illnesses frequently bring strong exudative breakdown with lots of mucus and discharge. The illness may be abrupt and dramatic, but the recovery is often equally quick and complete.

In contrast, a child with a classically small-headed illness pattern presents much more frequently with imbalances of digestion, like stomachaches, nausea, or cramping. We know right away from these symptoms that the metabolic–limb system is not in order. These illnesses—acute or chronic—all share the quality that there is too much awareness of digestive organs (experienced as pain or cramping) in a part of the body that should generally be unconscious. Our wakeful awareness should not properly extend down below the diaphragm, for when that happens, nerve–sense activity is entering into the realm of the metabolism. A second sign of this imbalance is that the digestion is easily overwhelmed and is unable to transform what has been taken in, with resultant symptoms like vomiting or diarrhea. These children may pick up every stomach bug that goes around. If they do get inflammations (usually less easily than children with a large-headed constitution), they tend to stay cool (without much fever), and the illness often drags on. It is, of course, possible for a small-headed child to get illnesses in the head and neck region, but the emphasis is different; there are more symptoms of pain, without many signs of hot inflammation—like a razor blade sore throat without redness. They may also take much longer to recover from an illness and thereafter stay quite pale.

Patterns of Eating

A child's patterns of eating and digestion also provide insight into constitution. It is helpful to consider eating in two phases—how aware we are of what we take in (a kind of nerve–sense digestion) and then how well we can embrace and transform that substance to make it our own (metabolic–limb digestion).

Some children naturally eat with gusto and give little consideration to what they take in. They do not have great concerns about food or strong preferences. Often when asked what their favorite foods are, they cannot even give a specific answer—not because they do not have foods that they love but because critical sensing is not a significant part of their eating process. They tend to love everything; they have not developed any antipathies toward food. It is, in fact, rare for them to get a stomach complaint, except sometimes from overeating. In these children the metabolic system is in good order. Appetite is good, though awareness of the process remains a little sleepy. This is true for many children with a classically large-headed constitution.

In contrast, when there is strong awareness around eating (a lot of sensing activity), then there are usually plentiful opinions about what is good and what is not. Another way to describe this might be to say that the child is "picky," but for many of these children avoidance of certain foods arises out of accurately sensing what can be handled by the metabolic system and what cannot. Their picky nature could reflect a healthy instinct about what should be avoided. There might also be strong sensitivities about combinations or textures of food. Meals are generally small—a child eats more like a bird—so as not to overwhelm the metabolism. There is very often an accompanying love of carbohydrates, especially white foods (rice, potatoes, noodles, crackers), as they are particularly easy and fast to digest. The resulting quick rise in blood sugar helps the child feel more at ease in the metabolism (see more on this in "Salt and Sugar" in chap. 15).

For children who experience early wakeful sensory maturation, the ability to transform food frequently becomes overwhelmed during the course of the day. This relates both to the child's dietary load (what kinds of food the child has eaten, and how much) as well as the sensory diet taken in (the number of things that had to be noticed or paid attention to). When dinnertime comes, there are scant metabolic forces left, so appetite for dinner is often small or nonexistent. Dinner is much more likely to be a successful meal when there is no background noise, when everyone can sit quietly and there is no rush. Quieting outer sensory demands allows more forces to be directed inwardly to support better metabolic order.

Patterns of Thought

There are similarly polar inclinations for how we take in sensory impressions and make them our own. Food digestion happens mostly in the metabolism and sensory impressions in the nerve–sense system;

they share related patterns. A nice way to gain yet another view into the balancing of blood and nerve is to see how a child retells a story.

Small children very naturally live into big imaginations, the kinds of pictures we hear in fairy tales. Fairy tales are special, because they describe true spiritual pictures. These spiritual pictures ring especially true for small children, because they are still very close to the experiences they had in the spiritual world before they were born. They live into those archetypes in a dreamy, mostly unconscious way. They hear the descriptions of death or transformation that are commonly part of a fairy tale narrative without being too concerned by them (like the loss of clothing in "The Star-Money" or a character being turned to stone in "Faithful John"), because they do not take the pictures too literally.[176] They are not experiencing the details but instead the bigger gestures of the story. When a child still breathes in sensory impressions in this way, the gestures of the story matter most. We might notice that for a child who lives in these big pictures the retelling varies a bit each time, sometimes with creative elaboration. The details may change in the narration (extra added events or citing six swans one day and nine the next), but we clearly sense that the child has taken in the images very deeply, and those images resonate within. This pattern of perception belongs more to a younger, dominant metabolic constitution.

An older child begins to hear a story differently. This comes predictably more to the fore with a six-year-old child (entering the seven-year change). Consistency and detail now become an important consideration, and the child will notice if the story changes from one day to the next. To varying degrees, plausibility also enters in: How would that happen? How would it be if I were doing it? How would I feel if I were doing it? A child may even get stuck on one particular detail of description and not be able to let go of it. Children need that question answered before they can hear anything more and will return to it if do not feel they have received a proper answer. This can be quite disruptive to the reverential mood created through story time, for the specifics are now suddenly held so tightly that the overall picture of the story is sacrificed. That kind of pattern of perception belongs more to a dominant nerve–sense system.

This progression—from an appreciation of the whole to a gradual understanding of the parts—follows the natural development of a child's evolving capacity for intellectualism. Mathematics in the Waldorf curriculum mirrors this development progression, as children first learn about the whole (one), which is then divided into parts (halves, quarters, eighths, etc.), in order to come to multiples. This progression from whole to part follows the archetypal progress of thought.

As individuals, we all constitutionally have different leanings. Usually one aspect feels more comfortable and natural—either we gravitate toward general picturing (which could be compared to deductive reasoning, starting with the overall principle and out of the wholeness finding specific application), or we prefer to begin with specific, concrete details (the starting place for inductive reasoning—carefully examining specific examples) until a pattern emerges. We think differently at different ages, but the preference for one or the other is an inclination we develop in childhood and carry with us through life.

The younger, more global way of taking in sensory impressions (particularly when it extends into grade school age), belongs to the large-headed constitution. Steiner described the large-headed child as "inattentive." We can see this because the child's sensing has not yet fully engaged with outside activity—it is still more inward. It is also reinforced by a certain metabolic self-contentment. Outside sensory impressions remain a little vague and soft. The strong metabolism works quickly to dissolve the details of sensory impressions. You can see the same kind of metabolic contentment in an infant who peacefully sits and watches the world, especially after a full feeding of mother's milk. The inattention of the large-headed child continues into later development, coloring patterns of thinking and sensing even when there is no immediate digestive load in the belly.

Another, related way we can understand this pattern of sensing comes in summer, when the whole world seems to expand. Children are eager to get out of school and let go of all of the academic content they have been working with. They need to stop taking things in so that they can digest what they have already experienced. Their forces move away from the thinking activity of the head and are redirected back to the limbs and to growth. It should be no surprise that children have tremendous growth spurts during this time of year. Children with a large-headed constitution could, for this reason, also be thought of as "summer" children. When summer arrives, everyone's feeling life moves toward expansion and relaxation. It is just not a good time to pin down details or to make nuanced decisions.

In June, we all (appropriately and predictably) become a little large-headed. We "cannot differentiate" and may be tempted to toss "everything together in a fantasy"[177] (another of Steiner's descriptions for the large-headed child). These summer-like children need big pictures and big ideas—through those they are able make a connection. Instruction that quickly goes to the details or always starts with them feels inaccessible to a child with a large-headed constitution. Their inattentive behavior stems from their lack of connection to information that feels too abstract and compartmentalized for their developmental stage. The more extreme this process, the more easily these children can be categorized as having attention deficit disorder (ADD). Placing these children on stimulant medication does increase their wakefulness and can perhaps improve academic performance in the short term, but it precludes the child's own developmental participation in the process. We need, instead, to help these children liberate their own forces from the metabolism so that they can begin to better sense the world around them and become interested in it. We could probably develop a pharmaceutical medication that would artificially stimulate children to lose their teeth earlier and earlier, but using it in children would not mean that we are all now truly physiologically ready to start abstract learning at an earlier age; we would only be fooling ourselves. In the same way, true therapies for the large-headed constitution help open a doorway so that children are encouraged to shift their own physiology. That self-engendered maturation brings much broader and long-lasting change. An anthroposophic approach to ADD meets the fundamental developmental need of the child in order to facilitate real growth and unfolding, as opposed to simple symptom management or suppression.

Children with a small-headed constitution can also often be considered to have attention problems (and may also be prescribed stimulant medications) but actually have a completely different experience of the world. Ritalin might be helpful temporarily because it brings focus, but for a small-headed child it really creates a kind of hyperfocus when such children are already too wakeful. Wakefulness is not the issue. Instead of not paying attention to facts and details (like the inattention of the large-headed constitution), for the child with an overly active nerve–sense pole there is no choice but to constantly react to all kinds of impressions. Attention is challenged by distraction. The small-headed child is pulled by too many sensory impressions—reacting too strongly to external impressions. Here stimulant medication can be particularly damaging in terms of side effects like anxiety, insomnia, and weight loss, because the wakening activity of the medicine only further exacerbates the child's underlying weakened metabolism. Stimulants bring some order to the flooding sensory impressions, but they do not aid the child in balancing the excessive nerve–sense activity.

For a child with such strongly developed sensing activity, impressions from a more peripheral activity (like a teacher standing at the front of the room and speaking) are quickly drowned out by more immediate and intimate sensations: temperature, clothing, blood sugar, ambient noise. Those can result in a brooding that comes from being affected by so many impressions. In order for a small-headed child to be able to pay attention to peripheral activities (like the teacher's instruction), more immediate bodily experiences and sensations have to be quieted. More of the body needs to be put back into the sleeping metabolic state, for when there are so many sensations it is difficult to prioritize which sensations deserve the most attention (and hence the distraction). As with tasting every ingredient in every food and being affected by it, the small-headed child is too often a servant to an ocean of sensations.

Always consciously carrying so many simultaneous details influences the way the child understands the world. Detail dominance explains why the small-headed child has "too little capacity for synthetic imagining" and thereby "cannot properly picture things." It is difficult for the child to gain a conception of the whole, because it requires surrender of the specifics. If we think again about Steiner's description that the small-headed child is a "little barbarian in art," this is probably because the layout, proportions, and relations of the picture as a whole suffer. It is hard to artistically integrate all the pieces when attention is too narrowly directed, if the need to look at the part makes us blind to the whole (see next page, table 6).

As the large-headed child is full of summer, the small-headed child is wintery, which brings clarity. At a certain point in fall when the weather gets cooler, we all become a bit more small-headed, and it feels good. We move beyond the expansion of summer and look at what needs to be done. Fall is a time when we almost universally feel the need to be practical, to get specific. Then winter comes, plant life dies down and retreats into the ground, and metabolic bounty is replaced by cool crisp weather and lengthening, dark nights. In winter it feels good to plan, to become more introspective—perhaps even a little brooding. We become more separated from the outside world during the cold season, and it helps us feel our boundaries. January and February are often times of sober reflection. We need the heightened inward consciousness of winter. Eventually comes a longing for growth and green plants and expansion again.

The wintery quality of the small-headed child benefits from warm sunshine and the dreamy inattention of the large-headed child from a little frost. These are relationships that begin to lead us into the realm of therapy.

Table 6: Patterns of illness, attention, and memory in the large-headed and small-headed constitutions

Large-headed constitution	Small-headed constitution
Illness patterns	
The nerve–sense system is not in order Hence the metabolism dominates These children tend to get a lot of inflammations of the head and neck (earaches, big tonsils, sore throats).	***The metabolic–limb system is not in order*** Hence sensing dominates These children tend to have problems with their digestion, be picky eaters, get stomachaches (easily vomit or get diarrhea).
Attentiveness and memory	
Remembers the larger pictures and images of a story but not the specifics. May instead be creative with the details or elements of a story. Can relate to the broader message or principle but may have difficulty knowing how to practically apply it to a specific situation.	Remembers the specifics, knows all the details. It can be almost painful for the child if those details are inconsistent or are told incorrectly. The child remembers specific examples but may miss the overall moral or message of a story.
Inattentive	Distracted

Chapter 15

Meeting and Guiding the Differentiation Process

The balance between sleeping metabolism and wakeful sensing has a very real impact in our lives. As with the movement polarity (feeble/maniacal), we all incline toward either a large- or a small-headed constitution. In fact, when people first learn about this polarity, there is often a surprised reaction at how accurately it describes a spouse, a child, or the difference between two siblings or two coworkers. While everyone does indeed exhibit a constitutional leaning, most of the time we do not need to be treated for it with a medicine. Learning about the polarities does not mean we need or want to "pathologize" the world. The question then arises: "How can we understand the difference between an inclination and true imbalance, a problem?" We could, of course, define some cutoff between "normal" and "ill." That is routinely done when diagnostic criteria are established for different developmental or psychological disorders, but that kind of black-and-white distinction can well deaden the quality of our observation. A better starting place might be to ask: "What are the different methods, the different levels of therapeutic activity that we can offer to a child, and which of these are appropriate for a given situation?" Particularly, for this polarity of blood and nerve, we can explore a whole range of support and intervention.

The first and simplest step is simply to observe and appreciate who an individual child is. That interest and intention are already a therapeutic step. It might feel too simple and almost mundane to say that we should be interested in who children are as individuals and the nature of their experience in the world. But to look at someone's individual needs (as opposed to broader developmental patterns) marks a threshold between pedagogy (which we can consider supporting and nourishing the developmental unfolding of all children) and therapeutic activity (which looks more deeply to recognize the individual inclinations and needs of the child in this incarnation). Steiner described how when we take on this step of individualized therapeutic intervention, we are doing the work of the angels.[178] We are working to balance what would otherwise be remedied only in the time between death and another birth.

Taking a child intensely into our observation and thinking activity is already therapeutic because it exerts a spiritual effect. It is part of what Steiner described as the "pedagogical law." The pedagogical law states that what we engender through conscious activity and insight works down into the rest of the body. This should not be considered a completely new insight, because in the first section we experienced how the spiritual stream (incarnating with intention) works to penetrate and transform the lower members. Through a kind of waterfall interaction, the formative activity of the "I"-being works down into the astral body, into the etheric body, into the physical body. What Steiner added to this picture when he described the pedagogical law is that what develops in our physical body is dependent on what is "living in the etheric body—in an etheric body." That "an" is very important, because it opens the door to the possibility of interpersonal spiritual physiology. It means that the etheric of a mother works not only on her own physical body but also on the physical bodies of her children (which is perhaps not so surprising). It additionally means that our etheric—as father, grandmother, teacher, therapist, or physician—will also influence the physical body of a child:

> Any one member of the human being is influenced by the next higher member (from whatever quarter it approaches) and only under such influence can that member develop satisfactorily. Thus, whatever is to be effective for the development of the physical body must be living in the etheric body—in an etheric

> body. Whatever is to be effective for the development of the etheric body must be living in the astral body. Whatever is to be effective for the development of an astral body must be living in an "I"; an "I" can be influenced only by what is living in a Spirit Self.[179]

The most common shared anthroposophic view of the human being includes four members: physical, etheric, astral, and "I," so this description contains a surprise—a fifth element. What is the Spirit Self? It is an aspect that is still very early in its development, arising out of the portions of the astral body that have been completely refined and purified by the "I." It is the aspect of our sensing and feeling life that has been fully penetrated through self-conscious, intentional guidance. One of the ways we cultivate our own Spirit Self is through learning to observe the laws of spiritual physiology and then bringing that knowledge to the needs of a child:

> And now you will be rather taken aback, for we come next to the spirit self of the teacher, and you will be thinking that surely the spirit self is not yet developed. Nevertheless, such is the law. The spirit self of the teacher must work on the "I" of the children.... How is the astral body of the educator to be "educated" for this purpose? Self-educated, too, as it must be today?... If teachers can feel their way right into this situation...if they are able themselves to feel the stoppage that the child feels, and able at the same time out of their own energy to evoke in their soul a deep compassion for the children's experience, such teachers will develop an understanding in their own astral body for the child's situation and will gradually succeed in eliminating in themselves all subjective reactions of feeling when faced with this phenomenon in the child. By ridding themselves of every trace of subjective reaction, sympathy, or antipathy, teachers educate their own astral body.... How can we set about acquiring this kind of understanding? By developing ever-greater interest in the mystery of the human organization.[180]

In this way the activity of observation and constitutional imagining brings therapeutic support to the "I" of the child.

In his description of the pedagogical law, Steiner sketched out the relationships (see table 7) indicating that the spiritual member of the teacher can work on the corresponding spiritual in the child, that is, the teacher's etheric body works on the physical body of the child.

Table 7: The Pedagogical Law

Child		Teacher
Physical	:	Etheric
Etheric	:	Astral
Astral	:	"I"
"I"	:	Spirit Self

These relationships are important because of the pathways of support they offer. They are also sobering because they show how our own spiritual and soul activity continually exerts an effect on a child's health. When we can approach a child with sincere interest (conquering our own patterns of reaction, boredom, or weariness), our Spirit Self waterfalls down into the members of the child's developing body. When we act dismissively or speak too brusquely (acts that spring unmediated from our astral body, for in that moment it is usually not our "I" that is speaking), we can exert a detrimental effect on the child's etheric and physical bodies.

As we now explore the more specific therapeutic offerings for a metabolic–limb system that is not in order (small-headed) or a nerve–sense system that is not in order (large-headed), we should look once more at Steiner's opening words for the faculty meeting of February 6, 1923:

> The teacher should have an instinctive feeling for each child, that is, for whether one of the three aspects of the human organism, the nerve–sense system or the rhythmic system, or the metabolic limb system, predominates, and for whether we need to stimulate one of the other systems in order to balance a harmful lack of balance in the other systems.[181]

With the liberation of forces out of the metabolism and the development of more wakeful sensing, the rhythmic system begins to develop in new ways during the grade school years. We can also think of the rhythmic system as the meeting place of the child's younger physiology with what will come later, where a child experiences the meeting of "past" metabolism with "future" sensing. In several places Steiner described actual currents within our soul life, one out of the past and one coming to us from the future, whose meeting point helps to define our feeling life.[182]

As has been described, the balance of this feeling realm colors children's learning styles. It is often helpful to consider the constellation of constitutions within a particular class, as one or two children with a very large-headed constitution among a class of predominantly small-headed children will strongly stand out and are often a source of concern. Including imaginative pictures and archetypes in the class lessons will invite the participation of these particular children and can sometimes help soften the class as a whole (even if it is not immediately satisfying to the children with small-headed constitutions). Or the reverse may be true, that a child with a very small-headed experience of the world may stick out in a more large-headed class and will need to be met with practical examples. Details give those more small-headed children concrete footholds, as staying too much in the realm of dreamy archetypes only frustrates them.

It follows, then, as a matter of course that in time it is also important for teachers to gain insight into their own constitutional leanings. Material always presented in a large-headed way—always beginning with the general principle and only gradually moving to the specific application—will feel very natural to some children and ponderous and inaccessible to others. Alternatively, an inclination to first bring many details but not always to move on to a broader overview or imagination will meet some children but leave others out. For each of us to look honestly at our own constitutions is a step of self-development, best taken up out of one's own questioning and observation. Learning about our strengths and imbalances brings the possibility to honor and accept our constitutional leanings, so that we can work to move beyond them and not be defined by them. That certainly contributes to the development of our Spirit Self.

Growing and developing children are not yet incarnated deeply enough to find balance for their inclinations (though we may sometimes expect that they should), so they depend on our interested and loving attention. Our devotion to them brings continuous fruits through the pedagogical law. For those children who seem stuck and limited by their constitutional leanings (so large-headed that they can never get to the detail or so small-headed that they cannot escape the distractions of the world's impressions) we are fortunate to be provided with additional therapeutic tools in the form of three realms of remedy: cold and warmth, salt and sugar, lead and silver.

Cooling and Warmth

Large-headed children have been described as summer children—the season when we all want to relax and expand, dissolve a little bit. Children who are too absorbed in their own metabolic process and too summery experience cool temperatures (particularly those directed to the head) as therapeutic. A cool cloth brings wakefulness and an immediate experience of boundary. It is most helpful in the morning, when we transition naturally out of the night's metabolic activity and waken into the world. We are stimulating a waking process by anatomy (the head), temperature (cool), and time (the morning). Per Steiner's description: "See to it that the child's head is cooled in some way... a cool wash in the morning."[183]

For the child with a small-headed constitution, who often tends to be too cool, too aware, and too wintery, a therapeutic application should instead be warm and directed to the seat of the metabolism (the abdomen); the child should be given "[a] warm stomach wrap two or three times per week, so that the child has it on overnight."[184] Bedtime application helps allow the child to release from the nerve–sense activity of the day and fosters the kind of metabolic warmth that allows for deep and renewing sleep. The therapeutic indication is a contrasting combination of temperature, anatomy, and timing: warmth to the abdomen at bedtime.

These outer applications are very simple, but with rhythmic application they can have very real effects. They are a gentle way to support the child's naturally shifting daily physiology.

Salt and Sugar

We take a further step of intervention when we begin to use substance. The two indications from Steiner—salt and sugar—are very common elements in our diet, but they relate to very different processes.

Beginning with salt: In the embryo-to-youth imagination, Steiner said of the large head, "I must compress it. I must also inwardly crystallize, so to speak, all that is still watery and fluid in the embryo, being part of the fluid body, so that it becomes the embryonic brain."[185] That compression comes about through hardening and shrinking the head pole. The boundary of the head and the activity of the senses is thereby refined. This awakens our capacity for objective sensing activity, something that is actually possible only through antipathy: "Formation of the head is breathed out of the cosmos through antipathy."[186] This shrinking and defining is accentuated by the activity of salt.

Do a small experiment and taste a pinch of salt. You will immediately become aware of how salt grabs your attention, wakens you, and defines a border for your tongue and mouth. Steiner described how the large-headed child needs salt. Giving the large-headed child a little extra dietary salt can be beneficial, perhaps a small pinch added to oatmeal in the morning. The salt process is also emphasized whenever we use the roots of a plant (like root vegetables).[187]

For the small-headed child, we need to bring the opposite experience. This is the realm of sugar. When we take a pinch of sugar in the mouth (especially after having just tasted something salty), we will experience how sugar smooths our sensations. Salt brings immediate consciousness to the exact border of the tongue, while a sweet flavor brings softer, happier feelings. Steiner said that for children with a small-headed constitution there is generally a problem with not receiving the "proper amount of sugar.... They become nervous and irritated when they have not had enough sugar.... When such little children have too little sugar for a period of time, their organism slowly decays."[188] It is remarkable how often children with a small-headed constitution are susceptible to low blood sugar. They often do well with natural sugars, like fruit, honey, or maple sugar (in moderation), particularly in the evening. Now an important consideration for both of these dietary recommendations is that most processed foods today are loaded with extra salt and sugar, so there is little worry about not being exposed to these things. The cravings of small-headed children often tend toward white, refined sugar, but these highly processed sugars do not bring about the metabolic health to which Steiner alluded.

For both poles, the child's need for either salt or sugar may not be related to insufficient dietary intake. Steiner instead explained that a child's challenge may be due to an inability "to properly handle salt" and that we can "help achieve the proper intake of salt by using a very dilute dosage of lead compounds."[189] Similarly, "the organism may, in a sense, refuse to properly process sugars. In that case you again need to assist the organism by giving a small dose of silver." [190] This brings us to the use of lead and silver as constitutional remedies.

Lead and Silver

Metals as remedies (as opposed to plant or animal substances) have a special relationship to the "I," so their use in constitutional treatments speaks particularly strongly to the individual child's pathway of incarnation. Their use brings a different, deeper level of therapeutic intervention, and for this reason they should be prescribed only by anthroposophic physicians trained in their application. Lead or silver really speaks to the child in a deep way. They are included in this general description of the polarity because they bring such archetypal pictures. Steiner emphasized how these two particular metals were part of spiritual schooling in the past and how they are able to balance the transition between the spiritual and physical worlds.

In a series of lectures about ancient mystery centers, Steiner described how lead and silver were considered not so much as earthly metals but as relating to much greater planetary processes. The metals were meditated upon, so that one might come into relation to the "speech of the metals," which could then tell one "of the most intimate relations existing between the metals and the human being."[191] Steiner described how these metals surround us all the time in the physical environment and in the atmosphere in very fine (nearly homeopathic) doses. The metals and their processes continually work into us through this very fine distribution.

Our interaction with lead develops and matures the nerve–sense pole. This allows us to perceive the physical world in an objective way, to be sensing it without being defined by it:

> In a crude, material sense, we cannot have lead in us; in the finer, more ethereal sense, we cannot live without it. For what would become of humankind if lead from the cosmos, from the atmosphere, did not affect us.... Without lead we would indeed have sense impressions; we would be able to perceive colors and musical tones, but with every perception we would become slightly faint, slightly out of our body. We would never be able to stand back from his perceptions and reflect in thoughts and mental

> concepts about what we perceived.... We should be unable to form any mental picture of our sense perceptions or retain any picture of them in our memory. It is the finely distributed lead in our brain that makes this possible.[192]

Lead relates to the planetary process of Saturn, described by Steiner as the force that brings us out of the spiritual world and allows us to experience the external world with the power of memory. For memories to be inwardly planted, impressions of the outside world must come into us and make their mark. To consciously meet and remember the outside world, we must (almost paradoxically) become separate from it. The boundary of the inner world and outer world becomes stronger as the nerve–sense pole matures. As with any dynamic process, it is possible for this lead-like process of independent sensing and memory to be taken too far. What would this look like? The lead process (in excess) would make the human being "completely estranged from the cosmos" and "would become, as it were, a hermit," completely cut off from our spiritual origins.[193] Through the incarnation process we must all, to a certain degree, work to become hermits from the spiritual world.

Bringing this picture back into our considerations of the large- and small-headed polarity, when nerve–sense maturation is too slow, the child needs to take a step away from the spiritual world. The child with a large-headed constitution has not yet come far enough along that pathway and stays too young. We can therefore see how a constitutional, homeopathic lead treatment assists the child in becoming more independent and therefore more objectively aware of the earth.

A child with a small-headed constitution, in contrast, has come too far into that state of being a hermit—too awake, too separate, too old too soon. It should come as no surprise that Steiner shared this with us: "Through the silver forces of the Moon, human beings receive the influence opposite to the lead forces from Saturn, and we are therefore not estranged from the cosmos."[194] Silver supports the missing metabolic vitality the small-headed constitution needs (much as in the age-to-youth meditation a sclerotic old man gradually fills with youthful vitality and starts to "ring"). Constitutional silver treatments help release children from the external conditions and demands of the physical world and make their sensing softer and a little younger.

This inclination to be overwhelmed by the outside world is exacerbated through early life experiences that demand strong sensing activity, like premature birth, repeated exposure to chaotic environments, frequent moves, as well as unpredictable, erratic, or abusive behavior from other children or adults. All of these situations require the child to sense too much, too early (whether through physical sensing, environmental sensing, social sensing, or a combination). This excessive early sensing is a shock. Shock and trauma disrupt the fourfold integration into the will, so that our metabolic system is never able to come into order. Silver acts as a balm for those traumatic disruptions. Steiner further described silver as "an excellent remedy for all diseases associated with karma."[195] Silver helps us in those situations when we need to be healed back toward the spiritual world and connect to our spiritual origins a bit more, when the conditions of our earthly life have become too much.

Chapter 16

Practical Applications of the Large- and Small-headed Polarity

The transition into wakeful sensing makes possible our capacity for abstract, intellectual learning. While the integration of spiritual and earthly streams predominates during the first seven years of life, the balancing of blood and nerve comes more to the fore during the grade school years, from roughly age six or seven (the change of teeth) to age fourteen (pubertal changes). This is a developmental period in which the health of the rhythmic system is particularly important. Both metabolic–limb system and rhythmic system activities are continuously taking place, but they find a particular developmental emphasis during their respective seven-year periods (see table 8).

Table 8: Major Developmental Activities of Birth to Seven Years and Seven to Fourteen Years

Birth to the change of teeth (0–7 years)	**Change of teeth to puberty** (7–14 years)
Overcoming the hereditary body, building healthy metabolic and limb activity	Differentiated activity of blood and nerve, balancing the rhythmic system
Willing	Feeling
Feeble/maniacal polarity	Large-/small-headed polarity

This seven-year emphasis is true, but it is important to point out that there are frequent situations when a process appears prominently outside the seven-year span in which it archetypally unfolds. For example, it is very possible to see a child with a strongly small-headed constitution in the first seven years of life or a very large-headed older teenager or a maniacal ten-year-old. In fact, from a therapeutic perspective, the polarities are often most striking when they show up outside their normal developmental emphasis. Consider a four-year-old child who is engaging in physical play and colliding with other children. This is perhaps not so unusual, but the same behavior in an eleven- or twelve-year-old would be more unusual and probably much more concerning. As another example, the self-conscious vulnerability of an early adolescence is awkward but somehow also developmentally appropriate, because a child's awareness of the outside world is growing in big ways. Seeing that same kind of raw, self-conscious vulnerability in a much younger child would be very out of place and could be a red flag for experiences of trauma. Knowing the appropriate windows for these developmental awakenings is very helpful for placing behaviors in the right context.

When we consider children from the perspective of large-headed and small-headed constitutions, it is important to look with fresh eyes. This is true because the way in which a child leans in one polarity (such as feeble or maniacal) does not predict what the process will be with the other polarities: a maniacal child could be either large-headed or small-headed and a child with feeble movement either small-headed or large-headed. Table 7 should not tempt us into thinking that the time frames for the polarities are fixed or that the polarities are mutually exclusive. As we explore later, it is very possible to see shades of multiple polarities within the same child, which allows for very individualized insight.

The next chapter looks at how observations of a large- or small-headed inclination have particular potency when we are considering aspects of first grade readiness and the timing of a child's entry into the more formal classroom setting.

Chapter 17
First-Grade Readiness
Observations and the Polarity of Differentiation

At six and a half to seven years, etheric forces that were previously directed almost exclusively to bodily growth in the metabolism become freed for activities of abstract thought and memory. Up until this point all children are archetypally more large-headed (with an incompletely developed nerve–sense pole), and all children become more small-headed as they enter the grades (better able to carefully observe and analyze).

A first and very classic measure of physiologic maturation considers whether a child can reach with one arm up over the head and touch the top of the ear on the opposite side.[196] If a child cannot reach all the way over, it is a sign that the child is still developmentally young and is not ready for first grade. This reaching is a measure of the relative proportion of the head to the limbs and of the relative large- or small-headedness of the child. When a child can successfully reach over the head and touch the opposite ear, there has typically been an accompanying awakening and maturation of sense perception. It is important that this sign not be used in isolation (for as with constitutional evaluation, first grade readiness needs to be guided by the overall constellation of signs and behaviors, not any single part of a checklist). We can understand this as a true measure of the young child's overcoming some of the large-headedness of early childhood (see table 9, pages 178–179).

A related sign of maturation is whether the child's body has begun stretching, so that the limbs and trunk become longer. For a child to grow into relatively more small-headed proportions, the limbs must experience significant growth (as the head obviously does not really shrink). This differentiated growth can be understood in relation to the now liberated etheric forces in the head. Earlier the head grew greatly in size, but now etheric forces that were previously used to grow the brain and sense organs are freed and instead move through them for sensing. Etheric forces in the metabolic–limb system continue to be involved in the transformation of physical substance and growth. Through this shift in etheric activity, the physical growth process of the head slows in relation to the growth process of the limbs. Trunk and limb lengthening suggest differentiated etheric activity.

Another important developmental sign that Steiner repeatedly linked with liberation of etheric forces is the arrival of new teeth. Just as the cutting of baby teeth suggests an infant's readiness for solid food, the appearance of adult teeth means that the child is ready to intellectually digest the outside world in new ways. This is a very good physiologic measure, as the child's maturation of inner organ development at age six or seven parallels the outer growth of adult teeth. Because this is a maturation process that emerges from the inside turning outward, it correlates well with the inner state of metabolic health. In other words, we can stimulate children to become more wakeful to the world before they would unfold such curiosity naturally, but we cannot make them grow new teeth from the outside through wakeful stimulation. It emerges only once a certain stage of inner metabolic maturation has been reached. That said, we should make subtle distinctions between the loss of teeth (having them fall out) and having new teeth grow in. This may sound like saying the same thing two ways, but they should not be lumped together, because some children now lose teeth at age five or five and a half years of age, when their etheric forces are clearly not yet finished growing the body and its inner organs.

If we look carefully at these children, the ones who lose teeth very early are often small-headed in their constitution. They are wakeful, more often small in build. Their nerve–sense system (through its catabolic forces) breaks down the roots of the baby teeth. What is striking,

Table 9: Summary for large-headed and small-headed constitutions

Between Blood and Nerve—the Polarity of Differentiation: This polarity is distinct from the will polarity of movement (feeble and maniacal). It instead speaks to possible one-sidedness of the feeling life, which develops between blood and nerve, a process that finds particular prominence as wakefulness emerges out of the metabolic dominance of early childhood. This is a useful lens for gaining insight into how a child inwardly processes an experience (in this middle feeling life), particularly in the elementary school years.	
This process is described through the polarity of large-headed and small-headed constitutions, presented by Steiner in *Faculty Meetings with Rudolf Steiner*, vol. 2 (Feb. 6, 1923, and May 2, 1923)	
Large-headed Stays young too long, too metabolic, cannot analyze, imaginative but inattentive, flighty	**Small-headed** Grows old too soon, too nerve–sense, weak constructive or synthetic imagining, brooding, irritated by external impressions
The nerve–sense system is not in order (hence the metabolism dominates).	The metabolic–limb system is not in order (hence the sensing dominates).
These children tend to experience a lot of inflammations of the head and neck (earaches, big tonsils, sore throats).	These children tend to have problems with their digestion, picky eaters, stomachaches (easily vomit or get diarrhea).
Attentiveness and Memory	
Remembers the larger pictures and images of a story but not the specifics. May instead be creative with the details or elements of a story. Can relate to the broader message or principle but may have difficulty knowing how to practically apply it to a specific situation.	Remembers the specifics, knows all the details. It can be almost painful for the child if those details are inconsistent or are told incorrectly. The child remembers specific examples but may miss the overall moral or message of a story.

<table>
<tr><th colspan="2">With Regard to First-Grade Readiness</th></tr>
<tr><td>May hold on to baby teeth a long time,
with adult teeth coming in around them</td><td>May lose teeth early (five years old), but has an empty space for a long time, as the adult tooth is not yet ripe enough to erupt</td></tr>
<tr><td>Reaching over the head to touch the opposite ear is a measure of getting sufficiently small(er)-headed.</td><td>Eruption of six-year old molars is a sign of organ ripeness, or real metabolic completion.</td></tr>
<tr><td>Looking for awareness and independence. Growing interest in the world around.
Is the child developing a sense of “I” (of the other)?</td><td>Looking less for signs of wakefulness than for signs of true physical ripening. A capacity for self-soothing, a sense of wellbeing.
Does the child have a healthy life sense?</td></tr>
<tr><td colspan="2">Therapeutic Realm:
What helps the child to feel more balanced in the body?
We can help with diet and outer application.</td></tr>
<tr><td>Large-headed: salt or root vegetables, cool water on the head in the morning.
Help the child awaken to the details, to be more exacting in observation.
Help them become a Sherlock Holmes and see all the details, not let things slip by unnoticed.</td><td>Small-headed: sun-ripened sugars, warm compress or hot water bottle on the abdomen at night.
Help the child relax enough to digest a sensory experience.
Help them be a little more like Miss Marple and wait until all of the elements have presented themselves and then gain the greater perspective.</td></tr>
</table>

however, is that sometimes these children will then have a gap in their teeth for a long time. It can take six to eight months (sometimes longer) for the metabolically mature adult tooth to grow in. So when there is early tooth loss, particularly in intellectually precocious children, we should not be fooled into thinking that they are fully ready for first grade. In these cases it is important to look for the true appearance of new teeth and also for the appearance of the six-year molars (which again, as new teeth, are an expression of metabolic maturation and are not preceded by any tooth loss).

Other children have a strikingly different pattern: at certain times they will almost have two rows of teeth, because the large adult teeth are growing in behind or in front of the baby teeth. It seems to be very difficult for these children to lose their teeth, and these children usually have a large-headed constitution. They exhibit strong, dominant growth (evidenced by the erupting adult teeth), but they lack the nerve–sense forces needed to break down the roots of the old teeth. They cannot dissolve the roots of their baby teeth and similarly will often struggle to think analytically. These teething patterns give an additional purview into constitution.

There are other structural and sculptural signs of development that are commonly considered signs of first grade readiness, which are more related to how well the child has claimed the inherited body. We saw in the polarity of the earthly and cosmic child that a lack of definition, a certain formable quality of the tissue, marks portions of the body that have not yet been fully penetrated (for the earthly child, limbs and trunk stay rounded and sculptable, whereas for the cosmic child, the head does so). We can also look more generally for sculptural changes as an expression of a certain completion of the first seven years. For example:

- The arch of the foot lifts, a marker of full penetration through the hereditary body and all the way out to the periphery and an overcoming of gravity.

- The knees and wrists can be seen as distinct portions of the limbs (sculpting), the fingers become longer and leaner (stretching) with visible knuckles (sculpting).
- In a related way, the rib cage and thorax become distinct from the abdomen. There is also generally loss of a younger child's "potbelly" abdomen, and the spine takes on an S shape—curving toward the front to create a hollow in the lower spine (lordosis) and arching toward the back in the upper spine between the shoulder blades (kyphosis). This differentiated activity of the spine grows out of the new dynamic that unfolds between the head and the limbs (as opposed to the more uniform shape of a young child's spine).

Other measures of first grade readiness are not physically perceived but express themselves through shifts toward wakeful interaction and activity. What starts as a fairly self-contained, body-oriented state of being grows into more parallel, social, and then intellectual interaction. Some examples of this progression include the following:[197]

- Play—A school-ready child shows increasing capacity for social awareness, for recognizing other's feelings and needs. Play becomes more goal-oriented, with steps of planning and the ability to visualize things without needing to collect material objects.
- Drawings and paintings—There is a shift from drawing as a purely exploratory and expressive activity (where the result mirrors inner experiences of the body and of the child's overall physiology) to an activity with intention. Again, the result is more goal-oriented. Picturing of the body also reflects the more complete penetration of the hereditary body, with figures colored in, the trunk more distinct, and fingers on the hands.
- Thought life—Causal thinking develops, memory becomes a conscious capacity (remembering things at will), and humor and riddles become accessible and enjoyable (the abstractions suddenly making sense).

These are all signs of an evolving small-headedness (as the nerve–sense system comes into better order). When these capacities arise out of healthy maturation, then they are accompanied by genuine enthusiasm, like the blossoming of a lovely flower. If they develop as splinter skills (capacities that have been cultivated artificially through imposed repetition or outside expectation), then the child often shows a certain rigidity associated with the activity. An example might be when a child is able to draw something in a stylized way—in abstract imitation—for which the details are correct but for which there is no accompanying story or imagination. Often only the lines of the figure are drawn and never colored in. Similarly, children may play out characters or story lines they have experienced (mostly through exposure to movies or other media), but the character's activity never evolves. The play is not really arising from the child's own imagination and curiosity.

Beyond physical markers and beyond social play, we can also look at first grade readiness in relation to the twelve senses. Through the seven-year change, children waken out of the lower senses (of life, movement, balance, and touch) and more into the world around them (toward the middle and higher senses). For the child with a large-headed constitution, a particularly helpful sign of that awakening comes when the child notices that a person is visiting the classroom (as an outside observer). The child may come to inquire about what we are doing and who we are, asking questions that come out of a genuine curiosity. This is an expression of early development of the higher senses of the child—particularly the capacity for really seeing another human being as an individual, the sense of "I." Seeing this growing social awareness in a large-headed child is a reassuring sign that the child is ready for work and learning in the grades. Children who are still fully absorbed with the metabolic activity of early childhood may well see a visitor and even ask the person to move so that they can get to a particular toy, but they do not yet encounter the visitor as another "I."

For the child with a small-headed constitution this social wakefulness is not such a good measure. We instead need to go to the other side of the circle of senses, to the life sense. Small-headed children will often notice a visitor's presence at four or five years of age, but they are watching out of nervousness. Social encounter is much more related to astral vigilance than to the curiosity of a liberated etheric sensing. The more appropriate measure for these children is to look to see if metabolic maturation has really been achieved and to assess the health of the life sense. How comfortable does the child seem in herself? Does the child show inner contentment, a healthy sense of wellbeing? Is there an inward, metabolic foundation, which the child can rely upon and not be overwhelmed by all the changing conditions and expectations of a grade's classroom? There are many children now who are very awake and will be able to keep up academically with the grade's classroom content but who will likely suffer emotionally and socially if they have not yet achieved that inner anchor. It is good to make sure that the anchoring activity of the life sense has matured and to not be fooled by isolated signs of intellectual development. We need more and more to protect children from too much intellectualization until they are able to inwardly digest what they encounter in the outside world.

Chapter 18

Building an Inner Foundation to Meet the Outer World

The Fairy Tale of Snow White and the Seven Dwarfs

If we take the polarity of blood and nerve and expand it to a societal level, we might ask: "What is the constitution of the world today?" This is a worthwhile question, because at certain points in constitutional observation we will have to seek to discern which parts of a child's behavior are related to constitution and which parts are simply related to the world we are living in. With ever-rising diagnoses of autism, attention deficit hyperactivity disorder, childhood bipolar disorder, depression, and anxiety, we must recognize that some aspects of these challenges relate to larger societal imbalances, not just constitutional inclinations. These societal illnesses are impacting the way we are able to connect with one another. We seem to be less and less good at it.

There have, of course, always been challenges in finding the best way to meet another person as a full human being. It is not fully innate. It is not a given. It is a skill, a capacity, that each of us has to individually develop. We have already explored one potential hindrance to fully sensing the other through the feeble and kleptomaniacal polarity. We have seen how incomplete development of the metabolic–limb pole limits our moral sensing. If we do not properly transform the hereditary body, then our sensing will remain either dulled and clumsy (like trying to hold a piece of glass covered in oil) or superficial and abstract (and therefore unable to develop true empathy).

A related, but perhaps even broader societal challenge arises when we cannot feel out into the world through what are known as the higher senses of hearing, word, thought, and "I." They remain unexplored if we are continually distracted by the need to feel ourselves inwardly (brought on by imbalanced senses of touch, balance, movement, and life). If our attention is continually redirected inwardly, our connection to the outside world cannot evolve, and without these higher senses our moral capacities are also blunted. What we ultimately are able to sense "outside" depends on how we feel "inside." The foundation that is laid down through the integration process of the first seven years metamorphoses into the outward social perception of older childhood.

When the lower senses are not in order, the metabolic–limb system is also not in order; we then all suffer from different shades of (small-headed type) distraction. Today many children experience difficulty finding the inward path to quiet wellbeing, whether or not their overall constitutional inclination is a small-headed imbalance. This has many academic and social ramifications, for the ability to sit and be instructed by a teacher, to listen to a piece of music, or to enter into real discussion and conversation all require that we are able to find a place of inner quiet. We need to feel well inside before we can properly attend to the world outside. When our demands for inwardly directed perception dominate, it is hard to notice the outside world. Think of trying to pay attention when you are ill or when you have low blood sugar or need to go to the bathroom—that is the same kind of process. Inward instability creates a (physiologically grounded) inability to look much beyond the point of our noses.

Now to have our sensing intermittently directed inward is normal and necessary. It allows us to stay connected to the needs of our metabolism and digestion. It helps us know when we need to pause to eat, to drink, to rest, or to go to the bathroom. At a certain point, however, we should be able to put our own needs aside. Children become better and better able to do this when they have moved, jumped, spun, slept, and digested enough that the lower senses are mature. If our inner sensory organs are not able to finish developing during the first seven years and they persist into older childhood and adolescence, they can become a true pathologic condition. A compensation takes place: what should unfold out of etheric maturation instead becomes a displaced astral activity, where we spend a lot of time trying to sense our wellbeing from the outside in. We do not feel our own wellbeing, so we invoke other senses as an alternative pathway for knowing how we are doing. In a child this creates a precociously wakeful but poorly consolable imbalance of the astral body.

This has become an almost pervasive illness in our time. It comes from not protecting and adequately supporting the fourfold integration of the hereditary and spiritual streams in the first seven years. Bringing abstract intellectual content too early—which should really enter into the child's life only after the change of teeth—robs the metabolism of its proper forces. Protecting a child from this imbalance may now stand as the most important task of early childhood education.

Knowledge of when our inner forces are ready to shift to the outer world is so important. Ignoring such archetypal rhythms exacts a price. We can gain a deeper sense for this cost by exploring sensory displacement in the language of archetypes. The fairy tale of Snow White and the seven dwarfs stands as an imaginative healing journey for such a precocious astral imbalance.

The fairy tale of Snow White is certainly widely known. It was popularized through the Disney adaptation and movie, though many of the true, spiritual pictures given in the original Grimm Brothers' story were not included in that presentation. So we have, in a way, to rediscover the story in order to see how it relates to the balancing of sense and wellbeing.

The story of Snow White has been examined by other authors with an anthroposophic insight. Henning Schramm, an anthroposophic pharmacist, described Snow White as a "copper" fairy tale.[198] Copper, as a remedy, bears a special relationship to the astral body. It helps guide the astral so that it finds a proper relationship to the physical body. It brings the astral body out of a head- and sensing-dominated activity (like anxiety) to a metabolically mediated activity (like rest, growth, and recovery).[199] That healing gesture runs throughout the story of Snow White. It provides us with spiritual pictures for recognizing overly developed nerve–sense activity in a child and then finding ways to help the child heal back into a more metabolically balanced state of being.

The story of Snow White begins, like the story of Iron John, with a description of Snow White's origins. She comes at the wish, the intention of her mother, a beautiful queen. We can observe right away that the story is full of queens—a beautiful mother, an evil stepmother, and eventually Snow White herself—all of whom can be recognized as different aspects of the same individuality. Right at the beginning of the story Snow White loses her connection to the mother's realm, her mother's death a picture of Snow White's transition out of the spiritual world when Snow White herself enters into an earthly incarnation. The mother's wish—for a child "as white as snow, as red as blood, and as black as the wood in this frame"—is a special picturing of our threefold existence in the body.[200]

The story then brings a second wife, the new queen, who we are told is beautiful, proud, and haughty. She cannot bear being second in beauty to anyone, and she has a "magic" mirror that, as is well known, tells her "who in this land is fairest of all."[201] Whenever she hears the answer, she is reassured, for "she knew that the mirror spoke the truth."[202] Her contentment is short-lived, however. For almost immediately the queen begins again to judge, inquire, question, and watch.

The essence of this second queen's activity is looking, being aware of what is present in the world around her. The queen's observation is different from normal observation, however. For her, looking outward is twisted and imbalanced in an unusual way, as her attention outward into the world is always ultimately reflected back to herself. She looks out but really is able to see only herself, her mirror a picture of her continually self-directed gaze. She does not properly connect with the outside world because her intentions are always ultimately tied to her own unmet inner needs and longings.

In fact, when the queen learns that Snow White is a "thousand times fairer" than she is, she becomes ill. The queen soon "took fright" and "turned yellow and green with envy.... The envy and pride grew ever greater, like a weed in her heart, until she had no peace day and night."[203] The queen summons a huntsman, orders him to take Snow White into the forest and kill her, and bring back her lungs and liver as a token of Snow White's death. The huntsman cannot bring himself to do this deed but instead allows Snow White to run away and in her place kills a young boar and brings back its heart and lungs. The queen's cook has "to boil them with salt, and the wicked woman ate them, supposing that she had eaten Snow White's lungs and liver."[204] The queen does this because she longs for a way to be like Snow White, but she cannot really come into Snow White's realm. In fact, the only way that she knows how to approach her is through destructive, death-bringing processes: she wants Snow White killed, wants her organs brought back, and then eats them after they have been cooked in "brine."

What does the queen represent? If we are able to release ourselves from a completely literal interpretation of the fairy tale and avoid simply placing the queen in an "evil" category, then we can consider these questions: What part of the human being is the queen? What part of our own development and physiology does she relate to?

A starting place is to consider the relationship between contentment (which she hopes to find by gazing into her mirror) and the envy that "grows like a weed in her heart." Contentment means that we are happy, satisfied within ourselves. We do not want anything more from the outside world—all that we need is in our possession. Envy is on many levels the opposite—with it we lose our contentment; we do not feel complete. We need something from the outside world, believing that only then will we feel truly happy and satisfied. With envy, we are caught in always gazing out; with contentment, our consciousness finds a healthy foundation within.

That may sound like a black-and-white distinction—envy is bad; contentment is good. But the experience of incompleteness, of longing, does have its proper place. It accompanies the growth that comes with biographical thresholds when we shift from one stage of life to another (like the seven-year change). We then experience an uncomfortable combination of expanded awareness—a greater capacity for sensing the outside world—without yet having the skills or security for really knowing what to do with that awareness. Whether the biographical shift that comes at the age of three, seven, nine, twelve, twenty-one, thirty-three, or fifty-six, there is an impetus to lean forward into new experiences and possibilities while simultaneously feeling worried, disoriented, and insecure because things are no longer as they used to be. Children in these transitions frequently exhibit burgeoning independence accompanied by regressive behaviors. In fact, sometimes a sign of looming maturation is an increase in younger, more dependent or regressive behaviors (wanting to sleep in a parent's bed again, sucking a thumb, acting like a baby), because these children can sense that their relationship to the world is changing, and they therefore long to connect to those earlier experiences that brought a sense of connection and contentment.

Those experiences of insecurity are generally temporary, however, because new growth unfolds as we loosen from the patterns and experiences of the past. That disorientation is a necessary ingredient. We need to lose hold of some of our previous foundations in order to create the space to build anew. We loosen so that we can reshape. Sensory envy is rightfully part of a growth process because it helps us look outside ourselves.

Of course, in excess, envy is not healthy. It is very possible for it to become one-sided. Then it stays too long and finds no counterbalance, no resolution. We find ourselves stuck in a place where we continually feel that we are incomplete and need something that lies outside ourselves. This is where the stepmother queen of the Snow White story lives. She longs; she looks and looks and looks but does not find contentment in the outer world. She is missing something. Her outward gaze does not bring her peace. She does not move into a new stage of growth. While it is easy to judge the figure of the queen as selfish and malicious, from a more archetypal physiologic viewpoint she is doing what the sense organs know how to do—she gazes outward, and when that is not enough she gazes even more. She is really stuck in the nerve–sense system. Our sensing physiology is essential, but if it finds no counterbalance, no inward anchor, it becomes pathologic. Unbridled sensing activity becomes destructive and devitalizing.

The activity of our astral body in the nerve–sense system should be full of envy. Its task is to continuously look out to see what is there. It would be a problem if our eyes suddenly became content and felt satisfied with what they had seen by lunchtime and therefore stopped looking for the rest of the day. We should be full of envious activity in our senses (in the head pole)—but it must be balanced by inwardly directed metabolism (of the limb pole).

The queen's envy is unhealthy because she can bring nothing to balance it. As her envy grows, it becomes evermore one-sided: "Envy and pride grew like a weed in her heart, higher and higher, so that day or night she no longer had any rest." Her nerve–sense activity grows so dominant that she literally cannot find any rest. She loses the balance between waking (the head) and sleeping (the metabolism). The queen seems to instinctively know that she needs to find a connection to the metabolism, to the inner organs, but she does this in a destructive way—she orders Snow White's death in order to harvest her lungs and liver. This feels a little shocking in its brutality, but we can understand her longing for the organs as a healthy instinct. The unconscious, metabolic organs could bring a balancing process to her envy. The queen, in her one-sidedness, does not have access to true inner organ function. She brings the activity of the nerves, which are by nature catabolic (breaking down) to the inner organs of liver and lungs (which bring anabolic, upbuilding activity). If we refer back to the differentiated interactions of the members of the human being, we can see that the astral body works in several different ways. It can act independently (which relates to sensing and breathing), through the etheric (which brings the pulse activity), or through the etheric and down into the physical body (which brings the blood process). The queen knows only how to work through the uppermost astral pathway. She cannot work cooperatively with the etheric and physical. When the queen does try to come down into the realm of the organs, it is through a nerve–sense activity, and that can bring only destruction—as she calls for Snow White's death and then cooks the organs (in brine!) and eats them. The queen's powerful nerve process becomes more and more pathologic the farther it moves down the body: it begins as an (appropriate) envy of the senses, then brings a one-sided imbalance to the feeling life so that she can find "no rest" and eventually an actual death process when she enters into the metabolic realm of the organs.

Now let us consider Snow White. The princess Snow White is also beautiful and in time grows more beautiful than the queen. She has something that the queen does not have—she is youthful. More than that, she is able to balance her nerve–sense activity. She is able to come into healthy connection with her inner realm. It is a special birthright from her mother, that Snow White should have skin as white as snow (a picturing of the nervous system), lips as red as blood (the metabolic–limb system), and hair as black as ebony (relating to iron and its relationship to the rhythmic system[205]). Snow White brings a possibility for experiencing the world as a truly threefold human being.[206]

The threefold nature of our existence allows us to engage with the outside world in richer ways. When we move out through the upper senses—from hearing, to word, to thought, to the "I" of the other—we must be able to fall asleep to ourselves. We must feel grounded and confident enough with our own experience of the body that we can surrender our inner sensing. The queen cannot do this. She looks outward, but her intention and orientation are always directed back toward herself, her magical mirror a picture of the blindness her imbalance demands. She looks out but can really only perceive herself.

The queen's inability to surrender her nagging self-awareness is healed by Snow White's journey. Snow White's meeting with the dwarfs is a pathway out of isolated nerve–sense envy into a true connection with the inner, metabolic realm.

If we begin with the outwardly directed higher senses and then move down and around the circle of the twelve senses, we come more and more into body-oriented activity. Most inward, most body-directed is the life sense.[207] The life sense has been previously described as the connection to our sense of wellbeing. It connects by acting as a doorway to the unconscious processes continuously carried out in our inner world. Those sleeping physiologic activities were described by Steiner as the "life processes." The life sense allows us to perceive the actual working of the life processes and creates the counterbalance to fretful, "rest"-less, outwardly directed sensing activity.

The life processes themselves are largely unconscious but dynamic. They are always in motion, always shifting in their relationship to one another and to the circle of twelve senses that stand around them. That relation of the life processes to the senses is a "microcosmic" human picture of the "macrocosm" that surrounds us:

> The human being, the mobile human being, must be pictured as having twelve separate sensory zones through which pulses a mobile, sevenfold life. If you ascribe the signs of the zodiac to the twelve zones, then you have a picture of the macrocosm; if you ascribe a sense to each zone, you have the microcosm. If you assign a planet to each of the life processes, you have a picture of the macrocosm; as the life processes, they embody the microcosm. And the mobile life processes are related to the fixed zones of the senses just as, in the macrocosm, the planets are related to the zones of the zodiac. They move unceasingly though them; they flow through them. Thus, you see another sense in which the human being is a macrocosm.[208]

There are seven life processes. In them, the astral body works with and through the etheric and physical bodies. The life processes make possible our digestion—of food, thought, experience, and interaction. They are our constant companions, but they work so continuously that we do not consciously recognize them. Our life sense is the gateway to this sleeping aspect of our experience:

> The sense that we shall call the sense of life involves processes that lie still more deeply embedded in the human organism. This sense exists within us, but we are accustomed to ignore it, for the life sense manifests itself indistinctly from within the human organism. Nevertheless, throughout all our daily waking hours, the harmonious collaboration of all the bodily organs expresses itself through the life sense, through the state of life in us. We usually pay no attention to it because we expect it as our natural right. We expect to be filled with a certain feeling of wellbeing, with the feeling of being alive. If our feeling of aliveness is diminished, we try to recover a little so that our feeling of life is refreshed again. This enlivening or damping down is something we are aware of, but generally we are too accustomed to the feeling of being alive to be constantly aware of it. The life sense, however, is a distinct sense in its own right. Through it we feel the life in us, precisely as we see what is around us with our eyes. We sense ourselves through the life sense just as we see with our eyes. Without this internal sense of life we would know nothing about our own vital state.[209]

In our fairy tale, Snow White makes a journey from the wakeful realm of the queen into the dark and unknown wilds of the woods. She charts a journey inward, moving away from the activity of the senses into the limbs:

> The poor child was now all alone in the great forest, and she was so afraid that she just looked at all the leaves on the trees and did not know what to do. Then she began to run. She ran over sharp stones and through thorns, and wild animals jumped at her, but they did her no harm. She ran as far as her feet could carry her, and just as evening was about to fall she saw a little house and went inside in order to rest.[210]

She stops when it becomes dark.

Snow White leaves the realm of daytime consciousness (the twelve senses) and comes to a completely different place. She finds a cottage in the woods, in the dark, which she enters "to rest." This will be the place where she sleeps—first on her arrival, then three more times to heal from the poisonous intrusions of the queen. The cottage, the house of the seven dwarfs, is a beautiful picturing of the activity of the seven life processes whose cooperative work transforms the outside world and allows it to come to rest. The dwarfs bring restorative life activity when we visit them:

> Inside the house everything was small, but so neat and clean that no one could say otherwise. There was a little table with a white tablecloth and seven little plates, and each plate had a spoon, and there were seven knives and forks and seven mugs as well. Against the wall there were seven little beds, all standing in a row and covered with Snow White sheets.
>
> Because she was so hungry and thirsty Snow White ate a few vegetables and a little bread from each little plate, and from each mug she drank a drop of wine. Afterward, because she was so tired, she lay down on a bed, but none of them felt right—one was too long, the other too short—until finally the seventh one was just right. She remained lying in it, entrusted herself to God, and fell asleep.[211]

By visiting the plates, cups, and then beds of each of the dwarfs, taking just a little of what they have, Snow White finds rest. She spends time with each of them. Her hunger, her thirst, and her fatigue (all expressions of an imbalanced life sense, a disordered inner world) are relieved.

When the dwarfs return home in the evening, they light "seven little candles" and encounter Snow White. They can tell that things are not as they should be and in turn speak to the changes of the "chair," the "plate," the "bread," the "vegetables," the "fork," the "knife," the "mug," and finally the "bed." They are astonished to find

Snow White, but they do not attack her or try to hurt her. Instead, they bring their candles and admire her beauty. They decide not to wake her but to allow her to continue to sleep in the bed. The seventh dwarf, in turn, "had to sleep with his companions, one hour with each one, and then the night was done," as they continue their cooperative, restorative work.[212]

Steiner's own descriptions of the seven life processes brings very similar images. Each life process lends a step to the transformation. In fact, every bit of food and drink, every social interaction, every sensory impression we take in must come into the company of each of the life senses for it to truly become our own:

> What I am talking about now is the very life that flows through us. That inner life also differentiates itself within us. It does so in the following manner.... First of all there is breathing, a manifestation of life necessary to all living things. Every living organism must enter into a breathing relationship with the external world.... The second process we can distinguish is warming. This occurs along with breathing, but it is a separate process. Warming, the inner process of warming something through, is the second of the life-sustaining processes. The third process that sustains life is nourishment. So here we have three ways in which life comes to us from without: breathing, warming, nourishing.... At this stage, the life processes take us deeper into the internal world. We now find processes that re-form what has been taken in from outside—processes that transform and internalize it.... The purely inner process that is the basis of the re-forming of what we take in from outside us can be seen to be fourfold. Following the process of nourishing, the first internal process is the process of secretion, of elimination.... Excretion and absorption are two sides of the processes by which organs of secretion deal with our nourishment. One part of the secretion performed by organs of digestion separates out nutriments by sending them into the organism. Whatever is thus secreted into the organism must remain connected with the life processes, and this involves a further process which we

> will call maintaining. But for there to be life, it is not enough for what is taken in to be maintained, there must also be growth. Every living thing depends on a process of inner growth: a process of growth, taken in the widest sense. Growth processes are part of life; both nourishment and growth are part of life. And, finally, life on earth includes reproducing the whole being; the process of growth only requires that one part produce another part. Reproduction produces the whole individual being and is a higher process than growth.[213]

The life processes are breathing, warming, nourishing, secretion, maintaining, growing, and reproducing. They are our beloved, but mostly unrecognized companions. They quietly guide and support the activities of our inner world (see fig. 7).

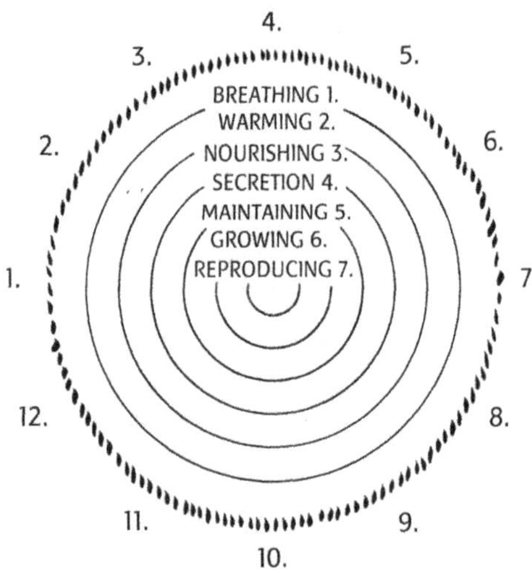

Figure 7: The life processes, within the circle of the twelve senses[214]

In the story, when Snow White awakens and tells the dwarfs that she has fled into their realm to escape the stepmother queen, it is agreed that she may stay with them in their cottage if she will cook, make the beds, wash, sew, knit, and "keep everything clean and orderly." This she does during the day, when the dwarfs take their picks and shovels and go back to their mines in the mountains (a picture of even darker and more hidden metabolic realms).

Much of the rest of the story is devoted to the queen's visits. The queen looks in the mirror, after thinking she has eaten Snow White's lungs and liver, but finds she is not the fairest: "Then she thought, and thought again, how she could kill Snow White, for as long as she was not the most beautiful woman in the entire land her envy would give her no rest."[215] The queen decides she must journey across seven mountains to the realm of the seven dwarfs.

The queen's encounters bring illness to Snow White. With the first visit she brings a bodice lace, offered as a pretty ware. When it is given, the queen (now an old woman) "pulled so quickly and so hard that Snow White could not breathe."[216] This is what happens when there is a cramping in the rhythmic system. We all can experience this, for if our thinking and sensing become too active, our breathing similarly becomes too formed—just consider what happens if someone jumps out unexpectedly and frightens you. You take in a deep and sudden breath, but you do not let it go. Only gradually are you able to properly breathe out, and that happens only when you are able to let go of your vigilance. In the story the dwarfs come and find Snow White in this contracted state, and they are frightened to see her motionless, as if dead. They find the tight bodice lace and cut it. The dwarfs help her to surrender the queen's vigilance. Through this first encounter the dwarfs help Snow White find balance relating to her breathing and the rhythmic system.

The queen returns a second time. Snow White has now been warned by the dwarfs not to let anyone in, but when the queen comes as a different old woman, she tempts Snow White with the simple phrase: "You surely may take a look." The looking (which belongs to the gazing and sensing of the queen's world) allows entry to the queen, who now gives a comb for the head.

Whenever the independent astral activity of the sensing process (the activity of the queen) is physiologically misplaced into the realm of the metabolism (the land of the dwarfs), it brings pain. Pain can, in fact, be understood anthroposophically as an astral activity that inappropriately takes direct hold of the physical body, without the mediation of the etheric.[217] A similar kind of excessive astrality can also be seen in the plant world, though when the astral body penetrates too far into a plant, the result is not pain but poison.[218] When the queen's independent astral activity comes to find Snow White this time, it brings poison. A poisonous comb is put in Snow White's hair, its forces so strong that she falls down, unconscious. Snow White must immediately go to the realm of sleep and abandon all sensing activity when she is confronted by the comb. The seven dwarfs again come and find her and are able to remove the poison comb. They again help to bring her back to balance—the first time removing a lace from the rhythmic system, now a poison comb from the nerve–sense system.

The third encounter with the queen confronts the metabolic–limb system with a poisoned apple. Snow White is deceived into thinking it is safe when she sees the queen eat a bite out of one half of the apple, but when Snow White takes her own bite into her mouth she falls down dead. The queen laughs loudly, saying, "This time the dwarfs cannot awaken you."[219] The dwarfs find her, without breath. They mourn her but recognize that she should not be buried deep in the ground. Instead, they place her on the mountain in a glass coffin, and "one of them always stayed with it and watched over her.... Snow White lay there in the coffin a long, long time, and she did not decay, but looked like she was asleep, for she was still as white as snow and as red as blood, and as black-haired as ebony wood."[220]

Twice before the queen has come. The tight lace and poisoned comb could be healed by the dwarfs. Both episodes stayed in the alternation of daytime and nighttime consciousness, of the wakefulness of the senses healed over by the restoring activity of the life processes. This restoration is something we do every day—generally in proper measure so that we do not become stuck in the envy, the breathlessness, or the poison of the queen's hypervigilance.

With the poisoned apple a new step must be taken. Snow White must find a new element to overcome the third attack by the queen, and this comes through the imagination of the king's son. He has been journeying through the forest and comes to the dwarfs' cottage to spend the night. The prince sees Snow White in her coffin:

> "Let me have the coffin. I will give you anything you want for it."
>
> But the dwarfs answered, "We will not sell it for all the gold in the world."
>
> Then he said, "Then give it to me, for I cannot live without being able to see Snow White. I will honor her and respect her as my most cherished one."
>
> As he thus spoke, the good dwarfs felt pity for him and gave him the coffin.[221]

The king's son also ventures into the realm of the dwarfs, but instead of gaining what he needs through envy and manipulation he is given Snow White as a gift.

When the coffin is carried away, a stumble frees the piece of apple from Snow White's throat. She revives, sees the king's son, and agrees to marry him. They journey together to his father's palace (a connection back to the spiritual world). There, at their wedding feast, the queen comes to visit Snow White one last time after learning that she is alive and now "a thousand times fairer than you." But at the wedding feast it is the queen who is now transformed:

> The wicked woman uttered a curse, and she became so frightened, so frightened, that she did not know what to do. At first she did not want to go to the wedding, but she found no peace. She had to go and see the young queen. When she arrived she recognized Snow White, and terrorized, she could only stand there without moving.
>
> Then they put a pair of iron shoes into burning coals. They were brought forth with tongs and placed before her. She was forced to step into the red-hot shoes and dance until she fell down dead.[222]

With this final encounter the wicked queen's machinations, her torment, and her envy are put to an end.

Who or what, we may ask, is the king's son? The king's son is part of all of us, as is the wicked queen, the seven dwarfs, and Snow White herself. They are all elements of our existence as human beings. The stepmother queen can be pictured as the dominating, envious, astral sensing activity of the head; the seven dwarfs can be understood as the transformative activity of the life processes, through which the astral body senses the activities of the etheric. The king's son—one who acts with devotion, who receives the gift of Snow White from the life processes, and who brings such a strong warmth that it transforms the wicked queen (with red-hot slippers)—can perhaps be best understood as an expression of the "I"-organization. It is the "I" that brings order to the other three bodies, the "I"-organization's warmth—its glowing red iron shoes—that finally makes the queen "dance" with her limbs and force her activity down into the metabolism so strongly that her isolated sensing activity must die.

The fact that the third encounter happens in the metabolic–limb system is significant, with the eating of a poison apple (digestion) that is dislodged by movement (of the limbs) and ending with red-hot slippers for dancing (a strong limb and warmth process). This third encounter is not just a balancing step, like the night's hygienic balancing of a day's wakeful activities. This is a therapeutic step. It is only through the metabolism, through the warmth, guided by the "I" that we transform. Indeed, it is only in the will that our true capacity for healing can unfold.[223]

A last important question then remains: Who or what is Snow White? Snow White, as suggested at the beginning of the story, stands as an imagination for the balanced threefold human being—"as white as snow, as red as blood, and her hair as black as ebony." It is Snow White alone who is able to begin in the realm of the wicked queen, who journeys to find the dwarfs and lives among them, and who then ultimately joins and partners with the king's son. She has the capacity to live in different realms, in different activities. Snow White's beauty and "skin as white as snow" do belong to our nerve–sense astrality, but she can move beyond them. Through a "marriage" with the "I"-organization, one-sided sensing activity is transformed. That is in many ways the essential task of our age.[224] We all must consciously strive to remain a healthy, threefold human being in today's sensory-dominant world.

The story of Snow White and the seven dwarfs serves as a reminder that we are all, regardless of our constitution, being aggressively pushed into a queen-like, envious gazing relationship with the outside world. There is so much to see, too much to actually keep track of. Our environment is also increasingly filled with virtual sensory experiences specifically designed to make us envious for even more outer experiences. The overpowering technological and commercial influences so prevalent in our society are not designed to satiate us. They want the exact opposite, for us instead to never be full, to always hunger and thirst for more. They want to connect us so strongly with the sensing part of our being that we forget about ourselves and become reliant on what the outside world can give us.

Having too much of our life dominated by sensory-rich activity brings illness. For the young child such an influence is particularly challenging and damaging because it disrupts the activity of the life processes. If a child is unable to develop the activity of the life processes in the first seven years of life, the window for archetypal development is in many ways lost. Supporting the formation of a healthy, secure inner world after the age of seven becomes not just a pedagogical task, but a therapeutic intervention. In medical practice it is far more common to prescribe a silver remedy than a lead remedy—the majority of children need constitutional support to help them heal, away from overwhelming sensory experiences; much less common is the need to be awakened into greater encounter and sensing wakefulness.

The march toward ever-earlier introduction of academic material into the life of the small child is as one-sided as the queen's envy and anger. We too often lose connection to the dwarfs, to the life processes, not appreciating what lives in that hidden realm. The resulting imbalance offers us an opportunity to discover such archetypal wisdom anew, to work to find our connection to the dwarfs, and sometimes even to heat the iron slippers that we must take up for deeper transformation.

When we can consciously build a healthy balance between blood and nerve, we find a rich feeling life. Our capacity to meet what comes from the outside world and make it our own feeds us. It keeps us interested in learning about the outside world in new ways. That nourishment of our feeling life is essential, for it creates the foundation for the powerful exploration of connection that marks the developmental movement of adolescence and young adulthood.

Part Three

The Polarity of Connection: Between Point and Periphery

In reality, all connections with the outer world that begin to make their appearance at puberty are fundamentally of the same nature. We should really speak, therefore, not of sexual but of earthly maturity. And under earthly maturity we have to include the maturity of the senses, the maturity of the breathing—and another subdivision will also be sexual maturity. This gives the true picture of the situation. Human being, then, reach earthly maturity. They begin to take again into themselves what is outside and foreign to them; they acquire the faculty of being sensitive and not indifferent to their environment. Before this time, they are not susceptible to the other sex, neither are they susceptible to their environment. Thus do human beings form and develop their third body, which is active in them until the beginning of the twenties.[225]

Chapter 19

From Breathing to Waking and Sensing

Development breathes. We may have the impression that development moves with a steady progression and trajectory, but in truth it is always shifting. In the first seven years of life the child is moving between heaven and earth, working to find a balance between cosmic carelessness and earthly inertia. Balance comes through exploration, usually overshooting, then pulling back, trying again, making adjustment. We build a middle space through experiencing the extremes.

Development also comes in spurts: phases of rapid change (with accompanying feelings of liberation and disorientation) followed by times of quiet consolidation. When we look with a broad enough lens, we see that alternating developmental emphases are completely appropriate. Change needs to be followed by consolidation, which then needs to evolve through further change. A complementary counter-swing of development almost always follows. In much the same way, initial breaths into the body—into growth and formative activity—are eventually complemented by exhalations (such as the liberation of etheric forces) toward thought and sensing activity.

The blossoming wakefulness of the nerve–sense system in the early grades is healthy, because it emerges out of the rich metabolism of early childhood. Such an emphasis on thought and sense unfolds naturally when it is built on a foundation of movement and digestion. When development unfolds in this way, the grade school child is not only ready for the thinking activities of reading, writing, math, and memory but also excited to explore them. The child is ripe for that next step. There is something of a developmental boomerang here, a lawfulness for growth that makes sure that when we go very deeply into one kind of activity, we will naturally be led into its complement.[226]

That keeps us balanced. The physiology of the senses needs the physiology of metabolism. We need to be able to digest what we will later take in.

Once this shifting begins, then we spend the rest of our lives working to find a healthy balance between sensing and digesting. That balancing is eternal. We shift back and forth all the time. A good example of this activity can be experienced during a conversation. It is really only with grade school age that a child becomes able to participate in a conversation. A child at this point can take in what another person is saying (by listening and sensing), work it through (with contemplation, a kind of digestion), and then respond. This is different from the purely imitative, mirroring activity of a younger child, because when there is a step of digestion, we add something of our own making to the interaction. A productive exchange has that quality—each person's participation adds something, so that the process builds and builds and what eventually comes into being has grown beyond what was there at the start. Of course, there are lots of discourses where that does not happen, and they have a very different quality. That is usually because there has not been much breathing between listening and digestion. One variation is when one person waits for the other to finish speaking to say what one already knows (no listening). Alternatively, there are times when one person listens and listens but then takes a very long time (hours, days, months) to take in what was said and only then replies. That drawn-out process may bring profound digestion and analysis, but the other person may no longer be there to hear the answer. In between lies the space a grade school child is working to create—a capacity to sense, to digest, and to respond as one unified process.

We can consider the developmental task of the grade school years to be this balancing between blood and nerve. Working to find that equilibrium bears fruit, for Steiner described this grade school age as a time of particular health. It is the period when heart rate and respiratory rate come into archetypal balance, with a refined ratio of four heartbeats to one breath. The child finds an inner physiologic harmony. In his foundational educational lectures, *The Foundations of Human Experience*, Steiner indicated that a primary task of Waldorf education is to teach children how to "breathe."[227] He was not referring to a need to teach breathing techniques for relaxation. Breathing in this context is a much broader developmental activity, of finding and supporting an inner physiologic balance between blood and nerve. Each breath is truly a mediation between the two poles: with exaggerated nerve–sense activity (which comes when we are startled) we breathe in, and with every exhalation we emphasize our metabolic–limb activity (like a yawn as we prepare to go to sleep). By the time children reach the older elementary years, they are much better able to modulate their own activity. They can move between nerve–sense-dominated activity and metabolically dominated activity from one moment to next. They can move between sensing and self-contentment and have the capacity for both analysis and synthesis. The grade school child enters an archetypally balanced phase of development, between seven and fourteen years, by developing the freedom to inwardly move between both activities.

In addition to breathing, Steiner described a second essential task of education, and that is to help a child learn how to "sleep." That indication again needs to be understood as a much larger physiologic process than just learning how to fall asleep. To begin with, the processes of both sleeping and waking must be considered, for they are two halves of a whole cycle. The turn of each day shares these two process. Waking is a small incarnation process and sleeping a small excarnation process. The astral body and "I" work into the physical and etheric bodies in the morning, then release from them in the evening. Such a cycle of day and night is, of course, the archetype, but the sleeping process finds expression in other alternate time spans as well. A related, much longer cycle is the process of incarnation and excarnation, into and out of an earthly body (a lifetime rhythm). Then there is a cycle that moves much faster—the alternating that occurs when we become more and then less attentive to our environment, more and then less connected to what is around us. We move from inside to outside and back again. As we will see, these movements of the "I" and astral body also relate to the older child's process of learning how to properly wake and sleep.

This moving, shifting connection with the outside environment comes into rich activity with puberty. It is a third major developmental movement. Connecting to the outside world follows the maturation of inner alternation between blood and nerve (described through the large-headed and small-headed polarity). It is a new step but follows and builds upon the sensory maturation that preceded it. Attentive connection necessarily depends on the health of the nerves and senses—a person cannot properly sense the outside world if the senses have not been properly crystallized. If we place this change in the context of a larger, overall progression we can say that a child needs the more large-headed metabolic dominance of early childhood as a foundation for waking into the small-headedness of school-readiness. Then the sensing "windows" that are created through maturation of the nerve–sense pole serve as portals for more dynamic interaction with the outside world. (If we put this in the context of children's drawings, the child must first have a house, then build windows into the house, then in time gaze through the windows to see what is outside.[228]) When these windows begin to appear (in the early elementary grades), children notice things differently and more objectively than they did before, though their activity is still mostly receptive. As wakefulness increases, the primary connection to the lower senses shifts. The change of teeth marks a transition from development directed mostly to touch, balance, movement, and life out to the middle senses that are more connected to feeling (smell, taste, vision, and warmth). Then, with adolescence, a child observes more and more through the four higher senses (hearing, word, thought, and "I"), which allow us to connect more deeply with those around us.

Puberty, the end of the second seven-year period, comes about through a birth of the astral body. Astral forces, freed from their inner, formative activity, now well up into consciousness. The major physiologic marker is not a change of teeth (as it was with the birth of the etheric) but an outer differentiation of the body through sexual maturation. This process of male and female differentiation is a new step. The physical changes that came at the end of the first seven-year period brought an inner physiologic differentiation: a relative shrinking of the head in proportion to lengthening limbs, adult teeth, and six-year molars. Those changes are outwardly quite uniform, because they come in the same way for both boys and girls; the lengthening of the torso and the development of a distinct chest and abdomen are also common for both sexes. If we did not see the face or genitals of a seven- or eight-year-old child, we would likely still not be able to tell if the child was a boy or a girl. In early adolescence, however, the astral body brings shifting, contrasting changes—an embodiment of polarity. Pubertal changes bring physical development that cannot really be fully understood outside of one sex's relationship to the other and to the outside.

When we go through the pubertal process, we are no longer complete within ourselves. Physically, we need another human being of the opposite sex for processes of reproduction to be possible. Emotionally, the adolescent child is not complete as an individual being because there is such a powerful expansion into outer awareness. The feeling life extends far beyond one's own body. Great pantheons of song, story, poetry, and film are dedicated to this particular shift, when we are suddenly able to feel closer to our peers and at the same time more isolated from them than was ever previously possible. We need the outside world in a way that we did not before.[229] This astral "birth" wakens an adolescent into a whole new experience of inside and outside.

This astral awakening to the outside world plays out on a smaller level with each day's waking process. Every night the "I" and the astral body separate from the body, and each morning they enter in again.

Morning reentry makes possible wakeful consciousness. Usually we are not aware of the transition from one state to the next—either we are awake or asleep, in fairly black-and-white terms. There are some gray areas, like the dreams that come in the early morning hours before waking, when the astral body has entered in just enough that we may move, speak, even remember the details of our dreams but are not yet awake enough to consciously connect with the world around us. Another gray area is the times when we are still awake but so tired that we fleetingly disconnect (often with a jerk or a flopping head) and lose our connection with the outside world. Waking and sleeping feel distinctly differentiated most of the time, like flipping a light switch on and off, but those states are only the extremes of a much larger daily ebb and flow. We are, in fact, carried by tides of wakefulness, which slip out through the head and the senses in the evening and then begin anew—entering through the limbs—with each morning's waking:

> At the moment of falling asleep, the astral body leaves the human being through the head. Actually, the astral body leaves us through everything that is a sense organ, but because the sense organs are concentrated chiefly in the head, the main part of the astral body goes out through the head. But as the sense of warmth, for example, is distributed over the whole body, and the sense of pressure, too, weaker radiations also take place, in every direction. The whole process, however, gives the impression that at the moment of falling asleep the astral body passes out through the head.... Now let us turn to human beings as they awake. When we observe them at the time of waking, we find that the astral body approaches through the limbs—actually through the tips of the fingers and toes at first—and then gradually spreads through the limbs. Thus at the moment of waking the astral body comes in from the opposite side. So, too, the "I," only now the "I" does not envelop the astral body but on returning is enclosed by the astral body.
>
> We wake from sleep and as we do so the astral body and the "I" stream into us through the tips of the fingers and toes.

> In order to fill the human being entirely, as far as the head, they really need the whole day; and when they have reached the head, the moment has come for them to leave again. You will realize from this that the "I" and the astral body are in constant, perpetual motion.[230]

This movement cannot be captured so cleanly with charts and graphs, however, because the astral body and "I" connect so quickly that we are usually not even able to consciously participate in the process, yet carry on so steadily that they carry us in and out of the spiritual world for a whole lifetime of nights and days:

> At this point you may raise the question: Yes, but if that is so, half an hour after waking from sleep we have in us only a small part of our astral body (and here I include the "I," as well) as far as the wrists above and as far as the ankles below. And that is actually so. If we wake at 7 o'clock—I will assume we are persons of decorum—and stay awake, then at 7:30 the astral body will have reached about as far as our ankles and possibly our wrists. And so it goes on, slowly, until the evening.
>
> You may ask: But how is it, then, that we wake up as a whole person? We certainly feel that we wake as a whole, all at once... yet properly speaking, only our fingers and toes were awake at 7:15, and at midday most people are within the astral body only as if they are sitting in a hip bath. This is really so....
>
> In the spiritual world our astral body works through the whole space taken up by the body, even when it has actually occupied only the fingers and toes. That is the strange fact. Even when the astral body is only approaching it can already be felt throughout the body. But its reality, its substantiality spreads out only slowly. Understanding of this phenomenon is of the greatest importance, above all in enabling a true judgment to be formed of the human organization in health and disease.[231]

This rhythmic movement of the "I" and the astral body determines much of our capacity for conscious connection, but our level of wakefulness is not dependent solely on the presence or absence of the astral body and "I." It is also strongly influenced by the way these higher members move through the body and reach out beyond it. Certainly the way the astral body and "I" connect with the forces of the physical world is radically different in a toddler and a teenager, even when both are awake. This is because the teenager's astral body has largely completed its formative activity in the body. It is no longer so intimately connected with physical and etheric bodies and can therefore reach beyond them. With the "I," the astral body can reach out and grasp the world and its forces. This process, again, relates back to the miniature waking process we experience each morning:

> At the time of awaking, the astral body does certainly come in; the "I"-organization also comes in—yes, they come in, and one can perceive how astral body and "I"-organization enter and proceed to lay hold of the physical and ether bodies. But that is not all, for here we meet with a fact of human life that is of great importance.
>
> Take the "I"-organization. When, at the moment of awaking, the "I"-organization returns, it does not lay hold merely of the etheric body and physical body; within them it lays hold of the external world, or the forces of the external world.... The "I" slips into physical body, lays hold of the physical body—slips in so far that it makes the physical body light. Through the "I" gliding into it, the physical body loses its weight. Thus, when I, as an awake human being, stand upright, then for my consciousness—for my "I," or "I"-organization, which also has its physical expression in the warmth organism—gravity is overcome. There is no question here of the "I" coming into indirect connection with gravity. The "I" enters into direct connection, places itself as "I" right into gravity, shutting the physical body completely out of the process.... And you do not do this via the physical body; you yourself come into direct connection with the earth forces.[232]

This thought can be hard to grasp, because we are used to considering our physiology as confined within the body. Even for those activities that reach beyond our physical boundaries—the substance and liquid we excrete, the air we breathe, our speech and sound—it is still fairly easy to grasp them with spatial measures. For the astral body and "I" it is different. They do not wait quietly inside the body for light or sound, warmth or touch, to come to us. They move out and connect directly with those forces. Our wakeful activity depends not just on neurotransmitter activity but on direct spiritual engagement with the world around:

> The "I"-organization is directly connected with a part of the general heat through which we are continually moving as long as we live in the physical world.... The astral body is directly connected also with the forces of "light." ... Now the astral body is connected with this light; that is to say, it has direct relation—not indirect through the etheric body—with all that underlies sensory perception on the earth.... When we wake up, we not only come into connection with the light that is within us, but, turning aside as it were from the light that is within us we member ourselves into the light that streams through the external world. It is the same with the external "chemical forces" that are at work in the world around us. Into these, too, we member ourselves directly. And this is very important, for it means that while awake we are membered into a kind of cosmic chemistry.[233]

To summarize this progression of wakening activity, we must picture that, to begin with, there is a centripetal movement of the astral body and "I," from the spiritual world into the physical and etheric, making connection first with the fingers and toes. This bathing of the etheric and physical by the higher members ("as if they are sitting in a hip bath") continues inward, into the body. During our waking hours this inward movement from the periphery, through the limbs, is accompanied by a complementary, centrifugal sensing movement of the higher members, out through the head and sense organs. In this way the astral and "I" come into direct relation with the heat, light, and cosmic chemistry of the outside world. This charts a path of a

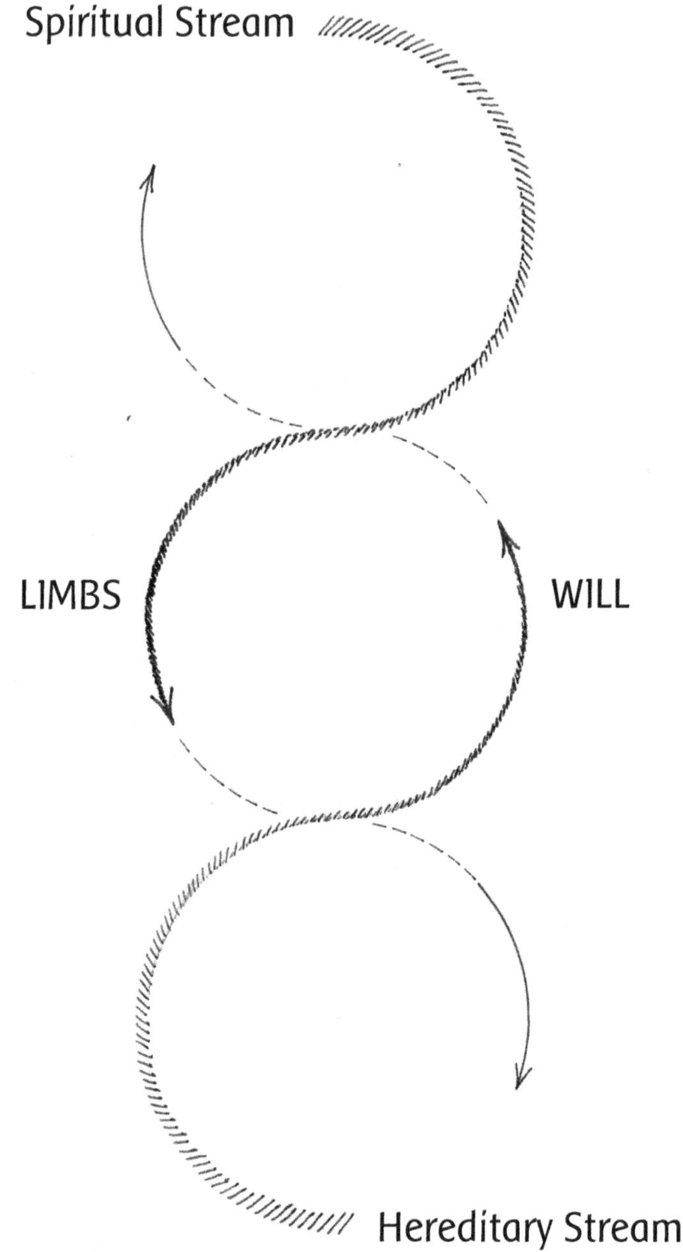

Figure 8: The meeting of the hereditary and spiritual streams in the metabolic–limb system

continuous inbreathing of the higher members connected to the limbs and a simultaneous exhalation through the sense organs.

That pathway follows an archetypal progression, one that links the first three seven-year periods and their related constitutional polarities. These developmental movements flow into one another, just as night follows day. For example, there is a mirroring between the meeting of the "I" and astral body with the etheric and physical bodies each morning and the meeting of the spiritual and hereditary streams in the first seven years of life (observed through the earthly–cosmic and feeble–maniacal polarities, related to the limbs and the will pole, see table 10). This is a process, a polarity of integration, as depicted in figure 8 (opposite).

> A second, intermediary step comes next. This is a process, a polarity of differentiated activity that expresses itself in a balancing of the inwardly connected limb integration and the outwardly directed sensing activity and the large-headed and small-headed polarity—the meeting of blood and nerve, of metabolism and sensing, related to the rhythmic system and the feeling life (see fig. 9, next page).

Now we can recognize a third step (fig. 10), which lives in the process of waking and sleeping and which creates a polarity of connection: the movement of the "I" and astral body (through and beyond the physical body) out through the senses and into the surrounding world and what can be described as the epileptic and hysteric polarity (used to help describe either an inhibited or an overflowing sensory connection with the outside world, which powerfully influences our capacity for conscious awareness and thought and is chiefly connected to the nerve–sense pole).

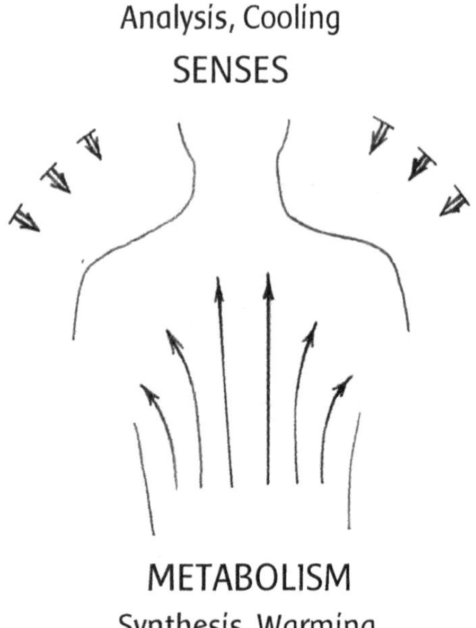

Figure 9: The meeting of metabolism and sensing in the rhythmic system

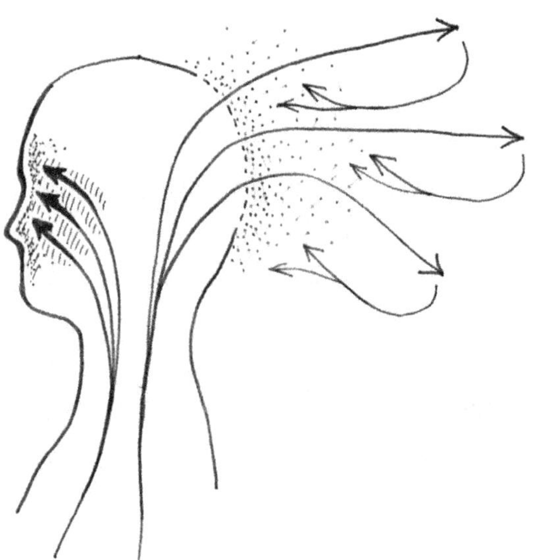

Figure 10: Polarities of outward connection through the nerve-sense system

Table 10: Major developmental activities of birth to seven years, seven to fourteen years, and fourteen to twenty-one years

Birth to the change of teeth (0–7 years)	**Change of teeth to puberty** (7–14 years)	**Puberty to adulthood** (14–21 years)
Overcoming of the hereditary body, building healthy metabolic and limb activity	Differentiated activity of blood and nerve, balancing of the rhythmic system	Relation of self and the environment, connection with the outside world through the senses
Willing	Feeling	Thinking
Feeble/maniacal polarity	Large-/small-headed polarity	Epileptic/hysteric polarity

Chapter 20
The Epileptic Constitution

> For a fifteen-year-old epileptic: "The first thing to do, therefore, is to see that the boy is placed where he will be sure of being treated in the way that is right and necessary for boys who are reaching puberty—that is to say, where care is taken to provide conditions under which such boys have their interest aroused in all the processes that go on in the world in which they find themselves.... We must try to bring it about that he is continually occupied with something outside himself and takes a keen interest in the objects and processes he finds around him."[234]

The quality of our conscious connection with the outside world through the sense organs carries special significance because we live in such a sensory-rich environment. Understanding the developmental progression and the associated sensory pathways for establishing a connection is very helpful. Every human being needs to develop wakeful sensing activity; that much is clear—but that is not enough. There needs to be a reciprocal ability to also shield our awareness.

The modern world expects nearly constant outward connection which is inherently unfair: we live in time that asks us to be observant, astute participants, while simultaneously bombarding us with so many impressions and demands that there is no way we can meaningfully make connection with all of them. So we are required, even from one moment to the next, to shift the activity of our astral body and "I"—at one point extending well beyond ourselves and, at the next, retreating safely within.

As with other physiologic activities, our greatest health lies in the ability to move between both extremes. Such flexibility allows us to be open and aware, yet somewhat simultaneously protected from the environment. This requires a real skill that comes only through maturation of the connection process. It may sound as if we are talking in contradictions, but it is very possible.

A good example would be when we are driving, trying to find the way to some new place in the middle of a huge thunderstorm with pouring rain. We need to be looking very closely for street signs or landmarks to guide us on the way, yet make ourselves oblivious to the pouring rain that thunders all around and obscures vision. If we were completely open and aware of every single raindrop hitting the windshield, we would be immediately overwhelmed. If we completely cut off sensing activity, we would miss the turn. As another example, think of a person in a crowded, noisy restaurant who is trying to have a meaningful conversation with a friend who is sharing something very important. That person is trying very hard to listen (to the friend) and not listen (to the background noise) at the same time. These kinds of situations quickly drain our energy for connection, and at a certain point everyone becomes overwhelmed from being so open. Then we have to disconnect just out of self-preservation. We stop trying to look for the right street sign and turn back, or we begin to just nod our heads indiscriminately when the friend is speaking without really hearing what she is saying. Fortunately, most of the time, we are not asked to walk such an acute sensory tightrope, and we can move more rhythmically between self and periphery. Our tolerance for these kinds of situations is influenced by how well rested we are (have we been able to sufficiently withdraw from the outside world?) but also by inherent, constitutional inclinations.

Each of us carries a sensory gesture into our relationship with the outside world. This can be described as being "thick-skinned" or "thin-skinned." Thick-skinned individuals connect less easily with the outside world and can therefore withstand much but thereby feel less. Thin-skinned individuals, in contrast, notice too much and cannot help feeling—and in many cases responding to—everything that comes toward them. One path of sensing may leave us numbed, the other a little too raw. We can understand them by considering the different pathways the higher members ("I" and astral body) may take as they pour forth into the environment.

The previously mentioned descriptions of how the "I" and the astral body move out past the physical body to connect directly with gravity, warmth, and light, were given as introductory thoughts for Steiner's description of an "epileptic" constitution. As with the other constitutional pictures, Steiner included a very specific behavior or quality (like movement patterns for feeble/maniacal, stealing for kleptomaniacal, or the proportions of the head and limbs for the large-headed/small-headed polarity), then expanded it into a much larger view of developmental activity. He started with a detailed description of how a particular spiritual process manifests. One has the impression that Steiner was speaking out of very specific perceptions. In this case he began with a description of the lungs:

> The lung may be so placed within the human organism that when human beings awake they are unable to make contact with the external world. Imagine we are asleep. While we are asleep something happens in our lung that has the effect that, if we were now to wake up we would come down into the lung but would not be able to get out again, to get through to the external world. Our "I" and astral body would need to press into the lung, to squeeze themselves into it, but they would be unable to come forth again. What human beings should be able to do, as you know, is to come down with the astral body and then come forth again into the world in all directions. The lung should be merely the way through. But in this case, the lung does not provide a free passage; it holds fast to the "I" and astral body—that is to say, it will do so if the human being wakes up. The unfortunate thing is that, when such a condition is present, we always wake up, for owing to the special way that the chemical processes are at work in such a case an infiltration of some substance in fine distribution enters the lung organization, having been blocked up in this way, and gets filled with a

> fine substance that has special affinity for it. The lung is then irregular; consequently, the human being wakes up. But how? We wake up without gaining consciousness. To gain consciousness, we would have to come forth from the lung, for we can acquire consciousness only when we have succeeded in penetrating right though. If we have merely come in, we wake up; if we succeed in pressing our way through, we gain consciousness. In the case we are considering, we stop short; we remain in the organ, and sleep that is healthy passes over into pathological unconsciousness. We wake up, but remain unconscious.[235]

This description challenges us to expand our understanding of the relationship between the body and the conscious mind in several different ways. These aspects are worth considering in some detail because they necessarily stimulate us to embrace a truly holistic understanding of constitution.

To begin with, we are told that a disturbed organ process (an organ that is not the brain) may limit the way in which we are able to wakefully participate in the world. This introduces a whole-body physiology of sensing and perceiving. What is conventionally attributed solely to neurological or psychological functioning, we are told, is in fact also dependent on the health of our inner organs. We must be looked at as a whole human being: an "infiltration of some substance" (a physical quality of an organ) influences and blocks our full consciousness in the waking process. This is the ultimate body–mind connection. In fact, the functional link between them is so intimate that it almost becomes inconsequential as to whether one starts from the side of the mind or from that of the body, because they meet each other in the middle.

Steiner went on to state that this description of a stuck lung process is an "exact description" of the condition of an epileptic patient, of a person who suffers from seizures. This is another challenging imagination to take hold of, not only because it is a spiritual description of the seizure process but also because we are taught that what we usually view as the illness, the pathologic condition (a seizure) is an expression of the higher members working against a subtle underlying imbalance:

> You see, we have come in this way to an exact description, drawn from within, of the condition of the epileptic.... Epileptics are able to enter with the "I"-organization and astral body into the physical body and ether body. That they can do, but they do not come forth into the physical world; they are held fast within. Let us consider, then, how it will be if the astral body enters the lung and is held fast there, unable to get out again. The astral body will remain pressed against the surface of the lung; astral body and "I"-organization will be, so to speak, dammed up, or congested, beneath the surface of the organ. This condition then manifests outwardly as a seizure. This is what seizures really are. Every time a seizure occurs, an inner congestion is taking place at the surface of some organ. These congestions are found, above all, in the brain, but we know how the parts of the brain are related to the other parts of the body; congestion in the brain may be caused entirely by the fact that congestion is present in the liver, or in the lung, in which case the cerebral congestion is only a projection, or feeble copy, of the congestion in the bodily organ. Whenever a seizure occurs, this congestion of "I"-organization and astral body within an organ can be observed.... Nothing of any real value can be said about seizures if we do not know that, at the surface of some organ, astral body and "I"-organization are being terribly squeezed and crushed. They cannot get out; they try to make their way out; they push but are held back.[236]

We are challenged to pull ourselves back and not get stuck on the specific symptoms, to learn to see symptoms not as the pathologic conditions themselves, but as potential expressions of a larger imbalance. This is not an easy task, because often, at a basic level, we really just want the troubling behavior (the symptom) to go away, and we do not trouble ourselves so much about the cause. Steiner was asking us to recognize that the fit, or seizure, is really part of the overcoming of an infiltrative substance in an organ. It is an exaggerated compensation that can indeed be damaging for the brain, but from a larger spiritual perspective we should recognize that the moments of seizure are not the actual disease. The seizure is a response to a larger imbalance. Whenever we can enlarge our sphere of consideration to move more upstream, to consider that the current behavior or symptom may actually be a response to a different imbalance, we open the door to understanding children's development on a more global level. Steiner was showing us how to begin with a specific symptom (like a seizure) but then work to place it within a whole physiology of consciousness:

> Suppose you have an organ with its ether body within it. For each single organ there is a definite relationship that should exist between physical body and ether body, on the one hand, and astral body and "I" on the other.... This relationship is, within limits, variable, but if it exceeds a certain limit of variability (and this again can be individual for the particular human being), we have abnormality, a state of illness; in some organ astral body and "I"-organization will be present, but in such a way that they cannot fill it in a right relationship. This will mean that they are unable to extend beyond it.... When the astral body and "I" are jammed and squeezed in this way in an organ, then there is too much astral body, too much "I," in that organ; there is not a proper amount but a surplus—with the result that the organ cannot help feeling the astrality. If the organ has in it the right and proper amount, it does not perceive or feel the astrality; it does not sense the presence of astrality within it. But if there is in an organ an activity of astral body and "I"-organization that does not belong there, then the organ is bound to feel it. If something is there in the organ that does not pass into consciousness, if there is congestion, so that a great amount of astrality and "I"-organization is present that does not go over into consciousness, then a seizure takes place. The very description I have given contains an indication of the accompanying phenomenon—namely, a disturbance of consciousness. Disturbance of consciousness is

> bound to occur whenever this congestion happens in an organ that is in any way connected with consciousness.[237]

We have just moved from an isolated neurologic process to a description of the whole way a child may relate to the outside world. This means that whenever a child is showing a "disturbance of consciousness" we should look to see if it is part of an "epileptic process." When the physical/etheric and astral/"I" meet in dramatic congestion it creates an observable seizure, but there are many children who still experience this congested, blunted conscious connection with the world but who do not have clinical seizures. They are awake but remain, at a certain level, unconscious.

Chapter 21

Therapy for the Epileptic Constitution

Helping the Child "Reach Through" to the Outside World

Steiner's therapeutic indications for the epileptic constitution similarly ask that we not focus too much on the illness but think more broadly. The seizure process happens at a threshold, the one between wakefulness within the body and conscious connection extending outside the body. To understand the externally visible seizure process, we have to look within, for Steiner indicated that the actual problem behind a fit is a congestion that occurs at the organ level, inside. For therapy, to really help a child with an epileptic process, we must work to bring ever-greater awareness outside. We ease the congestion by encouraging a child to gain a more conscious relation to the outer elements. Steiner gave several variations and several examples.

The first relates to symptoms of vertigo that may accompany seizures. Vertigo is really a disoriented experience of the body in space (and a loss of the sense of balance). Steiner shared that it can be met therapeutically through accentuated experiences of gravity. This is important because some children experience a variation of the epileptic process in which experiences of vertigo predominate and "lapses in consciousness" are the lesser symptom:

> Find out, to begin with, whether the disturbances in consciousness are nearly related to the phenomena of ordinary vertigo.... If we should find that the lapses in consciousness are only brief, but that there are on the other hand very marked symptoms of vertigo, we would be able to know with certainty where the trouble lies. For in such a case, the "I"-organization and the astral body would be failing to enter into direct relation with the forces

> of balance.... If you find this to be the case, let the child do gymnastics or eurythmy, but always giving the child at the same time an object to hold, such as dumbbells or the like. Especially during the period between change of teeth and puberty, such exercises for balance are important. If you [first] give children two dumbbells of exactly the same weight...you can do something else. Have them hold a dumbbell in the left hand that is lighter than the one in the right hand, and again have them do exercises; then let them take a dumbbell in the right hand that is lighter than the one in the left, and once again do exercises. Then tie some object (it need not be particularly heavy) to one of the children's legs with which to walk about, so that the child becomes conscious of the force pulling on that leg. When walking in the ordinary way, children are unconscious of the force of gravity. It is, however, important for them to place themselves with their "I"-organization right into the force of gravity. When you attach something to their leg, they immediately become aware of gravity. You can then hang the weight on the other leg. Now, to make the activity come nearer to the mental or spiritual, let them feel movements that they make with their arms; let them think themselves into a movement of extending the left arm, and then again extending the right arm, and finally both arms at once. Another way of helping children to become conscious of gravity is to get them to lift one leg while keeping the other on the ground.... You get them to make movements in which they must learn to control their external balance.[238]

These indications work in the realm of gross motor movement, but they have a different character from the stirring movements that are so helpful for the child with the feeble constitution. It is very possible that beginning with large, repetitive movements (bringing the qualities of the eurythmy "R" and "L") will make it more possible for a child to reach through into a more successful, differentiated experience of gravity. These epileptic therapeutic exercises, however, are about conscious connection with gravity, which is a more mature skill than simple stirring movement. Steiner's comment that this is particularly appropriate between the "change of teeth and puberty" reinforces that. Further exploration of the differences between the feeble and the epileptic constitutions is included in the section on aggressive behaviors (chapter 25).

The Fluid Element

A second therapeutic pathway relates to the fluid element and the circulatory system, which manifests as symptoms of nausea or feeling sick:

> Good results can often be achieved also in the case of epileptics in whom you perceive that their circulatory system is disturbed, and that the whole way in which the fluids are circulating is really the cause of the phenomena. If you notice that in connection with the attacks of epilepsy (which take the form of seizures and perhaps vertigo), feelings of sickness or nausea are present, then you will know that you are dealing with an incapacity to combine properly with the element of water. In such a case it will be good to bring the watery elements as much as possible to the notice of such children before they receive it into their organism. Try to prepare their food in such a way that they tastes it quite specially. Something could also be achieved by letting such children learn to swim.[239]

When we first hear that there is a disturbance in the circulatory system, in the watery element, we might be tempted to think just of ways to increase the child's water intake, to be more conscious about hydration. The real therapeutic step, however, is to help the child feel through the body and out into the surrounding watery element of the outside world. To "specially" taste food is such an interesting and perhaps unexpected way to accentuate the meeting of our own inner fluid element, via secretions like saliva, with the outside world. We bring particular consciousness to what we are meeting as we eat when that special awareness can be cultivated. It we eat in a rushed or distracted manner, even if the food is quite rich or flavorful, we do not meet and truly acknowledge it. We can then easily finish a meal and not really have even noticed what we have taken in. Building special awareness—through varying flavors, textures, perhaps even through unique combinations—makes eating a discovery. That kind of reaching out, as a discovery, helps the child to practice reaching through a congestion in the physical and etheric bodies. To drink specially could also be part of that exploration, perhaps with a cup of tea. The tea would be special not so much because of the ingredients but because of the way the tea, as a fluid, is consciously met. It is sipped, with ceremony. A tea party might even be part of the therapeutic process.

The indication by Steiner about swimming should be similarly understood. Being in the water offers children a chance to feel they are in special relationship to the outside fluid element. There is a very real and legitimate medical concern around swimming and epilepsy that must be mentioned, as a child who has a seizure in the water loses control of the body and can drown. Steiner seemed to be aware of this, adding, "Learning to swim is very good for epileptics, only we must understand what is involved and be intelligent and sensible in the use of such a treatment." [240]

While holding the imagination of swimming as an archetypal way to be in conscious connection with the element of water we should expand our own picturing of fluid activities to include other more accessible, everyday experiences such as putting hands into a tub of water and stirring, working with wet clay, jumping in puddles, or wading in a stream. The most important element, again, is how consciousness is cultivated in that experience, how the watery element is specifically sensed and met.

The Airy Element

Brief mention is made regarding conscious connection with the outside air. This makes great therapeutic sense, as Steiner elsewhere described how we are most intimately connected with the outside physical environment through our breath:

> When cloudings of consciousness occur unaccompanied by any marked feeling of nausea, carefully regulated breathing exercises are not bad, in order to restore connection with the air.[241]

We can imagine that this could include speech, singing, blowing bubbles, whistling, or other activities that bring special consciousness to the outside air.

The Element of Warmth

Finally we come to the element of warmth, an essential experience in the life of all children:

> And to establish a right connection with warmth, we should accustom epileptic children—really all children, but particularly epileptics—to feel the warmth. It is, as a matter of fact, quite wrong to allow any children to go about half naked with nothing on their legs, and it is often the cause in later life (only, people do not know it) of irritation of the appendix and even appendicitis; for epileptic children it is a downright poison. Epileptic children should be clothed in a way that induces a tendency to sweat; sweating should always be mildly present in a nascent state. They should, in fact, be a little too warmly clad. That is real therapy.[242]

As we saw earlier, warmth is an essential process in the transformation of the hereditary body (through inflammation). Consciously cultivating and feeling warmth brings richer connection of the "I"-organism with the outer warmth processes and supports a simultaneous physiologic resculpting of an organ imbalance (like a lung that is too material, too dense because of a foreign infiltrate).

Table 11 summarizes the ways we can help a child come into more conscious connection with the outside elements.

Table 11: Pathways for bringing a child into a more conscious connection with the outside world

To Learn Control of External Balance

- For when there are symptoms of vertigo
- Holding dumbbells in the arms
- Working with differentiated weights (one arm holding a heavier weight), then switching sides
- Tying an object to the leg and letting the child walk around with it, then switching to the other leg
- Balancing on one foot
- Closer to the mental or spiritual: "Think oneself into a movement"

Bringing the Watery Elements to the Notice of the Child

- For when there is nausea or feelings of sickness
- Being stimulated to very specially taste food
- Letting the child learn to swim or come into connection with water

Restoring the Connection to Air

- Breathing exercises or other activities related to the airy element

Accustoming the Child to Feeling Warmth

- Clothing in such a way as to induce a tendency to sweat
- Being a little too warmly clad: "That is real therapy."

Chapter 22

The Point-and-Periphery Meditation

Overcoming our own hindrances to properly connect with the outside world is a universal human striving. It certainly does not end with puberty. In fact, in many ways, adult biographical development essentially depends on how we consciously develop our connections with the world. Are we stuck inside? Are we too exposed? What is this particular situation calling for? As with all healthy development, the answer is not fixed. It lies in building capacities so that we are able to move inward and outward, to recognize where we are and where we need to move.

Consciously working to refine our capacities for sensing the outside world marks a process of self-development—however humble. We practice connecting, then releasing. This practice of self-development informs our observation skills. If we learn to intentionally move our own astral body in particular ways, we may be better able to see an astral imbalance in a child. We reach out to connect to the child, but that recognition is not sufficient by itself. The outwardly directed therapeutic eye which recognizes a constitutional leaning in a child then needs to breathe back into itself, in order to gain an objective understanding of the underlying spiritual picture (through thought). We need to move out, then pull back in; both aspects must be present for us to be truly therapeutic. For example, if a child's sensing connection is stuck inside and we can feel it, then we step back to consider what might help the child and realize that fostering ways to better connect with the outside elements is important. We live into one gesture and then move to its counterpoint. The more flexible and practiced our inward life, the more we find we can breathe into a given situation and then imaginatively shift to the appropriate therapeutic gesture. In a beautiful way, the more we cultivate self-observation and self-directed meditative work, the richer our outer therapeutic offerings can become. Inner work resonates with outer activity.

A third essential aspect for inner work is genuine interest. We need it before we can really even enter this kind of expanded, then concentrated, consciousness. Steiner emphasized the importance of observation in service of the other and related the following situation:

> Suppose you want to be able to speak to some fellow human being from an intuitive power of vision. The things you need to behold in that person are by no means written plain for all to see.... What you need to do is to see through what lies on the surface, right through it to the real state of affairs.... You need to tell yourself with courage and with energy—not just saying it at some particular moment, but carrying it continually in your consciousness, so that it determines the very quality and content of your consciousness: "I can do it." If, without vanity, in a spirit of self-sacrifice, and in earnest endeavor to overcome all the things that hinder, you repeat these words, not only feeling them, but saying them to yourself over and over again, then you will begin to discover how far you are able to go in this direction.[243]

The starting place for such an "intuitive power of vision" is cultivating interest and enthusiasm in the other. Then we begin to breathe back and forth, and the process starts to come alive. We take what we have seen outwardly and begin to carry it imaginatively within us. We hold it as a question, and then an answer or insight can emerge. We move back and forth, in and out. It is hard to think of a more archetypal movement than this contraction and expansion, as we live with it continuously. Steiner gave us a special imagination to strengthen this capacity. It is known as the point-and-periphery meditation, which he introduced through the following sequence:

> Try to accustom yourselves to live your way every evening into the consciousness: In me is God. In me is God—or the Spirit of God, or what other expression you prefer to use. (But please do not think I mean just persuading yourself of this truth theoretically—which is what the meditations of the majority of people amount to!). Then, in the morning let the knowledge I am in God shine out over the whole day. And now consider! When you bring to life within you these two ideas, which are then no longer mere thoughts, but have become something felt and perceived inwardly, yes, have even become impulses of will within you, what is it that you are doing?
>
> First, you have this picture before you: In me is God. And on the following morning, you have this picture before you: I am in God. They are one and the same, the upper and the lower figure [Steiner drew a picture here; see next page fig. 11]. And now you must understand: Here you have a circle (yellow); here you have a point (blue). It doesn't look like that in the evening, but in the morning the truth of it comes to light. And in the morning you have to think: Here is a circle (blue); here is a point (yellow). Yes, you have to understand that a circle is a point, and a point is a circle. You have to acquire a deep, inner understanding of this fact.[244]

In this way outside becomes inside, and inside becomes outside. When we repeatedly live into the contrasting elements, we can find the possibility for entering into one movement while simultaneously holding the other. Expanding while contracting, contracting while expanding. We are both the point and the circle.

This meditative reorientation makes conscious the shifting activity of the higher members. We inwardly accomplish what the child does every day through the sleeping and waking process, but now we are able to intentionally accompany the movements of the astral and "I" in and out of the body. This brings greater vision, because we are not just carried along by the tides of waking and sleeping—we actively participate in them and learn to observe the process in others and also

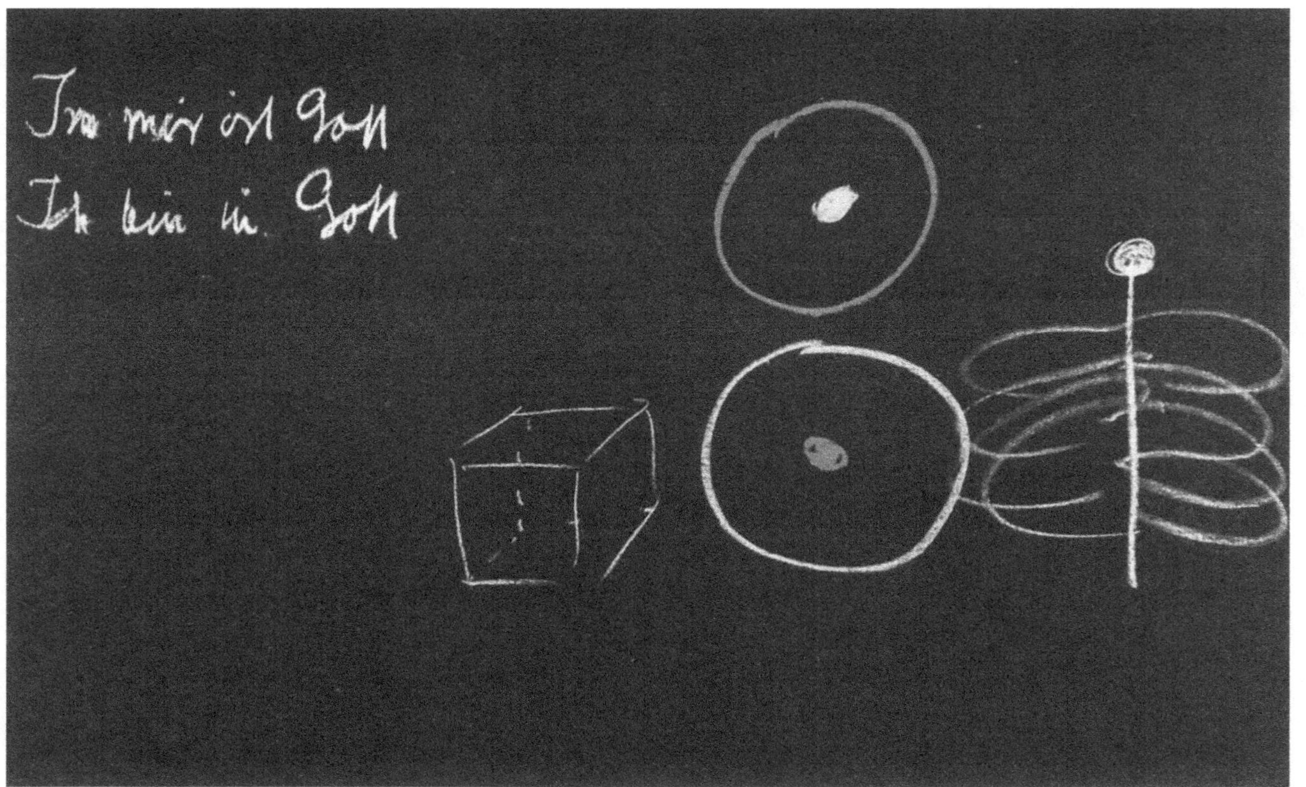

Figure 11: Steiner's blackboard drawing for the point-and-periphery meditation

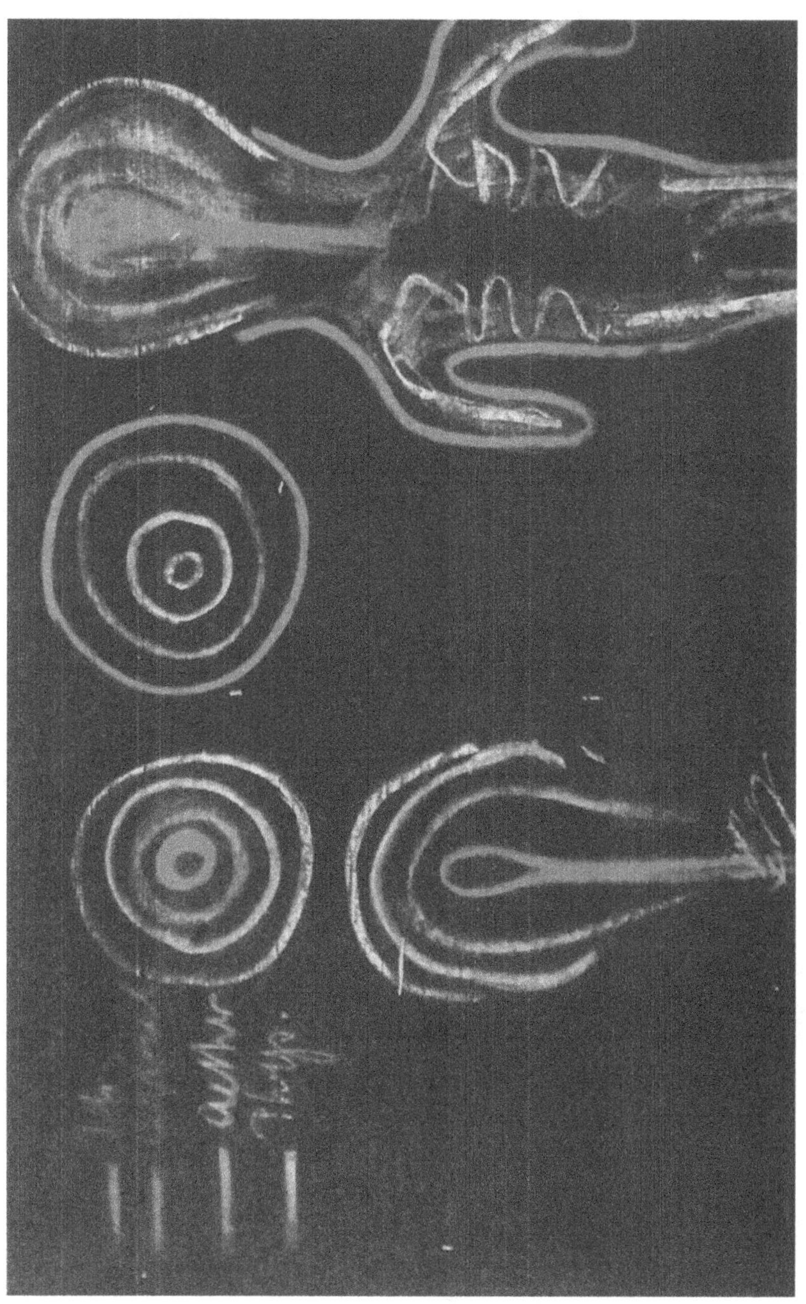

Figure 12: Point and Periphery in the Human Form

in ourselves. Steiner indicated that changes in sleep and dream life are, in fact, part of the path of esoteric development.[245]

This inward and outward movement can evolve in many different directions. Steiner's description of the meditation begins in a very spiritual place, the breathing back and forth between the human being and God, and then moves to the human form, differentiated into "metabolism and limbs" person and "head" person:

> You must, first of all, be quite clear in your mind that these two figures, these two conceptions, are one and the same, are not at all different from one another. They only look different from the outside. There is a yellow [lower] circle [fig. 11]; here it is, too [fig. 12]. There is a blue point [in the yellow circle]; here it is, again [fig. 12]. Why do they look different? Because that drawing is a diagram of the head, and this a diagram of the body. When the point continues on into the body, it becomes the spinal cord. It makes its way in here, and then the part it plays in the head organization is continued in the spiral cord [fig. 12].
>
> There you have the inner dynamic or morphology of the human being. Taking it as your starting point, you will be able, by meditation, to build up anatomy, a physiology. And then you will acquire the inner intuition that can perceive in how far the upper and lower jaws are limbs; for you will begin to see in the head a complete organism in itself, sitting up there on the top of the human being, an organism whose limbs are dwarfed and have—in the process of being stunted—turned into jaws. And you will come to a clear perception of how teeth and toes are in polarity to one another. For you have only to look at the attachments of the jawbones, and you can see it all there before you—the stunted toes, the stunted hands and feet.[246]

Then we go even further—taking an active interest in all elements of our interaction:

> But my dear friends, meditation that employs such pictures as I have been giving can never take its course in the kind of mood that would allow us to feel: "Now I am going to settle down to

> a blissful time of meditation; it will be like sinking into a snug, warm nest!" No, the feeling must be continually present in us that we are taking the plunge into reality—that we are grasping hold of reality.
>
> Devotion to little things—yes, to the very smallest of all! We must not omit to cultivate this interest in very little things. The ear lobe, the paring of a finger-nail, a single human hair—should be every bit as interesting to us as Saturn, Sun, and Moon. For really and truly in one human hair everything else is comprised; a person who becomes bald loses a whole cosmos! What we see externally we can verily create inwardly, if only we achieve that overcoming which is essential to a life of meditation.[247]

When we attain this, when we are able to find cosmic truth through devotion to the smallest details, we should celebrate. Steiner finished his discussion by calling for absolute enthusiasm when the process succeeds:

> Here was a girl concerning whom I told you that a kind of abnormality must have occurred in her development between the third and fourth year. You questioned the mother, and the mother confirmed that it was so. What did you do then? Please tell me, honestly and sincerely: what did you do, when the mother confirmed the fact? [Silence.] Please be esoterically honest and tell me the truth, you three: what did you do? [Silence.] If you had done the right thing, you would now be telling me: "We danced and jumped until we made a hole in the ceiling!" And the after-effect of this jumping for joy would still be expressing itself today—and not merely in words, it would be shining out from you like a light.
>
> That is what you need—enthusiasm in the experience of truth. This enthusiasm is an absolute sine qua non.[248]

Building inner flexibility brings enthusiasm and reassurance. It helps us know that we are doing the right thing, that we can meet the child with confidence.

When we behold with real interest and attention, focusing devotedly on a child, we ourselves are embraced in the periphery by the spiritual world. When we open to the periphery, to broader imaginations after having observed children with love, we open a space in which the children themselves can initiate a step of growth.

Children with an epileptic constitution need the most help moving from the point to the periphery. We support their congestion and astral pushing by pulling consciousness into more intimate relation with the outside environment. The opposite gesture—holding the periphery to create a safe inner space in which children feel that they can safely meet the world—stands as the most essential task and often the greatest struggle for children with a hysteric constitution.

Chapter 23
The Hysteric Constitution

Most children experience some anxiousness as part of such a developmental shift, especially if they are expected to just dive in before they really know what they are doing. In that kind of situation, we are not yet particularly comfortable with all the aspects of new activity and so get stuck—eager on the one side to take on new skills but also longing for things to just go back to the way they were before. The wish to return to an earlier stage and to a simpler consciousness underlies most regressive behaviors. Suddenly wetting the bed after moving to a new house or wanting to breast-feed when a new sibling arrives (after having weaned long since) are common examples. These regressive behaviors are usually transient and therefore generally not that concerning. They mark an honest hesitation or discomfort on the child's part, but they can usually be remedied with extra attention and reassurance.

There are some children, however, whose timidity arises not simply from the insecurity of a development shift. They instead experience a more pervasive displacement of sensing activity. They are always anticipating and frequently dreading what will happen next. This can be observed when a child's sensing activity extends too far beyond the boundaries of the physical body and temporally too much into the future. The resulting kind of anxious anticipation relates to what Steiner described as the "hysteric" constitution.

We can start building a very practical picture of the difference between the epileptic and the hysteric constitutions by watching how children navigate a developmental shift. Some children are steadfast and deliberate as they move into a new phase of life. Their developmental milestones typically come a bit later than average; they seem to need more time for most things. This might be the pattern for a child who does not speak at all and then one day speaks well, easily and fluently, or for a child who struggles with reading until one day in second grade it clicks and then—zoom—the child reads easily with interest. This kind of slow and even laborious pattern shows a pushing, pushing, trying to get through, and then it is done. By the time a child has successfully manifested a new capacity, the steps of learning are largely already complete.

A playful image of this could be watching young children (say, toddlers or those of preschool age) get ready to go outside in very cold weather. In preparation, they put on a pair of nice thick mittens before putting on the coat, or pull on boots before snow pants. Putting on mittens first makes putting on a coat quite a bit more difficult, as a hand with a mitten on it does not easily slip through the sleeve of the coat. Instead, a child has to push and push and push to get the mittened hand to work its way through until it finally "pops" out the other end. Getting dressed to go outside ends up being a long, challenging struggle, and in many ways it mirrors the process of the "I" and astral body working to overcome the congestion that comes from not being able to work through the etheric and physical bodies. The "pop" of the mitten is very much like the fit of a seizure, for a seizure is the overcoming of the congestion. Similarly, when a developmental process has had to be pushed and pushed to manifest, then seemingly suddenly (though this is not quite true, as there has, of course, been tremendous hidden work) the skill is there. It may be late, but it is now relatively complete. From Steiner's description of how the higher members must work to overcome such a congestion, we can appreciate how this kind of developmental pattern might be seen in a child with an epileptic constitution.

Children with a hysteric constitution outwardly also seem to wait and wait, but their inner process is very different. Their waiting and delay come not from being stuck but from pulling back. They are reluctant to enter into an activity until they feel, with some degree of confidence, that they can do it perfectly (and therefore with relative safety). These children routinely watch and study a process for a long time before they will participate. They figure out all of the parameters of what is involved, and only when they feel fully informed and capable will they venture to join in. Their deliberateness comes not from needing to push hard and long in order to get through but from deliberately holding back. These children could perhaps be crudely grouped together with children who are slow due to an epileptic process, but only if we were using a purely external time measurement. It is true that, as a group, they are all not very good with transitions. They can take a long time but grouping them together in this way would ultimately not be a very useful categorization, because it does not help us really know what the child needs. Children with a hysteric constitution are actually engaging so much—on a sensory level—that they are overwhelmed. Their delay is actually more of a retreat.

The child holds back, because the world is being felt too much. Everything is felt, even before it happens. It is as if the child says, "I can feel all the aspects of the new situation that could go wrong, all the ways that it could be uncomfortable, before I even engage." Waiting to engage is a protective measure, though waiting until things can be done with absolute security risks a kind of paralysis. Instead of pushing a mittened hand through the coat sleeve, this way of approaching the world is much more like getting into cold water—like entering an alpine lake where the water is too cold to be really comfortable. It takes a lot of little steps to get into the water, and the bottom is not quite even, with unexpected rocks, sucking mud, or even a darting slippery fish. Entering the water is particularly hard at those places where the water comes up against our most sensitive spots—groin, ribs, nipples, underarms, and neck—because we can feel the cold water so acutely in those spots. For a very sensitive child, whose sensing is not held back but instead continuously spills over into the surrounding environment, the whole world feels this way. Every activity, every encounter, is filled with unpredictable rocks and mud and icy water, making it feel as if life is better lived in the warmer shallows or, perhaps better yet, by just staying on the shore and not getting in at all.

That image fits the process of a hysteric constitution, in which the astral body and "I" continuously overflow. Steiner introduced this as the polar experience to the epileptic constitution:

> But now you will easily see that we may also have a quite different state of affairs. Instead of an organ whose surface holds back within the organ the "I"-organization and the astral body, we could have an organ whose surface lets too much through—an organ that does not, as it were, keep back sufficient for its own use. Here the astrality, with which is associated the "I"-organization, is not dammed up, but tends, on the contrary, to overflow the organ. The surface becomes, as it were, porous for the astrality and the "I"-organization; they "leak" out of the organ. With imaginative consciousness we do actually see rays streaming forth from the organ. In an organ that "leaks" in this way you will always find also the physical correlate of secretion; even where the secretion is not strikingly present, you will find that it can occur and can be detected.... When a human being is affected with this condition in childhood, the condition can be healed only if we are able to hold fast the astral body and "I"-organization—bring them back, as it were, into the organ.[249]

Steiner described a spiritual picture of overflowing astrality. We are told that a "porous" organ allows the higher members to continually "leak" out and that its physical correlate is secretion. It is aided through helping the child learn to "hold fast" the astral and "I."

Steiner portrayed the hysteric constitutional (like the epileptic) through a progression: first a precise spiritual description, then its relation to physical symptom (secretion instead of seizure), then an expansion into the much broader process of sensing the world and experiencing outside elements:

> Let us see what it is we really have before us in young children who are said to be suffering from hysteria. They have difficulty

making contact with the external world.... They have difficulty in correctly taking hold of the equilibrium that belongs to the fluid element, of the equilibrium associated with air, of the differentiations in warmth, in light, in chemical action, and in the universal cosmic life. But instead of grasping all of these too weakly, as is the case with the epileptic, these children take hold too strongly; they put their astral body and "I" into their whole environment—into weight, into warmth; they seize hold of all the elements more intensely than is really possible for a so-called normal person. What is the result?

You have only to remind yourself how it is with you when you have grazed your skin at some spot. Suppose you then grasp some object with the sore surface, where the skin has been rubbed away. You know how it hurts. The reason you are so sensitive is that you come up against the external world too vigorously there with your inner astral body. We are able to contact the external world with our astral body and "I"-organization only in moderation. Children who, from the first, bring their astral body right out—such children will in a subtle way touch and take hold of things as though they had been wounded. Nor will we be surprised to find in them this hypersensitivity, or hypersensitive response, to the world around them. Human beings in this condition are bound to feel their environment much more keenly and much more intensely; moreover, they will have a much more powerful reflection of their environment within them.[250]

Steiner then built a whole psychological portrait, with sensory, social, and emotional consequences:

And now ideas will begin also to arise in children that are painful in themselves. It comes about as follows. The moment they begin to develop will in any direction, they have to reach out into something in regard to which they are hypersensitive. As soon as the will begins to develop, a strange condition arises in the conscious part of them. They become superconscious of the will unfolding; in other words, the unfolding in the will causes them pain. Pain is present in a nascent state as soon as the will begins to appear, and children will try to hold back the pain.

> This happens with great intensity. They grow restless and struggle when trying to do things, because they are trying to hold back the pain.
>
> Here, you see, I have given you descriptions of inner conditions that find their outlet in life in a clearly recognizable way. Children want to do something but feel pain and cannot do it; instead of the soul life flowing out into action, they have a terribly powerful inward experience, in the face of which they shudder—they shudders at themselves. Now, however, it may equally be a question not of an outward action but of a concealed or disguised action in thought—for the will lives also in the sphere of thought. When it is a matter of an action in the thought life, when it is ideas that should unfold, it may be that in certain forms of illness these ideas, at the moment they should develop, evoke anxiety and fear and are unable to arise in the mind. Every such idea that evokes fear the moment it should come to consciousness—every such idea simultaneously causes the life of feeling to develop below it; feelings surge up, and depression invariably sets in. Feelings that are not comprehended, not taken hold of by ideas, give rise to depression; only those feelings are not of a depressing nature that, as soon as they arise, are immediately apprehended by the life of thought and ideation.[251]

We come to a very exact explanation of the kind of childhood fear and anxiety associated with profound boundary challenges. The world is felt so acutely that the unfolding of will "causes pain" with resultant anxious powerlessness. Unfolding a deed or a thought brings pain. The pain cannot be understood or contextualized, and so children's encounter with the world and their feeling life are largely abandoned. Their whole psychological gesture is to hold back.

Steiner then brought a physical expression of this abandoned boundary: bed-wetting. Nighttime bed-wetting (nocturnal enuresis) is another manifestation of the unmet or unheld boundary of inside and outside. The physical, inside/outside boundary of the body generally comes into consciousness in concert with increased physiologic astral activity at two and a half to three years of age. With that astral maturation, children learn where their body/bladder ends and where the outside world begins. They now feels: I have an inside and an outside. This comes after the "terrible twos," when the answer to all questions or requests is "No!"—a very appropriate response for identifying and reinforcing what is "me" (what I want) and what is not (what belongs to the outside world). If the world is not met because it is felt too strongly, if there is a constant hysteric avoidance that prevents any real engagement, then that boundary cannot be properly built. The astral and "I" never properly anchor into the physical and etheric:

> A phenomenon in a child, which brings the complex of symptoms to expression with somewhat rude plainness, is nocturnal enuresis. It is perfectly obvious, but only in the light of what has been explained will you see the phenomenon of bed-wetting in a child in the right perspective, for it originates with the condition we have been describing. Whenever you have a case of bed-wetting, you can assume that the astral body is running out, or overflowing. As a matter of fact, secretions and excretions of every kind are always connected with the activity of the astral body and the "I"-organization. These must therefore be in order if we want the secretions and excretions to be in order.[252]

Then Steiner turned back once more to the soul experience of the child, for herein lies the most essential aspect of the child's experience:

> Now it is through the physical body that the "I"-organization and the astral body are connected with the four elements (as they are called), while in the etheric body the "I"-organization and astral body are more connected with the higher elements, with a part of the warmth, with the light, with the chemical ether and with the general life of the universe. If now we may borrow from the physical realm a word which can be most expressive when we extend its application to the spiritual...let us take the word *soreness* and speak of children having soreness of soul. Children are sore in the soul, and such soreness on the part of children is a concept that embraces all accompanying phenomena. If it cannot be made better by means of curative education, then, when they

> attain puberty, either the feminine or the masculine form of this soreness will appear. The feminine form will have the character of *hysteria,* as it was called when there was still a true perception of it. The masculine form will have a different character. We shall be able to speak about that, too; we shall find that it assumes quite other forms.[253]

We receive further indication of these "other forms" as soreness of soul extends from an immediate reaction into a broader physiologic state:

> Wherever therefore you have a case where the conditions are the opposite of those found in epileptic or epileptoid trouble, you will always have to give your attention to the excretions. And you will find you need to observe particularly how the child sweats. Whenever you want to bring something home to a child, to call up ideas in that child, then watch carefully to see whether the inner soreness of soul, which is experienced at the origination of an idea, does not express itself in conditions of sweating. There is a certain difficulty here. In the ordinary way, one might imagine that when something like sweating had been stimulated by an inner condition of soul, the sweating would be noticeable immediately afterward. It may be in some circumstances but it is not necessarily so.... What arises as the result of it is first "digested" in the human being and will sometimes then take the strangest paths within the human being, appearing not at all quickly but, curiously enough, only after some time over the next three or three and a half days.[254]

Steiner elaborated on this process of a delayed sweating and related it to the much greater threshold experience of being born into the body and dying out of the body:

> Now everything that is caused by expansion of astral body and "I"-organization is connected with what meets us in the normal expansion of astral body and "I"-organization at death. When it is a question of congestion, the opposite condition from dying

> sets in. In epileptic phenomena there is the attempt to dam up life within the organism, to imitate, under abnormal circumstances, the process of creeping into the physical organism when the descent to earth takes place. But in the condition of which we are speaking now, we have to do with an imitation of what happens at death. After death the astral body and "I" expand at the same time as life flows away, and it is with an imitation of this condition that we are here concerned. When once we are able to feel this, we come to acquire, little by little, something that is important in the observation of such cases. We actually acquire an organ of smell for what is present in the child; we smell this outflow. For it can really be smelled, and it belongs to the esoteric side of our work to acquire this perception and to experience how the aura of these children has a different odor from the aura of normal children. There is actually something faintly corpse-like in the auric sweating of these children. Such a fact can help to bring it home to you that we do indeed have here a kind of imitation of death; the accompanying phenomena of "dying" appear in the sweating that occurs for one reason or another. Such phenomena can appear in the course of the next three days, approximating to the period during which the backward review after death takes place, when the astral body and "I"-organization are expanding.[255]

This is a challenging indication—to come to a place where we can observe the "auric sweating" of a child. It is perhaps easier to approach this by contrasting it with the other constitutional pictures that have been given that relate in some way to melancholy, sadness, or depression.

We have learned that for the child with a heavy, unpenetrated hereditary body there is a shade of melancholy, regardless of the child's temperament. This comes as part of the feeble constitution. In such a child, we observe that the melancholy comes out of the experience of heaviness, out of the child's experience of wanting to unfold the will, yet being unable to get the limbs to do what is intended. Gravity is certainly part of that melancholy, but in terms of the child's feeling life, he is generally interested in the world and wishing to participate. It is the inability to fully take hold of the hereditary body, the physical body, that brings melancholy frustration.

In contrast, the brooding that comes when the metabolic–limb system is not in order (the small-headed constitution) arises through being "easily irritated by external impressions."[256] It is accompanied by a certain digestive weakness. This brooding, this irritability, comes from not being able to fully work through what has been taken in. It is experienced mostly in the feeling life. There is no problem with the sense organs—sensing activity is accurate and exacting and often precocious with the small-headed constitution.

The soul-soreness of the hysteric constitution is yet again different. It brings a depression and anxiety that comes from avoiding engagement. It is conflicted; since there is pain involved with any unfolding of the will, the goal becomes either to fully preempt pain (by not engaging at all) or to shift so as not to feel the pain (by lifting out of the body). It shows up in different ways. First, we might notice that the child does not engage, does not move, and only watches. While intently watching, the child often simultaneously avoids all eye contact. This looks a lot like a deer in the headlights, with dilated pupils and nervous sweating. This is very highly active non-engagement. Things are frozen because there does not seem to be a safe place to go to, so the best is not to move.

Another, less dramatic expression is when a child is exceptionally ticklish. Some hysteric children cannot stand to be touched or examined because they are so painfully ticklish. In fact, when this is the case, you can explore their astral overflowing by moving your finger in a ticklish motion from several feet away and then slowly getting closer to the body to see when they begin to laugh and squirm. There are some children who can be tickled from across the room. How then to examine the belly of a child like this? With slow, deep, steady pressure—nothing sudden or unexpected (we will come back to this picture in chapter 24, "Bringing Therapeutic Support to the Hysteric Constitution").

Now, how do we observe such "auric sweating?" This is perhaps best observed in someone who has experienced trauma. Trauma injures the sensory boundary with the outside world. When the boundary is lost and now brings a continuous experience of pain, there are two broad categories of compensation. One is to become hypervigilant, to seek to always observe everything that is going on so that one will never be caught off guard again. The other pathway is to dissociate from the body, and this is related to the "faintly corpse-like" smell of the aura. For if I am not in my body and I do not reach out of it to the boundary, if I stay back, then I will not feel the pain even when it comes. The body is partially abandoned. This can develop to the point where almost nothing feels good in the body, and because one cannot be safely housed in the body, there is a desire to "die" a little bit, to leave the body. We then observe an anxiety or depression that is wounded and a little bit toxic—it is different from (feeble) melancholy; it is different from (small-headed) brooding. In an adolescent or young adult this hypersensitivity can shift from fear into exaggerated risk taking or exaggerated sexuality but always with an undertone of pain. Boundary violation is accepted because, at a certain level, the boundary of inside and out has already been abandoned.

Another expression of hysteria worth noting is explosive episodes of mirth and hilarity. This comes from holding back for so long. The child gets to a point where it is no longer possible to contain the feeling life, and so it pours forth. Like nervous laughter before an exam or a crude joke at a funeral, these hysterics often come after great stress or sadness:

> Observe carefully how the condition alternates between depression on the one hand and on the other a kind of excitement or mania, outbursts of mirth and cheerfulness. What is the cause, when they occur in these forms of illness, of such alternation between states of depression and mania? Owing to the inward soreness, there is a perpetual longing not to let the will come to expression. If the will fails to unfold in the life of ideas, then

> conditions of depression arise. But when this has been happening for a long time and children can no longer restrain themselves but must give vent, there arises—because the inner soreness is repressed and the children can now flow right out, together with the astral outflow—an enhanced feeling of wellbeing. So in this way we have alternating conditions of sadness and hilarity, which, when they occur in a child who has also the other symptoms of sweating and bed-wetting, should be carefully watched.[257]

The earlier hysterical process can be supported and healed, the better, for this constitutional leaning does not necessarily resolve with time alone. The child needs guidance and protection to continue stepping forward into life.

Chapter 24

Bringing Therapeutic Support to the Hysteric Constitution

Very often when a child approaches the world with such hypersensitivity, parents and other adults lovingly make it their work to protect the child. This is, of course, an appropriate instinct, but facilitating avoidance does not necessarily help the child learn to better encounter the world. More protection does not always beget better encounter. So what should we do? How can we help children learn to shift their astral body to make engagement less painful?

Steiner presented a forthright but loving therapeutic gesture for us to hold. He told us how to help stimulate boundary through a special kind of engagement. He warned us that shocks that arise out of unconscious patterns can indeed be damaging but that consciously crafted and directed shocks and surprises help the child to consolidate the astral body and that these shocks will have a positive effect on glandular secretion. We can help by lovingly, consciously engaging with the child (who by nature seeks to not engage):

> How am I to treat such a child?···Suppose you are a very nervy teacher.... Anything in the environment that may cause even a slight shock to the child—if it originates in the unconscious, in the temperament of the teacher—must be avoided. And do you know why? Because the teacher must be capable of inducing shock consciously and deliberately; shocks are often the very best remedy for these conditions! They take effect, however, only if they do not proceed from unconscious habit but are given consciously and deliberately, the teacher watching all the time to observe the effect on the child.... Having first tried to bring children to do as much as they are capable of doing with their particular constitution, then try, at a certain point, to bring the

> work into a quicker tempo. This will mean that the children are then obliged to let not the feeling of soreness, but the anxiety connected with the soreness, recede, because you are there in front of them and they cannot help getting into a state of anxiety on that account. The fact that the children are at this moment compelled to come into a state of anxiety, compelled to enter an experience that has been promoted artificially and is different from the previous one, brings it about that they strengthen and consolidate within them the "I" and astral body, which are trying to flow out. If you repeat these things systematically with children over and over, a consolidation of "I" and astral body will take place. But you must not grow tired! You must do the thing over and over again, preparing your whole teaching so that, as it proceeds, at certain moments it simply takes a new turn.... By such means you will find that you can work very strongly indeed upon glandular secretion, and therewith on the consolidation of the astral body in children.[258]

Steiner went further, saying that we must work with children, engage them, and inwardly help children to do what needs to be done. We must seek to meet them inwardly, in their place of discomfort, and then from that soul-soreness guide them through into deed:

> Suppose we are faced with depression in a child. The first step will have been taken the moment such children feel that we are strongly united with them inwardly—that we understand them. But because we are dealing here with a kind of hypertrophy of thought and will, what the children need is more than simply sharing their sorrow. If we are merely dejected and sorrowful with such children—that is no good to them! We cannot help them unless we ourselves are competent to cope with the depression we are experiencing with them and are able therefore to give them effective consolation, so that they feel comfort and relief.... A constant idea in such children is that they think they should do something, and yet they cannot do it. It is a complicated idea, but we must be able to study and understand it. They should do something and cannot do it, but they have to

> do it nevertheless—and then it turns out differently from how they would have liked. Examine the soul life of such children and try to get hold of the idea in their soul. One could express it in the following words: "I want to do it. I cannot do it. And yet I must do it.... That is why it turns out differently from what it ought to be."[259]

We connect with the child's depression so that we really feel it, then ourselves inwardly move to push past it. Because of the waterfall effect described by the pedagogical law, our Spirit Self and "I"-being can work down into the child's overflowing astral body and give it form. We help children come into a new experience that allows them to move past the primacy of their astral experience. Going back to our earlier analogy, it is perhaps like seeing someone sticking just a toe into icy water, recognizing that it would be better and less agonizing to just jump in, and then we lovingly decide to dive into the water, too. It is empathy, imbued with moral fortitude. We can gently, but firmly support children at that moment of painful decision when they would otherwise become paralyzed inwardly:

> The whole of a child's illness is really contained in this complex of ideas. Such children detect in themselves the peculiar constitution that consists of the out-flowing astral body and "I"-organization. It manifests in the astral body kind of working outward into the world—"I will do it." But they know that then they immediately come up against the external world and its reagents. Here is the soreness; here it hurts. The children are forced to perceive: I cannot do it! Then they know that it nevertheless has to be done. They feel: I have to reach out with my astral body into the agents of the world. But I have no control over what I take in hand, I am so unskillful with my out-flowing astral body. The thing turns out different, because I am not in full control; the astral body flows out too strongly.... We have to put forth all our efforts to discover these inner, unconscious complexes of ideas in children. Now suppose the moment comes when such a complex shows itself to you. You notice it. As a

> matter of fact, it is there almost every time a child is about to begin some outer activity or even in the way of thought; it is nearly always there. If you intervene at this moment by gently helping in what such children have to do—doing it with them, feeling, as it were, every movement of the child's hand in your hand, then such children will feel that the second stage is being corrected for them by what you are doing. Naturally they are not helped at all if you simply do what they need to do for them. You must intervene only reflectively. Say, you get a child to paint. You do not paint yourself, but sit nearby and move your paintbrush, accompanying with your brush each movement the child makes. The child will have the idea that you are providing gentle guidance in forming ideas, while thus, with love in your heart, you do what the child must do. The fact that you are nearby in this way—the child will feel it like a gentle caress in the soul. Even down to intimate details of this nature, we will be able to find, if we practice a really careful observation, the right thing to do.[260]

This approach requires us to recognize the difference between "sympathy" and "empathy." We must understand the child's experience but not be captured by it. Table 12 summarizes Steiner's therapeutic indications for a hysteric child.

Through consciously directed pedagogical encounter we can repeatedly show the pathway for a child to heal this soul-soreness from the inside out. Children must find their own capacity for gathering and consolidating the astral body, for as they grow older we are less and less able successfully to hold back all painful encounter with the world.

Table 12: Supportive measures for the hysteric constitution

Bringing consciously directed "shocks"
· Bring activity into a quicker tempo. · "You must do the thing over and over again, preparing your whole teaching in such a way that, as it proceeds, at certain moments it simply takes a new turn." · Humor is also a very good technique for bringing shocks.
Working to make sure that children feel how we are strongly united with them inwardly, that we understand them
· "Children need more than that we simply share their sorrow. If we are merely dejected and sorrowful with them—that is no good to children." · "If you intervene at this moment by gently helping in what the children have to do—doing it with them, feeling, as it were, every movement of their hand in your hand, then they will have the feeling that the second stage is being corrected for them by what you are doing." · "Say, you get children to paint. You do not paint yourself, but you sit down near them and move your paintbrush, accompanying with your brush each brush movement they make. They will have the idea that you are gently guiding them in forming their ideas, while thus, with love in your heart, you do with them what they have to do."

Chapter 25

Aggressive Behaviors toward Other Children

"[There are] children who are not accessible to moral influence, who, for example, readily become violent during their attacks—for epileptic attacks may disguise themselves as outbursts of violence of which the child has afterward no memory."[261]

Aggressive actions are particularly challenging behaviors to work with, whether they come in the form of hitting, crashing, yelling, biting, or scratching. These interactions are socially hurtful—whether or not physical injury actually occurs—and force us to ask questions about what individual behavior patterns should be allowed or tolerated and when the general social health of a group needs to be protected.

Aggressive behaviors also make us fearful, and this is especially true for parents of the other children, the ones who are on the receiving end of the interactions. In recent years a great deal of attention has been paid to how to confront bullying behavior and other under-recognized forms of abuse, with the result that many parents and teachers are protective and proactively confronting aggression. How does all this fit with a constitutional understanding of the child? Well, it means that we are asked to hold competing and sometimes contradictory priorities—to do everything possible to ensure that no one gets hurt and, at the same time, to meet the individual needs of the children who are striking out and help them to find better ways of interacting with the outside world. What is the right approach?

One philosophy is zero tolerance. This means not tolerating any kind of aggression and clearly communicating that hurting another child is not allowed. The inward gesture needed to accomplish this kind of discipline is a form of antipathy. This is not necessarily bad, because we, in fact, need the process of antipathy any time we want to create a boundary. That word itself, antipathy, may bring negative images to mind, perhaps implying that we no longer like the child. That is not what is meant. It is used here as a description for the developmental step of objectifying a process, a step that is inherent in the maturation of the senses (very much the therapeutic gesture for a large-headed child, such as cold water on the head in the morning or homeopathic treatment with lead). Making clear boundaries helps a child learn the boundary of appropriate social behavior. To be able to state clearly to a child that hitting, kicking, or hurting another human being is not a way we can act with each other—that should indeed be a consistent and enforced message. But that approach alone is frequently too one-sided. If that is the only message given, then a child often learns to suppress the behavior—and while aggression sometimes comes out of true ill will, it is more usually tied to broader constitutional challenges. As a one-size-fits-all approach, zero tolerance may blind us to individual constitutional needs. Expecting a child to continually suppress strong sensory needs sets the child up for failure, when those needs either finally spill out or coalesce into an inner pool of anger or resentment.

On the opposite side of strong boundary is an approach that lives in full sympathy. Here the priority is always to love and accept children and to work to help them express and channel all feelings of frustration, isolation, or anger. This approach brings gifts, because we do need to regularly help children find good ways to express what they are experiencing inside. This loving connection will, however, sometimes only enable the behavior, as when a parent explains that a child is just angry or tired while the child is violently striking the parent in the face. Very often this kind of provocative aggression comes from children's lack of perceptible boundary or secure connection—they strike out until they encounter a boundary—in this case, the face and the parent's reaction. Allowing children to act out whatever they feel may be rooted in a deep love for them, but it does not necessarily help children know how to be in the world. In fact, in the classroom setting, a bubble of social isolation often develops around children who are provocatively aggressive or manipulative. The other children feel that there is no consistent way to navigate interactions with such a child, so they keep their distance. These children can become pariahs in the class, reinforced by a cycle of provocative aggression, social retreat by the other children, more provocative interaction, and so on.

A third possible pathway works to combine elements of both antipathy and sympathy. It works with the imagery of point and periphery. A breathing between extremes helps to define a therapeutic space for interaction. It is helpful to describe it in three discrete gestures—one of sympathy, one of antipathy, and a third balanced between the two. We can also name them as distinct steps: "acknowledgment," "boundary," and "pathway." Formalizing them in this way helps us recognize which element needs particular emphasis. (Does this child need more boundary, more acknowledgment, more pathway and direction?) In many ways it parallels the much broader steps of constitutional assessment, which we can also break into three steps: Where is the child out of balance? What would be the opposite constitutional process? (This often translates into the appropriate therapeutic gesture). Then, as a last step, we decide on a pathway from where the child is now to where the child needs to be. We briefly look at how these steps can be used as a way to communicate about very basic behaviors and then explore how they may lay a framework for building constitutional approaches for aggressive actions.

No child automatically knows the right thing to do. All small children are continuously working to discover the right way to be in the world. Transitions are particularly hard, because the child is asked to enter into new activities or situations and to find a whole new set of social anchors in order to know the right way to act. Transitions are also the time when aggressive behaviors very commonly come out, like getting ready to leave a place or switch to a new activity. These three steps can be particularly helpful with those transitions.

The first step, *acknowledgment,* lets children know that they are being met, regardless of behavior: "I can see that you are angry" or "You seem worried" or "You are very tired." Acknowledgment is a good first ingredient because it can help avoid escalation. If the first response children always hear initially is "Stop it!" or "Be quiet!" it communicates that what they are doing is not right, but it does not help children know what behavior would be better. If only a boundary message comes, it becomes frustrating and shaming for children as individuals, particularly if that poor behavior is rooted in a constitutional sensory need. An element of acknowledgment creates a little breathing space; it helps children identify their mood or behavior (by naming it) and potentially, in time, also better learn what they actually need inwardly. "You seem very tired" could help them learn over time that when they act this way it usually means they need to rest.

"Are you hungry?" might signal that a child is not feeling well and needs to eat something. This opens a space to connect with the life sense, which, when disturbed, makes us feel unsettled or unwell. Fatigue and hunger are common contributors to irritable outbursts, though going into deeper self-analysis beyond those two categories quickly becomes too intellectual for most children. The acknowledgment step is not really meant to be a process of self-aware reflection or psychoanalysis. Rather, it is about meeting the children where they are. It is interesting that one of the most effective and, at the same time, surprising acknowledgments can be to simply ask, "Do you need some attention?" One might see the look of relief when the child says, "Yes." That is how acknowledgment helps to avoid escalation; it lets children know they are being seen.

The second step, *boundary*—which is easy to identify and all too frequently the first thing that comes out of our mouths—lets children know what is not allowed and what is not good. This step should be clear: "You may not hit me" or "We do not hit each other in this classroom" or "Screaming will not get you what you want." It does not warrant explanation or elaboration. Being clear and brief helps, as sometimes the boundary needs to be repeated several times to be heard. Boundaries need to be firm and consistent, even to the point of being boring. A moving behavioral target—when one's response changes from day to day—is hard to understand and hard to remember and usually unsettles children. A clear and consistent boundary is best.

The third step, *the pathway,* helps children know how to act to get connection or attention: "I will help you when you have stopped screaming" or "You may tell people what you need without hitting" or "If you are angry, come and get me so that I can help." Without this step, children must intuit the right ways to interact. Children generally do not yet have an innate moral hierarchy of behaviors—capacities for abstract thought before age seven and capacities for moral sensing before age nine—so most of their behaviors are based on imitation and effectiveness. It is developmentally inappropriate (if not developmentally impossible) for us to expect younger children to prioritize behaviors morally. We have to share with them good ways to connect and communicate. If that is lacking, children usually continue to do whatever gets the most consistent response, even when the response is negative. When children feel lost or lonely and bother someone—disrupting the whole group activity so that all (negative) attention is directed toward them—they suddenly know where they are and what they are supposed to be doing. Mission accomplished! Many children learn that negative attention is better than disorientation or loneliness. So this third step—*kind but direct instruction*—helps shift habitual patterns of provocative, socially destructive behaviors.

What follows are some examples of three-step communications that have proved helpful. There are, of course, many possible variations. In some circumstances, especially if a pattern of repeated debate or argument has developed, it may even be helpful to script out a response ahead of time. Then, when the moment comes, it is at the tip of our tongues. When these kinds of phrases are repeated often enough, they become boring, an antidote to the child's relying on provocative behaviors as a way to create interaction and attention:

> I know that you are angry (*acknowledgment*), but you may not hit your sister (*boundary*). I cannot help you when you are hitting people, so you need to stop (*pathway*).

> I am sorry that you are bored (*acknowledgment*), but I cannot help you when you are screaming (*boundary*). I will help you when I am finished talking on the phone (*pathway*).

> Yes, you are having trouble falling asleep (*acknowledgment*), but it is dark outside and it is time for sleeping (*boundary*). I will be very happy to see you in the morning when the sun is shining (*pathway*).

> You have a lot of crazy energy today (*acknowledgment*)! Let me just finish this (*boundary*). Then we can go outside (*pathway*).

These phrases may sound somewhat formal, but they are offered only as examples. It is important to put them into language that feels natural and used in a flexible way. Sometimes the boundary part needs to repeated. Sometimes the acknowledgment can be done nonverbally.

In some situations, the concerning behavior is not aggression but disruption. Many children today have become quite skilled at asking a series of questions that seem to need answers, but questions are frequently means of circumventing a boundary (one that captures attention). This is especially important to think about when it feels as if the same answer has been given over and over and the child is not listening—because, in reality, the child may not be listening. The questions are a hook to create more interaction or to gain orientation. The same three steps in answering are helpful here too; only now the boundary is about verbal connection.

> You have a lot of questions (*acknowledgment*). But we are just working quietly right now (*boundary*). Can you show me the next step you need to do (*pathway*)?

The last example helps us begin discussing constitution in aggression:

> I saw you hit your brother (*acknowledgement*). You may not hit him (*boundary*). Please go and tell him you are sorry (*pathway*).

Sometimes there is no good response for the pathway, no way to really give helpful guidance. This happens more often when we are needing to respond after the fact to an aggression. Then we say, "Go and tell him you are sorry." Apologizing may admittedly bring more consciousness to an aggressive interaction, but it cannot really make amends. If we find that we are repeatedly coming to this place where no amount of instruction seems helpful, then we need to look for a deeper cause. To do this, we can turn to the constitutional polarities we have already learned about.

When we start to use a constitutional lens, the initial step of acknowledgment gets bigger. It involves really looking to try to understand the underlying experience of the child who is the aggressor. A starting place is to ask, "How does the child act during transitions?" All of us, given the right circumstances, will devolve into socially unhealthy behaviors. They are our way for compensating (or decompensating) when we are out of balance. One helpful question to pose to parents: "When you are out late with your child at a social function and the child is becoming overly tired or overwhelmed, what does the child do that lets you know it is time to go home? What behavior lets you know that a meltdown is not far away?" Most parents know the answer to that question immediately—it is a universal parenting experience. Do children get wound up and find it difficult to stop? Do they suddenly explode into a tantrum or meltdown? Do children become restless, distressed, or uncomfortable? Or do they become increasingly irritable so that eventually nothing feels good? From a therapeutic perspective we can begin to find the roots of aggression by seeing how a child becomes unglued. Very often that process is predictable, so understanding its source helps us be proactive in our intervention.

Aggressive behaviors fall into two main groups: imbalances in the way we use and guide our limbs (which we can approach through the feeble and maniacal polarity) or imbalances in the way we sense and perceive the world (which we can approach through the epileptic and hysteric polarity). It is much less common for children with a predominantly large- or small-headed constitutions to express themselves through aggression. For this discussion we can therefore concentrate on the polarities of limb and sense. What happens leading up to an aggressive behavior is different for each constitutional type.

Epileptic Aggressive Behaviors

A child with an epileptic constitution can have "outbursts of violence of which the child has afterward no memory."[262] These outbursts are really a kind of fit, in which the astral body and "I" congest and build in intensity, then finally break through. That picture of congestion followed by a kind of bursting helps us characterize these children's aggressive behaviors as large and "explosive." The child is really unable to control what she or he is doing in the moment. It is not volitional, not planned, not specifically targeted, though it may be predictable. For these children a pattern is often observed: From the time of waking or arriving at school, the parent or teacher senses that things are "off" and that it is going to be a hard day. Simultaneously, there may be a sense of things building inwardly, an inner storm, while the child's outside connection and awareness of the world is dulled. In that building-up time it feels hard to reach the child. That dulled, disturbed consciousness is related to the congestion (in contrast to sensing that the child is not paying attention because of fatigue or distraction). Once a fit of anger or aggression starts, it is the kind that is usually best left alone until it has burned itself out, unless such children need to be moved or redirected to avoid hurting themselves or other children. It is generally not very helpful to reason with children who are having an epileptic-type fit or to coach them until things have begun to settle down. This is because the children's consciousness is truly disrupted. Afterward, they may have no memory of what happened or why they were upset. Many such children look and act much better and more at ease once they have worked through their explosion or meltdown. Whatever was building up has been released, and things are okay again.

For children who may have been on the receiving end of this kind epileptic aggression, such explosions can be pretty scary, because the behavior seems to come out of nowhere. The aggression was not necessarily related to a specific aspect of the preceding interaction. This is because the child with an epileptic constitution has been pushing from the inside out and was not that concerned about or even necessarily that aware of who happened to be there on the outside. A regular playmate will, of course, receive the brunt of these fits more often, but in general the anger and aggression coming from the epileptic process is indiscriminate, so that it is possible for many different children to be the recipient over time.

On these "off" days, children with an epileptic-type aggression may seek strong gravity experiences or spend a long time stirring mud or pushing or lifting. They can become upset when they have to transition away from such activity, because it has been helping them work through to a connection with the outside world. It is during that transition time, when the child feels disconnected and disoriented, that the need to break through becomes strongest. For these children the overall gesture is a congestion, a dullness in consciousness that then builds until it erupts into a (violent) outburst. It is not necessarily directed against any single child or particular to any single situation but may be predictable in terms of the pattern that something builds inside and then erupts outward.

Feeble Aggressive Behaviors

The pattern of aggression for an epileptic constitution shares some characteristics with the feeble child, but it is not the same. The feeble constitution can also exhibit seemingly big, physically aggressive behaviors, but they arise out of a different constitutional need. A child with a feeble constitution is similarly working to create a better connection, but the goal is really to penetrate and feel at home in the limbs, not to move out through the senses. That is an important distinction. There is no accompanying disturbance in consciousness for the feeble child. In fact, an important aspect of feeble/earthly experience is that such children are usually aware of what is appropriate; they just cannot implement it fully. The thought impulse does not get down into the limbs. The moral challenge for the feeble constitution is finding a way to really take hold and change a behavior that plays out through the limbs (like grasping an oil-covered piece of glass). These children are generally remorseful after there has been a collision. They may well understand what was wrong but paradoxically do the same thing again the very next day because they cannot yet fully take hold of their bodies.

Feeble aggressiveness comes out of play or movement that is too big. These children instinctively seek repetitive, gross motor movements as a way to bring all four members together for healthy will/limb function. They are rarely malevolent; instead, they are much more like a boulder rolling down the hill that crashes into whatever lies in its path.

These children's aggressive behaviors come out when they are able to enter into big body activity, which feels good to them (activities like recess, circle games, or free play). Their aggression tends to happen at the times of day when such gross motor activity is possible—like knocking someone down during a chasing game or getting too big in their movements, too excited during circle time and not being able to reign in their limb activity when everyone else has already come to a stop.

Transitions can also be hard for these children, but it is because it takes them time to stir their limbs into a new activity; once they are finally "in," they don't want to stop. They are just starting to feel comfortable and capable. They want to keep going, and they do not easily shift to something new. They are commonly the stragglers in the class. Their overall gesture is one of seeking big, repetitive, gross motor activity that then becomes too big or lasts too long and collides with other children.

Hysteric Aggressive Behaviors

Children with a hysteric constitution can also be aggressive, but with a very different flavor. They can hit, scratch, or yell, but it is usually because they are trying to protect themselves. Their basic gesture is one of holding back to avoid pain, and they will do what is necessary in order to preserve that protected space. Whereas children with feeble movement or an epileptic outburst become too physical and collide with those around, those who are soul-sore stay back. They react instead when someone else comes too close. Hysteric aggression may be more targeted than aggression from the epileptic or feeble constitutions. The hysteric child regularly feels pain and, in a way, instinctively knows what hurts and also what will wound other children. Hysteric aggressive behaviors lie not so much in the realm of gross motor explosion or collision; they come out more often as hitting, scratching, biting, or even saying cruel things. These children can have an uncanny sense about finding the chink in someone else's armor.

Hysteric children often seek out ways to protect themselves, such as finding places to hide or withdrawing from interaction. Transitions or free play can be particularly hard because everyone is moving at once, sensory impressions multiply and quickly become overwhelming, and the child is asked (though it can feel like being forced) to shift into another activity that requires new encounters and a new unfolding of the will (which is inherently painful).

Aggressive behaviors arising out of this protective reactivity may be directed toward specific children or be limited to the interaction of two children. Usually the child who is on the receiving end of the hysteric child's aggression is violating private space—perhaps unbeknownst to the child, like a jolly child with feeble movement who repeatedly runs into and knocks down a hysteric child, who then yells and scratches. This can look like targeted aggression, but it really comes as a response to the dynamic of interaction. Sometimes the aggression is preemptive, striking out in anticipation of when the other child is going to come too close. The child's overall gesture is one of aggression that arises out of a need to protect personal space and to avoid too intimate an encounter.

Maniacal Aggressive Behaviors

A fourth type of aggression comes with the maniacal/kleptomaniacal constitution. With these children we can observe that interactions have a feel of being inconsiderate. As we have learned, the child with maniacal movement is constantly striking out with fingers and toes. That movement is not really coming out of a deep-seated constitutional sensory need (like the pushing through for the epileptic, the repetitive gross motor movement for the feeble, or protection for the hysteric) as much from a superficial inattention. The limbs are not guided; the consequences of the limbs hitting others are usually not attended to, unless a kind of disconnected curiosity at the other child's reaction is provoked. To have moral perception, the limbs have to be penetrated. Because the child is only very superficially involved with what the limbs are doing, the child commonly does not notice if something is painful or distressing to another child. In fact, there is enough of a disconnection that once a reaction is elicited in another child (especially a very sensitive, hysteric child) it can feel fun to repeat it to see if the reaction will happen again. It is a little bit like the situation with a child who finds a toy that makes a noise when a button is pushed, and so the child pushes the button over and over again—only there is not enough moral perception to recognize that the other child is different from a toy and that repeated aggressive or manipulative behaviors are truly hurtful.

This kind of behavior can be widespread. (The limbs are not guided, regardless of whom they are directed to.) Alternatively, they can target specific children who are particularly reactive. This probably comes closest to the picture of what is considered ruthless bullying, because it can evolve into something that is repeated and intentional. The overall gesture is unguided and therefore potentially amoral limb activity, which can manifest in repetitive (widespread) provocation or targeted, manipulative provocation.

Chapter 26

Boundary as "Limitation" and Pathway as "Therapeutic Approach"

With these different constitutional patterns in mind (a step of acknowledgment) we can recast the step of voicing boundary to acknowledging limitation: "What is disturbing the child's activity or interaction?"—which could alternatively be phrased as "Where is the blockage?" Then we can also recast the step of pathway and, instead of telling the child how to behave, ask ourselves: "What will help the child be able to make that change?" We can usually find good clues for this last step, as a child has often already been engaging in a variation of that kind of activity, though potentially in a socially unhelpful way.

For the child with an epileptic constitution we have already built the picture of a congestion, a dullness in consciousness that then builds until it erupts in a (violent) outburst. That is the child's basic physiologic experience. We can now ask: "What is limiting the child's activity and interaction?" It is the congestion created when the astral body and "I" find resistance as they try to move through the physical and etheric bodies to connect with the outside world. What do children need to overcome this? They need to make good connections with the outside world.

So now, what should be done? Certain measures can help the child on a more continuous, constitutional level, and there are special therapeutic tools that can be applied in the moment. As continuous constitutional support, the child should be dressed warmly, "almost to the point of sweating."[263] Any time that the child becomes cool, the receptivity of the physical and etheric for the activity of the higher members is compromised. The child needs to strongly connect with the element of warmth. The child needs to experience a differentiated connection with the outside elements of gravity (earth), water, and air. This process needs to happen over and over again. It is not a process that can be changed with a one-time correction or communication, because it is a physiologic imbalance not an intentional misbehavior. Let us create an imagination for this process: Let us think of thick woods with lots of trees, fallen logs, and undergrowth, and we want to make a path through it to the other side. How many times would we need to walk through the woods before we successfully created a visible, passable footpath? Many, many days and many trips across the woods would be required. That is really the process the epileptic constitution has to work through to not be held back by the physical and etheric bodies. The more a child can be assisted therapeutically into creating that pathway to the outside world, the less the child will need to be pushing through, for it is that pushing that results in aggressive explosions. The therapy is really not so much about interventions that correct the behavior when it appears, but more about building support that helps children shift their own physiology.

That said, there are some techniques that help on those days when we can see that the congestion is building. Recognizing that process in its early stages is very helpful, because it offers time to be proactive and help shift course, instead of just being reactive once the explosion has happened. When the congestion is building, just asking the child to stop does not really help. Inwardly, the astral body and "I" are working terrifically to find a pathway through. Creating extra resistance—"Don't do that!"—will not help the congestion find its resolution. It might even make it worse, for with a process like this, when the whole child's organism is working to push through, it will not be solved until a path is found (which may well be an explosion of anger, even a fit, if necessary).

It is also important to remember that an inherent part of this congestion is disrupted consciousness. The child's activity is tied up inwardly, so subtle suggestions or corrections will likely not even be heard. This is less about willful disobedience than it is about disconnection. In fact, connection or instruction will likely be heard only when instruction provides a pathway that beckons and encourages the child to come out—through differentiated touch, through steady voice, through an invitation to specially sense the world ("Can you help me move this?" "Which one is heavier?"). Give these children something to do that helps them connect. If we are really worried about the consequences of an "explosion," then we can help the child work through this process in more isolation. The pathway becomes one not of "do not do that" but rather "do what you need to do, but let us do it over here." If the child has already exploded, immediate correction and reprimand probably also will have little effect. The child's consciousness has been so stuck and dulled that it may have no recollection of what just happened. Help these children land safely. Give them some time, perhaps shielded from other children. The other therapeutic indications for the epileptic constitution should also be considered.

Children with a feeble constitution are seeking big, repetitive, gross motor activity that becomes too big or lasts too long and then collides with other children. What limits children's interaction? It is their need for stirring activity that helps them overcome the gravity and melancholy of the hereditary body. What helps the child? Large, gross motor movement and spiritualized activity (such as painting or eurythmy) help. The child with a feeble constitution needs to be able to move. This process, like that for the epileptic constitution, needs to happen over and over. The challenge is that since there is a good possibility for the child to crash over into another child whenever there is an opportunity for large movement, there may arise the temptation to limit that child's participation. But movement is what these children need. Such a child must be allowed to be a rolling boulder.

How do you safely let a big boulder roll down the mountainside? One essential aspect is that you cannot successfully ask it to suddenly change course. Boulders do not change their path without a big obstacle in the way (which may be someone else in the class that the child ends up crashing into, or the teacher/parent who must stand in the way and be collided with). This means that asking a feeble child to continuously change activity is usually a prescription for conflict or collision. Quick transitions and sudden stops will not work well for such children. Creating time and space for them to use up their momentum, to keep going, and then loop back into the next activity will be much kinder. It is as if there were an open meadow the boulder can roll into and slow down as it comes down off the mountainside. Creation of these open spaces helps children avoid accidental collision and confrontation.

Moving now to children with a hysteric constitution, we acknowledge their experience as aggression arising from a need to protect personal space and avoid encounters that seem too intimate. It is these children's soul-soreness that limits interaction and creates defensive reactions. It is accompanied by a kind of inner contradiction, as they become lonely (every child's developmental impulse, guided by greater archetypal spiritual activity, is to find healthy ways to connect with the world) and, simultaneously, hugely fearful of contact. The bridge to safety and freedom from reactivity comes through creating safe spaces and times for interaction. A hysteric child regularly needs to be sheltered from too much sensory stimulation. A very large class size, a lot of noise, and abrupt, unexpected changes in routine or activity are unsettling. Consciously providing the child with the option of more protected space and activity (especially during more unstructured time) will help.

Aggressive or reactive behaviors usually come out when the hysteric child is feeling most overwhelmed and vulnerable. Confronting an aggressive behavior head on, especially if it is done with angry or disapproving overtones, will likely make things worse. If a child continues to be aggressive or defensive in the face of correction or even escalates, direct conversation may be too much. (In other words, correcting the child more harshly will likely not make the child stop.) An alternative, much more successful approach is to inwardly turn our gaze (sometimes even physically turning, too), so that rather than looking directly at the child, we stand more parallel and look at something together. This method of communication works better to diffuse the tension that is always felt by a child with a hysteric constitution. This is close to Steiner's indication for painting, that the child's hand should be guided by the teacher, though the teacher should not do the painting for the child. Looking together, with parallel gaze, helps the child push through the pain of interaction and calms that acute soul-soreness.

Direct touch is probably also not a good way to redirect the child with hysteric reactivity. When the child is already feeling hurt or violated, touching the child may bring even more aggression (think of a cornered cat with its claws out). Safe touch is probably strongly desired by the child, but to be safe it needs to be initiated by such children themselves. Uninvited touch from the outside, especially when perceived as rough, will likely prolong and escalate the confrontation. This can be a challenge when we, as adults, may ourselves be reactive—even resentful—toward a child's aggressive behaviors. Strong or reactive touch could fall into the category of "unconscious" shocks that Steiner described as being so harmful for the hysteric constitution.

Over the long term, creating ways for the child to overcome such hysteric reactivity is very helpful. There is only so much protection and buffering that can be brought to the child, and as the child gets closer to the seventh year it is essential that the child find safe, loving experiences to connect with the outside world that are self-engendered. The child can learn this through therapeutic guidance. These experiences can fall into the category of consciously directed "shocks" or shifts that Steiner recommended (like a change in tempo). One example of this might be helping the child to pet a small animal, like a rabbit, that suddenly jumps or shifts unexpectedly. That jump will startle a hysteric child. If an adult is there to quiet the reaction and say, "See, the rabbit is jumpy, but look how much she likes it when you gently stroke her back," then the reaction is successfully moved through.

Overcoming such reactivity takes time and many repetitions. Humor is also a wonderful way to provide a consciously directed shock that helps these children surrender some of their vigilance.

A teacher or parent's accompaniment for hysteric aggressions needs to be much more companionable than for the epileptic or feeble constitutions; epileptic children need space and activity to let them finish pushing through to connection, and on some level this has to be accomplished on their own. The feeble constitution needs space and movement to really gain good momentum and levity and then the space to allow that to fully play out. Those can be done away from other children and away from adults. The hysteric child, however, needs to be consciously held in conflict from the side; to be present, holding the space, allowing the child to push through the pain. A strong, loving, and almost unflappable relationship during aggressions is often most successful. Warm companionship that reassures and encourages the child to keep pushing through to real engagement is the best long-term gesture.

Aggressive behaviors from a child with maniacal physiology arise out of unguided and therefore potentially amoral limb activity. The limbs strike out because they are not consciously penetrated. That superficiality of interaction can bring social interactions that manifest in repetitive, widespread provocation (with everyone within arm's or leg's reach potentially affected) or targeted, manipulative provocation (with the dominant head activity curious about the reaction, but the heart and feeling life not active enough to sense whether the behaviors are hurtful to the other person). What is the limitation for this child? The child's activity is guided too much by the head, so that the feeling life stays cold and the morality of the limbs never develops. What does the child need? The child needs to become a truly threefold being in whom thinking works cooperatively with feeling and willing.

Steiner indicated that the cosmic child is helped through invoking strong feeling. This is the situation in which direct correction and even confrontation over hurtful behaviors can be helpful for aggressive behaviors. We, of course, need to tell the child with an epileptic, feeble, or hysteric constitution that hitting, crashing into, kicking, or biting other children is inappropriate behavior and is not tolerated, but it is with the maniacal and kleptomaniacal constitution that consciousness needs to be brought right down into the activity of the limbs.

Asking children not just to apologize but also perhaps to see that the other child is upset or crying, or asking children how they think the other person feels can bring out more of that strong feeling. This feeling aspect is particularly important when we give a correction not to hit, and then the child protests when getting in trouble for kicking. A very literal interpretation of rules or boundaries is a sign that the feeling life is not yet awake. As a very specific therapeutic activity (for more extreme behaviors), asking these children to hold their feet while they are being corrected over a behavior, or holding or squeezing their hands and feet from the outside may allow better connection with moral sensing (following Steiner's indications about "holding the feet").

As there are times when maniacal aggressive interactions evolve into truly intentional provocations or taunting, direct and clear boundaries need to be voiced and enforced. The child may not stop until an outside force intervenes. Remember that the therapeutic eurythmy sequence of the maniacal child ends with "A" and "U"—the formative, quieting, and penetrating activity of the vowels. What for the hysteric constitution would be a devastating reprimand or correction may just be scratching the surface of real feeling life for the maniacal child. Pausing to create space for moral sensing, a kind of guided gazing into the well, may well be more effective than simply voicing rules. The more we understand the roots of a behavior, the better we can effectively meet and redirect it. We can then find ways to assist a child in moving beyond socially destructive or socially distressing behaviors to instead find more meaningful and constructive connection with the world around.

Chapter 27

Fairy Tale Images for the Pathway

This process of consciously guiding and supporting an act of transformation stands at the heart of many different fairy tales. To round out our considerations of the epileptic and hysteric polarity, we will therefore consider one more set of imaginations, particularly relating to the figure of an old woman. She—whether witch or fairy godmother—figures prominently in many "therapeutic" quests.

The old woman in a fairy tale often has magic. In some stories she uses it to cast dark spells, in others to bring benevolent protection—but in both extremes her influence provokes or encourages a step of development in the main character. In the story of Snow White, the evil queen's machinations drive Snow White to find the dwarfs and to overcome the pathologic one-sided nerve–sense astrality. In another well-known fairy tale, Dame Holda (or "Mother Holle"), an old woman, waits at the bottom of a well. She sets forth tasks for both the industrious and lazy sisters who come into her land, and then she rewards them in relation to the level of their kindness and generosity. In both of these stories, the old woman must be encountered before there can be a transformation.

To work therapeutically with children we must, in certain respects, become the old woman. Our task is not to coddle and not to ignore, but instead to journey with the child in order to find the right pathway for transformation. Images for some of these transformative tasks have already been considered, such as serving the king as cook, gardener, or warrior or reverently watching and guarding a golden well so that nothing will defile it. For the epileptic and hysteric polarity we will consider yet another story, one with an old woman who lives far off in the mountains. It is the Grimm tale of "The Goose-Girl at the

Well." The old woman exists in a magical realm and clearly is more than what she appears. The goose-girl's story gives us a chance to step into another set of imaginative gestures. Those pictures can be helpful for our dream life, our own process of waking and sleeping. We learn at the outset that the old woman is not afraid of hard work:

> There was once upon a time a very old woman, who lived with her flock of geese in a waste place among the mountains, and there had a little house. The waste was surrounded by a large forest, and every morning the old woman took her crutch and hobbled into it. There, however, the dame was quite active, more so than any one would have thought, considering her age, and collected grass for her geese, picked all the wild fruit she could reach, and carried everything home on her back. Any one would have thought that the heavy load would have weighed her to the ground, but she always brought it safely home. If any one met her, she greeted him quite courteously. "Good day, dear countryman, it is a fine day. Ah! You wonder that I should drag grass about, but everyone must take his burthen on his back."[264]

Young children are all working to take the burden on their back and find the right pathway to come into life. Indeed, in the next scene, the old woman meets a "handsome young man" who so far has met no one in the forest. It is reminiscent of the huntsmen meeting Iron John in the woods, an encounter with the physical body:

> He [the young man] suddenly perceived the old witch kneeling on the ground cutting grass with a sickle. She had already thrust a whole load into her cloth, and near it stood two baskets, which were filled with wild apples and pears. "But, good little mother," said he, "how canst thou carry all that away?"
>
> "I must carry it, dear sir," answered she, "rich folk's children have no need to do such things, but with the peasant folk the saying goes, don't look behind you, you will only see how crooked your back is!"
>
> "Will you help me?" she said, as he remained standing by her. "You have still a straight back and young legs; it would be a trifle

> to you. Besides, my house is not so very far from here, it stands there on the heath behind the hill. How soon you would bound up thither."[265]

We discover that the young man's father is a rich count (again, a picture of the royal heritage a child carries when leaving the spiritual world), but this does not stop the young man from agreeing to the old woman's challenge. He replies, "Farmers aren't the only people who can carry something, I'll take on your load." It is not an easy task, however, and he quickly finds that the burden is much more than he imagined:

> "No, it is not light," answered the count, and pulled a rueful face. "Verily, the bundle weighs as heavily as if it were full of cobble stones, and the apples and pears are as heavy as lead! I can scarcely breathe."
>
> He had a mind to put everything down again, but the old woman would not allow it.
>
> "Just look," said she mockingly, "the young gentleman will not carry what I, an old woman, have so often dragged along. You are ready with fine words, but when it comes to be earnest, you want to take to your heels. Why are you standing loitering there?" she continued. "Step out. No one will take the bundle off again."[266]

The young count journeys with her into the mountains. He must watch his step as "the stones rolled out from under his feet as if they were alive," and beads of sweat soon stand out on his forehead. When he decides he simply cannot go on and must stop to rest, the old woman responds, "Once we get there you may rest, but now you must keep going. Who knows what advantage you may derive from it!" He even struggles to throw off the pack, but it is stuck on his back "as firmly as if it had grown there." In spite of the burden and in spite of his fatigue, he pushes on in order to make his way. As he walks, he hears:

> "Don't get angry, dear sir," said she, "you are growing as red in the face as a turkey-cock! Carry your bundle patiently. I will give you a good present when we get home."
>
> What could he do. He was obliged to submit to his fate and crawl along patiently behind the old woman. She seemed to grow more and more nimble, and his burden still heavier.
>
> All at once she made a spring, jumped on to the bundle and seated herself on the top of it; and however withered she might be, she was yet heavier than the stoutest country lass.
>
> The youth's knees trembled, but when he did not go on, the old woman hit him about the legs with a switch and with stinging nettles.[267]

Finally, the young man makes his way up the mountain. As they arrive, they meet the old woman's geese, and the untidy woman who cares for them. This "goose-girl" addresses the old woman as "Mother" and asks, "Did something happen to you? You stayed away so long." The old woman responds in a most remarkable way:

> "By no means, my dear daughter," answered she, "I have met with nothing bad, but, on the contrary, with this kind gentleman, who has carried my burthen for me; only think, he even took me on his back when I was tired. The way, too, has not seemed long to us; we have been merry, and have been cracking jokes with each other all the time."[268]

And the old woman now says to the young man, taking his load and looking at him in the friendliest way:

> "Now seat yourself on the bench before the door, and rest. You have fairly earned your wages, and they shall not be wanting." Then she said to the goose-girl, "Go into the house, my dear daughter, it is not becoming for thee to be alone with a young gentleman; one must not pour oil on to the fire, he might fall in love with thee."

> The count knew not whether to laugh or to cry. "Such a sweetheart as that," thought he, "could not touch my heart, even if she were thirty years younger."[269]

The young man's task—as given by the old woman—is to push and push, even when the load seems impossible. He must overcome that resistance. This is a helpful image of the task for the epileptic constitution. But in the story it is a special task, a therapeutic task, for the young man's arduous journey makes it possible for him to come into relation with the outside world in a new way. The old woman, who seemed to only taunt and mistreat him (beating his legs with a rod and with nettles), at the end of the journey treats him in a completely different way. When they reach their destination, the old woman takes his load and looks at him "in the friendliest way." This is very much a picture of the epileptic constitution's pushing through the resistance of the physical and etheric bodies and overcoming it. Working with the burden of his journey brings the possibility to "fall in love with you." He is able to relate to the outside world in a new way, for we love only what we can truly see and connect with. This brings us to the character of the goose-girl.

The first description of her in the story comes as she approaches with the geese: "Behind the flock walked, stick in hand, an old wench, strong and big, but ugly as night." There is little about her to entice the young man, so he leaves the old woman and the goose-girl on the mountain, "and set[s] off without even once looking back at the beautiful daughter." He is, however, given an emerald box, which he is told will bring him luck.

The young man travels out of the wilderness to a big city and there learns the true value of the box. He encounters that city's queen, who collapses and weeps when she sees the box:

> "Of what use to me are the splendors and honours with which I am surrounded; every morning I awake in pain and sorrow. I had three daughters, the youngest of whom was so beautiful that

> the whole world looked on her as a wonder. She was as white as snow, as rosy as apple-blossom, and her hair as radiant as sunbeams. When she cried, not tears fell from her eyes, but pearls and jewels only. When she was fifteen years old, the King summoned all three sisters to come before his throne. You should have seen how all the people gazed when the youngest entered, it was just as if the sun were rising."[270]

This youngest daughter of the city's queen is striking. Her beauty radiates out to all. She has no guile; she does not hide. Everyone can see immediately how lovely she is. It would be hard not to notice her. Such beauty, in the language of a fairy tale, often belongs to the astral body—for the beauty of shape, proportion, and color all arise out of the sculptural archetypes and activities of the astral forces. Light, too, shines continuously from this third daughter—"It was like the sunrise." The astral body works down into the physical body via the "light ether." These images of exceptional beauty and light, which all can see, suggest a capacity of the girl's astral body to extend well beyond the borders of her body—it can fill an entire room.

This beauty is also accompanied by a very unusual process: she cries. Not with tears but with pearls and jewels. A very unusual kind of excretion, such that all can see the depth of her emotion! As we see in the next part of her story, her outward (astral) beauty and radiance also bring vulnerability. The queen of the city continues:

> The King spoke, "My daughters, I know not when my last day may arrive; I will today decide what each shall receive at my death. You all love me, but the one of you who loves me best, shall fare the best."
>
> Each of them said she loved him best.
>
> "Can you not express to me," said the King, "how much you do love me, and thus I shall see what you mean?"
>
> The eldest spoke. "I love my father as dearly as the sweetest sugar."
>
> The second, "I love my father as dearly as my prettiest dress."
>
> But the youngest was silent.

> Then the father said, "And thou, my dearest child, how much dost thou love me?"
>
> "I do not know, and can compare my love with nothing."
>
> But her father insisted that she should name something. So she said at last, "The best food does not please me without salt, therefore I love my father like salt."
>
> When the King heard that, he fell into a passion, and said, "If thou lovest me like salt, thy love shall also be repaid thee with salt." Then he divided the kingdom between the two elder, but caused a sack of salt to be bound on the back of the youngest, and two servants had to lead her forth into the wild forest.
>
> "We all begged and prayed for her," said the Queen, "but the King's anger was not to be appeased. How she cried when she had to leave us! The whole road was strewn with the pearls that flowed from her eyes.
>
> The King soon afterward repented of his great severity, and had the whole forest searched for the poor child, but no one could find her. "When I think that the wild beasts have devoured her, I know not how to contain myself for sorrow; many a time I console myself with the hope that she is still alive, and may have hidden herself in a cave, or has found shelter with compassionate people. But picture to yourself, when I opened your little emerald book, a pearl lay therein, of exactly the same kind as those that used to fall from my daughter's eyes; and then you can also imagine how the sight of it stirred my heart. You must tell me how you came by that pearl."[271]

This picture of the third daughter is a helpful imagination for the hysteric constitution, with its striking astral radiance and vulnerability. Her struggle to find expression for her love and her choice of "salt" give us spiritual pictures for the therapeutic experience she must find.

Why salt? Salt does indeed make food taste better and for this reason has long been prized, but its inclusion in the story may be part of a much deeper picture. For salt (as a substance but even more so as an archetypal alchemical process) brings boundary. If we put some salt on our tongues, we are immediately aware of the boundary of the tongue. Put on enough salt, and we can taste and feel the boundary of the tongue for several hours afterward. Salt makes us more aware. It is related to the crystallizing forces of the nerve–sense pole; we have already heard from Steiner how the large-headed constitution cannot properly handle salt. For large-headed children (who still have an incompletely developed nerve–sense system), a lead treatment helps them to better handle salt and to properly finish forming the sense organs. Such reinforcement of boundary brings more awareness, but awareness is only one side of boundary.

For the hysteric constitution the image of salt plays perhaps a different role. For when the bag of salt is tied to her back, the third daughter leaves the city, and this is her first step toward going off into the forest. It is in the woods that her mother, the queen, prays that the girl has "hidden herself in a cave and found shelter with charitable people." The girl does find charity in the form of an old woman, who assigns her chores and tasks her with caring for the geese, and through this process the third daughter is transformed. Her radiance changes so dramatically that now no one can see her beauty, and the count, when he first meets her as the goose-girl, thinks, "Even if she were thirty years younger, she couldn't stir my heart." There, in the woods, in the mountains, away from all the people of her father's court, the third daughter finds an experience of boundary that protects her enough so she can live safely in the world. She still acts as a daughter in her new role, but with a gentle, nonthreatening encounter:

> Soon afterward the daughter also entered. But the old woman scarcely thanked her, and only shook her head a little. The daughter sat down beside her, took her spinning-wheel, and twisted the threads as nimbly as a young girl. Thus they both sat for two hours, and exchanged never a word.
>
> At last something rustled at the window, and two fiery eyes peered in. It was an old night-owl, which cried, "Uhu!" three times. The old woman looked up just a little, then she said, "Now, my little daughter, it is time for thee to go out and do thy work."

> She rose and went out, and where did she go? Over the meadows ever onward into the valley. At last she came to a well with three old oak-trees standing beside it; meanwhile the moon had risen large and round over the mountain, and it was so light that one could have found a needle. She removed a skin that covered her face, then bent down to the well, and began to wash herself. When she had finished, she dipped the skin also in the water, and then laid it on the meadow so that it should bleach in the moonlight and dry again.
>
> But how the maiden was changed! Such a change as that was never seen before! When the gray mask fell off, her golden hair broke forth like sunbeams, and spread about like a mantle over her whole form. Her eyes shone out as brightly as the stars in heaven, and her cheeks bloomed a soft red like apple-blossom.
>
> But the fair maiden was sad. She sat down and wept bitterly. One tear after another forced itself out of her eyes, and rolled through her long hair to the ground. There she sat and would have remained sitting a long time if there had not been a rustling and cracking in the boughs of the neighboring tree. She sprang up like a roe which has been overtaken by the shot of the hunter. Just then the moon was obscured by a dark cloud, and in an instant the maiden had put on the old skin and vanished, like a light blown out by the wind. She ran back home, trembling like an aspen leaf.[272]

The king's third daughter journeys to the mountains to create a new skin. While she is in that skin she is big and "ugly as night"—so protected that she cannot be fully seen. In that protected space she is able to do many tasks for the old woman, independently and without fear. When she sheds her skin, she is once again as radiant as the sun, but she cries pearls of sadness that fall to the ground (a kind of soul-soreness). In that exposed state she hears even the tiniest rustling of a tree and reacts, "springing like a roe." Then quickly she puts her skin back on, still "trembling like an aspen leaf," and runs away. When she returns to that exposed, astral state, her sensitivity overflows, with its vulnerability.

The young man, we next learn, has experienced the encounter quite differently. For the goose-girl their encounter under the moon was a process of exposure, then retreat. For the count's son's it is curiosity, then a searching and longing:

> He could see that it was the goose-girl, whom he had seen before in the house of the old woman. "Oho," cried he, "there she comes, and if I once get hold of one of the witches, the other shall not escape me!" But how astonished he was, when she went to the well, took off the skin and washed herself, when her golden hair fell down all about her, and she was more beautiful than anyone whom he had ever seen in the whole world. He hardly dared to breathe, but stretched his head as far forward through the leaves as he dared, and stared at her. Either he bent over too far, or whatever the cause might be, the bough suddenly cracked, and that very moment the maiden slipped into the skin, sprang away like a roe, and as the moon was suddenly covered, disappeared from his eyes.[273]

When the young count sees her shed her skin, he immediately recognizes her inner beauty. Her true being is revealed to him, and in this magical realm of the old woman's mountains and meadows he is able to find her when many others cannot (including the third daughter's father and mother, who now begin to search for her). He has a capacity for leaning and looking, working to make connection.

After this encounter the young count guides the city king and queen to the old woman's house, and when they come into the house the goose-girl gazes specifically at him:

> When she perceived him, she became as red in the face as a moss-rose; she herself did not know why.
>
> The King said, "My dear child, I have given away my kingdom, what shall I give thee?"
>
> "She needs nothing," said the old woman. "I give her the tears that she has wept on your account; they are precious pearls, finer than those that are found in the sea, and worth more than

> your whole kingdom, and I give her my little house as payment for her services."
>
> When the old woman had said that, she disappeared from their sight. The walls rattled a little, and when the King and Queen looked round, the little house had changed into a splendid palace, a royal table had been spread, and the servants were running hither and thither.[274]

With this step, the young count and the goose-girl (really a princess) are united. They have both journeyed, taking quite different paths, but through the old woman's gifts find their way to return to a kingly realm. The young man, the count, has learned to push through to see her; the goose-girl, the third daughter, has learned how to shield herself in order to let herself safely be seen. The story finishes with a hint of the old woman's wisdom and benevolence:

> This much is certain, that the old woman was no witch, as people thought, but a wise woman, who meant well. Very likely it was she who, at the princess's birth, gave her the gift of weeping pearls instead of tears. That does not happen now-a-days, or else the poor would soon become rich.[275]

We emulate the well-meaning wise woman when we can work to create a proper pathway. Then the gifts can come. Working between point and periphery we can help both epileptic and hysteric children find a healthier and more satisfying connection with the surrounding world.

Table 13 summarizes the contrasting gestures and therapeutic process for the epileptic and hysteric constitutions, while incorporating some of the language and imagery from the fairy tale of the Goose-girl at the Well.

Table 13: Summary table for epileptic and hysteric constitutions

In the language of the fairy tale...the contrasting pictures and processes of the epileptic and hysteric polarity	
"No, it is not light," answered the count, and pulled a rueful face. "Verily, the bundle weighs as heavily as if it were full of cobble stones, and the apples and pears are as heavy as lead! I can scarcely breathe."	When she cried, not tears fell from her eyes, but pearls and jewels only. When she was fifteen years old, the King summoned all three sisters to come before his throne. You should have seen how all the people gazed when the youngest entered, it was just as if the sun were rising!
Epileptic Process	**Hysteric Process**
"The human being wakes up, but remains unconscious. You see, we have come in this way to an exact description, drawn from within, of the condition of the epileptic.... Epileptics are able to enter with the "I"-organization and astral body into the physical body. That they can do, but they do not emerge into the physical world; they are held fast within.... Astral body and "I"-organization will be, so to speak, dammed up, or congested, beneath the surface of an organ. This condition then manifests outwardly as a fit. This is what fits really are."[276]	"They have trouble making contact with the external world.... Remind yourself how it is with you when you have grazed your skin at some spot. Suppose you then take hold of an object with the sore surface where the skin has been rubbed away. You know how it hurts! The reason for being so sensitive is that you come up against the external world too vigorously there with your inner astral body.... Children who, from the first, bring their astral body right out—such children will subtly touch and take hold of things, just as though they have been wounded.... People in this condition are bound to feel their environment much more keenly, much more intensely; moreover, they will have within them a much more powerful reflection of their environment."[277]
The epileptic–hysteric polarity mirrors the daily process of waking and sleeping and finds expression in variations of wakeful connection with the world through the senses.	

Part Four

Bringing the Pieces Together

Chapter 28

Helping Children with Attention or Memory Problems

Attention problems are a widespread concern in the classroom. An initial approach to attention-deficit disorder with and without hyperactivity (ADHD/ADD) was presented in the section on the large- and small-headed constitutions in relation to a child being either inattentive (related to too much metabolism and an incompletely developed nerve–sense system) or distracted (relating to insufficiently developed metabolism and too much sensing activity). That polarity of blood and nerve activity and its potential imbalance serve as a useful foundation for considering the process of wakeful awareness. We can now, however, expand that duality into a larger picture and consider the situation through the lens of multiple polarities, for we will find that residual imbalances in the way a child has incarnated into the body may disrupt the way consciousness is liberated through the head pole to meet the surrounding world. More simply stated, we must feel good in our body before we can properly attend to the outside world. Tracing the major developmental movements, working from the metabolic–limb system up to the rhythmic system and then from the rhythmic system into the nerve–sense system allows for a broad survey of any given child's constitution. The insights we can gain in that process actually make the terms *ADD* and *ADHD* seem comparatively hollow, as we recognize that they too often become a catchall diagnosis. As psychiatric diagnoses, they acknowledge there is an "attention" imbalance, but beyond broad recommendations for stimulant medication they offer relatively little in the way of individualized therapy or insight. We can develop much more specific and therefore generally more effective therapeutic perspectives and treatment plans through a spiritually inclusive understanding.

The process begins by following the sequential, developmental steps that have been described up until this point, to see if any particular process has become stuck or too one-sided (which is really the definition of a constitutional inclination—that a process falls too far to one side). Observing a child begins to feel more like "trying on" different developmental processes to see if they fit the child's behavior. (For example, does this child move maniacally? Is the child's consciousness blocked or interrupted?) The following pathway is offered as one possible means for following, stepwise, the general developmental progression. With practice this process of "trying on" becomes a much more fluid, imaginative, and less formal process, one that breathes back and forth between open observation and thoughtful consideration.

First impressions, inspirations, and intuitions are also great gifts and should not be discounted, though they are not always predictable. This progression can be reliably turned to as a starting point as well as a means for corroborating other kinds of more intuitive impressions.

The Will

We begin with the meeting of the earthly/hereditary and spiritual streams. This is the dominant process for the first seven years of life. When this process of integration is incomplete, a child must devote continued energies toward that will process, which in turn diverts energies away from how the child learns to relate with the outside world. So a first set of questions to ask is this:

> Does the child engage well with the outside world through the limbs? Are the limbs enlivened? How far out into the limbs can we see these children penetrate their physicality? To the neck? To the shoulders? Upper arms? Elbows? Forearms? Wrists? Fingers?

The answers will justifiably be different, depending on the age of the child, but they quickly give a general impression about the process of integration. Then, moving beyond that measure of penetration into the limbs, we can look to see:

- Does the child move too little or too much?
- If there is too little movement (which could indicate a feeble constitution), look further to determine the answers to these questions:
- Do we see the heaviness of the earthly/feeble constitution? Is it difficult for the child to overcome that resistance?
- As part of that process, is the child repeatedly seeking out big, repetitive, gross motor movement?
- Is the child clumsy or viewed by others as physically aggressive or destructive?
- Can the child understand and follow moral instruction or rules/guidelines for social interaction (or, alternatively, is it like trying to hold a piece of glass covered in oil)?

If there is too much movement (which may suggest a maniacal constitution):

- Is there an accompanying superficiality of engagement and a constant striking out with the fingers and toes?
- Do limb movements seem intentional and guided, or are they largely disconnected from the children's thinking pole?
- Do these children feel the consequences of their actions, or is the feeling life largely left out of the interactions?
- Do they steal or randomly take possessions from others? (If so, then one should think also about the kleptomaniacal process.)

Incomplete integration of the earthly and the spiritual streams can continue to strongly influence movement patterns and moral habits well past the age of seven. The dominance of these processes beyond their developmentally appropriate window has definite consequences for the successful shift into later feeling and thought capacities. A child gets stuck in still trying to sort out the process of healthy limb awareness and activity. Looking at the limbs through the feeble/maniacal pole is particularly helpful when an "attention" problem includes an aspect of "hyperactivity" (ADHD as opposed to just ADD).

An incomplete integration process plays out not only through movement patterns but also through the maturation of the four lower senses. Touch, balance (vestibular sensing), self-movement (proprioception), and the life sense also relate to this will realm. It is very common—on both sides of the polarity, with either too much movement or with not enough movement—for a child to spend a lot of time creating self-stimulating activities, invoking those senses in order to better unite the four members.

As a reminder, at a basic level, this is a process of trying to get the spiritual and hereditary streams to better fit together through the process of limb activity. The child self-stimulates through the lower senses in order to feel more oriented in the body. That sensory seeking and repeated stimulation are really attempts to finish sculpting the inward-sensing process. Only when that inner anchoring has reached sufficient maturity can the child begin to direct attention outward. Up until that point it is very common to see a child anchoring inwardly (through stimulatory activity of one or more of the lower senses) to be able to concentrate on something outside—for example, a child will need to constantly bounce the foot, rock back and forth on a chair, or lean on the desk, in order to pay attention to what is happening in the classroom.

With this view in mind, we can ask:

- Does the child seek strong *touch* (either continuous superficial touch or very strong, rib-cracking touch)? Or does the child consistently avoid touch?
- Does the child seek *vestibular* (balance) input, through (either quick and fast or big and crude) rocking, leaning, spinning? Or does the child avoid those activities altogether?

- Does the child have difficulty modulating movement? Does the child instinctively *seek to go into movement* all the time (invoking the sense of self-movement)?
- Given the chance, does the child happily engage in bigger and bigger movement? Are large gross motor activities preferred while smaller, fine motor activities are difficult (feeble constitution)?
- Does the child have difficulty coming to rest? Does the child seem largely unconscious of the constant movement (maniacal constitution)?
- Does the child seem to be able to come into contented restfulness inwardly? Is the child connected to his or her own state of *wellbeing* (life sense), or does there seem to be a disconnect from healthy sensations of needing to eat, to drink, or to rest?

Seeing the child in movement or free play allows a good opportunity for observing the level of integration in the metabolic–limb system, through patterns of movement and sensory-seeking behaviors.

The Feeling Realm

The next step lifts our view up to the rhythmic system, to the balance of blood and nerve and a consideration of how this interplay affects the way such children orient themselves toward the world. This is the realm of the large-headed and small-headed polarity, and so we can begin with this question:

- Does the child's physiology seem to be dominated by metabolic–limb activity or nerve–sense activity? Or, conversely, does either the metabolic–limb pole or the nerve–sense pole seem out of order?

We can determine this more specifically by looking to see:

- Is the child warm or cold? Red-cheeked or pale?
- Does the child tend to always synthesize (a kind of lumping together and oversimplification) or does the child always

lean toward analysis and start any consideration by placing emphasis on specific details (and only with difficulty coming to an overall synthesis)?

These observations help us gain insight into the child's basic feeling orientation. These inclinations may or may not result in attention or memory problems, as every child has a starting orientation of being either large-headed or small-headed. But most children will, over the course of the elementary school years, be able to move beyond that inclination, that is, a large-headed child may always need to first develop a big picture understanding but out of that overall perspective can then move into specifics; a small-headed child may first need to grasp the basic facts, see the nitty-gritty, and only then will start to understand the way that these facts relate to each other through examples.

For some children the inclination remains so strong that the child has difficulty finding its counterbalance. We can ask:

- Is the child unable to analyze, to break things down into details (suggesting a nerve–sense system that is not in order, with sense organs that need to be further "crystallized")?
- Or is the child unable to synthesize and cannot escape the details? Is the child unable to let go of the specific details to come to an overall, relational perspective? (The metabolic–limb system with its building activity is not in order.)

Then, out of this overall consideration, we can ask these confirmatory questions:

- Are the children flighty and inattentive, occupied with and not yet awakened from their own metabolic activity? (They are still too young and therefore large-headed.)
- Or are the children distracted and brooding, waking too soon into an active sensing life? (They are precociously awake and therefore small-headed.)

For specific therapeutic steps, please refer back to chapter 15.

Thinking and Sensing

The third step is to follow the child's process of conscious connection with the world. This is the realm of the epileptic and hysteric polarity. This process necessarily builds upon the earlier steps of forming healthy metabolic–limb activity, then balanced, rhythmic activity between blood and nerve. If there is a major imbalance, it is important to work to address those developmentally "earlier" processes, as it is very possible that a thinking or sensing problem will improve when a child liberates the attention that has continually been directed to these earlier development tasks. So before we look specifically at the epileptic/hysteric polarity, we should consider:

- Are these children well centered and grounded enough in themselves that they can let go of the body and direct their focus toward sensing the outside world? (If not, more therapeutic work may need to be done in the metabolic–limb and rhythmic systems before the sensing process can be addressed.)

Then we can ask:

- Is the child's conscious connection repeatedly interrupted? Does the child have to continuously push through the physical and etheric bodies to break out of a dulled sensing (epileptic process)?
- Or is the child so open to the world that sensory connection is actually painful and there is a continual pulling back, defensively, in order to limit encounter and minimize the child's soul-soreness (hysteric process)?

Figure 13 attempts to show how we can imaginatively move through from willing to feeling to sensing. Then table 14 summarizes particular qualities of the attention challenges as they relate to the feeble/maniacal, large-headed/small-headed, and epileptic/hysteric polarities.

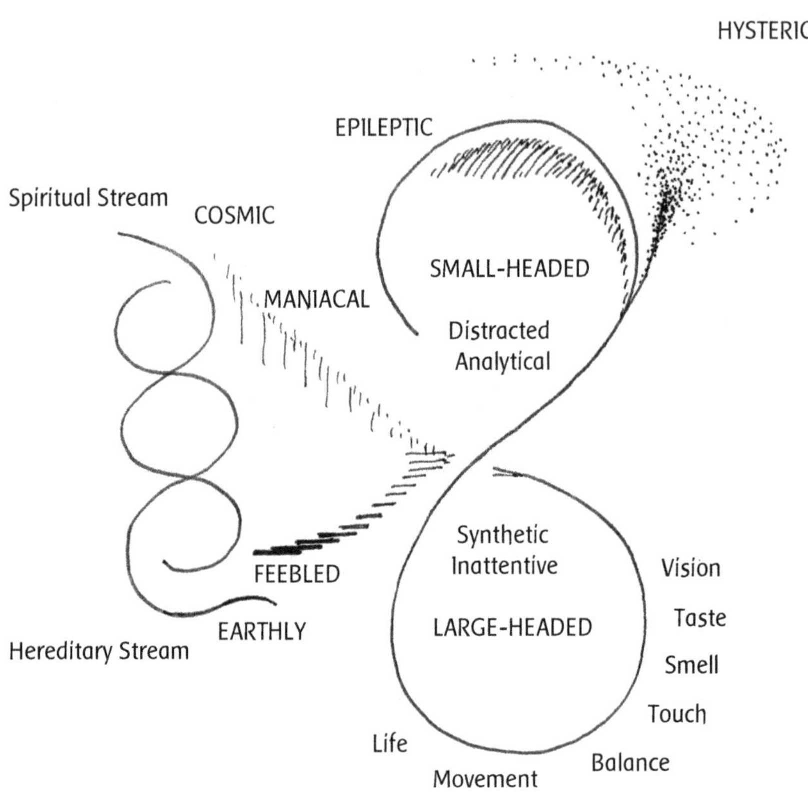

Figure 13: Tracing the developmental progression through the constitutions

Table 14: Patterns of attention and memory for the different constitutions

Constitutional inclination	**How it influences processes of attention and memory**
Earthly / Feeble	Most activities have to be warmed into. Just as large, gross motor repetition allows the child to penetrate the limbs and the will sphere, so too do processes of thinking and memory need to be refreshed and reviewed. Thinking works better after the limbs have been moved, and instant recall—without that warm-up—may be a challenge.
Maniacal / Cosmic	Factual intelligence is generally not the root of the problem—challenges more often instead relate to whether attention can really be harnessed for the task at hand, that is, there may be tremendous recall regarding abstract facts or concepts but far less capacity for really engaging with the present activity or interaction.
Large-headed	Wakefulness is still soft and often dreamy. Stories and pictures are much more alive than facts. Memory relates more strongly to the feelings engendered when something was experienced than to the particular details. Learning happens more through understanding principles or archetypes than through practical examples. The child has trouble analyzing.
Small-headed	These children have an excellent capacity for details. They notice details so strongly that they may even brood over them (especially when something does not fit). Attention can be distracted away by other more acutely experienced thoughts or impressions. Finding the larger picture, relational understanding, and artistic expression may all be a struggle.
Epileptic	Consciousness is interrupted, because the "I" and astral body lose contact with the outside world when they are held back. They must push through the density of the physical and etheric bodies. Time and connection are lost in chunks, though there may also be a continuous, overall diminution in the level of consciousness.
Hysteric	Sensing is always happening, though contact with the outside world may frequently be abandoned. The child retreats to limit the amount of contact. Participation and recall may seem poor, though it is often this defensiveness that underlies the lack of engagement. In the extreme the child may even seem dissociative.

Considering these six foundational patterns gives insight and orientation for many different situations. They follow the archetypal progression from bodily growth to outward connection. We now take an additional, complementary step, which is to instead consider the pathway of an impression as it comes from the outside into the child's awareness. We can again follow several steps or phases, from initial wakeful awareness to a more inward stimulation of the feeling life and then to a final settling of an impression as memory within the metabolic regions of the body.

For this inwardly directed pathway we must first look to see whether the child is attentive. Is the child able to direct energies outward to attend to the world? If not, then we should go back to the inside-to-out developmental pathway of the three polarities just described. If the child is attentive, then we need to look differently.

This question of attentiveness—of whether the windows to the outside world are really open and receptive—is important, because if there is a problem with memory or recall, we may commonly (though potentially incorrectly) assume that the child was not paying attention. There are definitely children who are attentive, who are able to successfully quiet the experience of their body so that they truly can attend to what is happening in the immediate environment around them, but they later cannot recall it. They may be totally captivated by a story or presentation, without distraction, but it all disappears. This means that something happens to the impressions once they pass through the gateway of the senses.

We can contrast the pathways in this way: the wakening developmental progression we have already traced from healthily integrated will (feeble/maniacal) to differentiated feeling (large-/small-headed) to conscious connection (epileptic/hysteric) works from the limbs up. It moves centrifugally, from the center to the periphery. A complementary pathway starts in the head and works down. It follows the transformation of impressions to memories and flows inward and downward. The movement is centripetal, from the periphery of the body to the inner world.

Impressions that come in through the sense organs properly start as purely objective representations of outside phenomena. Many different impressions (hundreds, thousands, probably even millions) come in through the gateway of the senses each day, many more than we consciously recognize or comprehend. Most of them do not enter far enough in to have much meaning. What determines whether an impression will be memorable? One essential step is that an impression moves beyond the pure objectivity of the senses and enters into the feeling realm of the rhythmic system. Feeling is an important part of memory—we remember interactions or encounters much better when they are accompanied by a feeling, good or bad. We also look or listen differently when feeling arises, for then more of our being participates in the interaction. Feeling is an important intermediate step in the process of digesting a sensation in order to make it a permanent part of our physiology.

Taking this process one step further and following the pathway using the language of the four members, we can say that the largely body-free activity of the "I" in the sense organs shifts down to cooperatively work with the astral body (as evidenced by feeling). As the impression works further down in the body and more into the activity of the metabolism, the process becomes a cooperative activity of "I," astral, and etheric forces. We actually hold our lasting memories within the etheric body. It is our memory body.

We can see this progression in Steiner's lecture "The Invisible Man within Us."[278] The "I"-being, involved in all steps of physiologic activity, is differentiated by its varied, cooperative interaction with the other members. As an impression moves from the sensing process of nerve to the dual activity of "I" and astral that underlies respiration, to the threefold cooperation of "I," astral, and etheric (to pulse), the process becomes less conscious and more related to our metabolic organ activity and memory, as shown on page 302, figure 14.

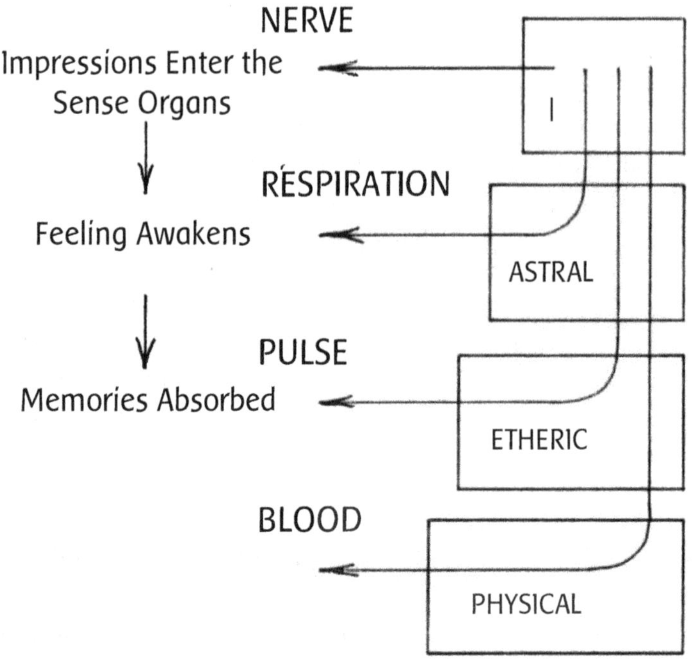

Figure 14: The pathway in, from sensory impression, to feeling, to memory

This kind of waterfall movement, down out of conscious sensing into increasingly cooperative activity with the astral and etheric, is met by a continuously active, opposing current. That opposing current works in a loosening, dissolving way and is what allows us to forget. In the middle the two currents meet. Their interaction determines the quality and longevity of our memory. This is how we are able to remember a telephone number long enough to dial it or remember historical facts and dates for an examination the next day but forget by the end of the week. The formative laying down of memory is continuously buffered by a dissolving and loosening stream.

This middle realm of remembering and forgetting lives between the polar activities of blood and nerve, whose potentially one-sided expression we learned about through the large-headed and small-headed polarities. The mingling of remembering and forgetting lives in the rhythmic system and is colored and influenced by our feeling life. We have already seen how a small-headed child, who is nerve–sense dominant (owing to metabolic–limb activity that is not in order) very often has an excellent memory for details. The activity from the head pole is very strong. In contrast, a large-headed child, with dominant metabolism, quickly melts away details and may fail to appreciate why those details are even considered so important, for they are so quickly gone. This is not to say that the large- and small-headed polarity is the polarity of memory—it is only one aspect of the process. For it primarily describes the upward liberation of metabolic etheric forces into sensing etheric forces and the proportional maturation of the nerve–sense system that occurs with that liberation in the early grade school years. The process of liberating forces up into thinking, however, does bear some influence on how memory comes down.

Steiner characterized a distinct downward pathway for impressions. He described the formation of memories as an imprinting process that relies on an actual crystallizing process, a "salting" process. This process is then met and mediated by glandular absorption. Steiner placed the process in the context of listening to a story:

> We could call what is happening the impression of the spiritual into the physical. A kind of incorporation of what we observe and comprehend during a story is necessary. Something akin to a physical phantom must develop and then impart itself into the whole organism. The organism is filled with delicate salt deposits. Not coarsely, of course. A salt phantom is imparted into the whole organism, and the necessity arises to dissolve it again through the metabolism.
>
> This process takes place when children read or listen to stories. When we believe ourselves to be occupying the mind and spirit in our lessons, we really evoke metabolic processes.... The children must be interested in the subject. Genuine interest is connected with a delicate feeling of pleasure that must always be present. That feeling expresses itself physically in very subtle

> glandular secretions that absorb the salt deposits caused during reading and listening. We must endeavor never to bore the children. Lack of interest, boredom, leads to all sorts of metabolic problems. This is especially the case with girls. Migraine-like conditions are the result of one-sided stuffing of material that must be learned without pleasure. The children are then filled with tiny spikes that do not get dissolved. They tend toward developing such spikes.[279]

For the child to experience a "delicate feeling of pleasure" the activity of sensory impressions must move out of the thinking realm and into the feeling realm—not just because we are so much better able to remember what stirs our feeling life but because it provides for the proper absorption (through a dissolution) of the salt crystals. The imprinting of impressions is shown in figure 15.

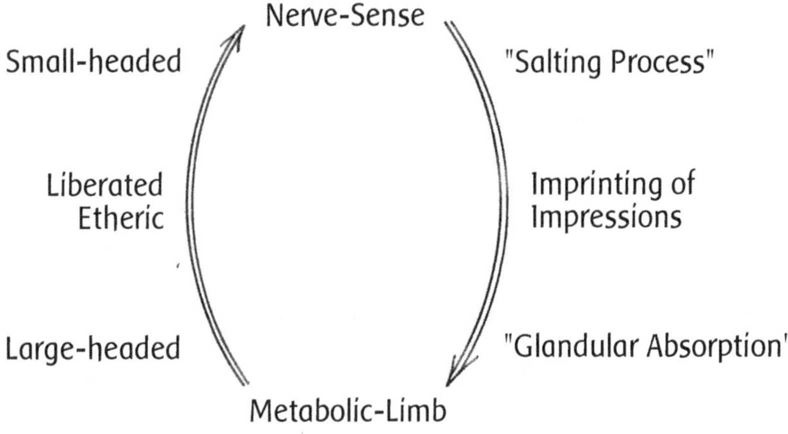

Figure 15: The imprinting of impressions

This process of absorption and dissolution is influenced and supported through specific activity. That is an aspect of pedagogy that is perhaps unique to Waldorf education—the recognition that for a child to develop in a healthy way, not only the sensory activity of memory must be stimulated, but its balance as well (see fig. 16):

Eurythmy and singing lessons can be said to be working in the opposite direction, engendering an organic process that is quite different. All the organs connected with these activities contain spirit. When the children are doing eurythmy they move, and during the moving the spirit in the limbs is streaming upward. When we ask the children to do eurythmy or to sing, we liberate the spirit. The spiritual, of which the limbs abound, is liberated—a very real process.... In singing, eurythmy, and physical education we spiritualize the children. They are quite different beings at the end of the lesson; there is much more spirit in them. But this spirit wishes to consolidate, wishes to remain with the children. We must not allow it to dissipate. We can prevent it from dissipating quite simply and effectively by making the children sit or stand quietly at the end of the lesson. We should try to maintain this calm for a few minutes. The older the children, the more important this will be....

But both, spirit and matter, contain something that is more than either of them, a higher element. We must say that if this higher element is brought to a state of calm, it is matter; if it is brought into movement, it is spirit.[280]

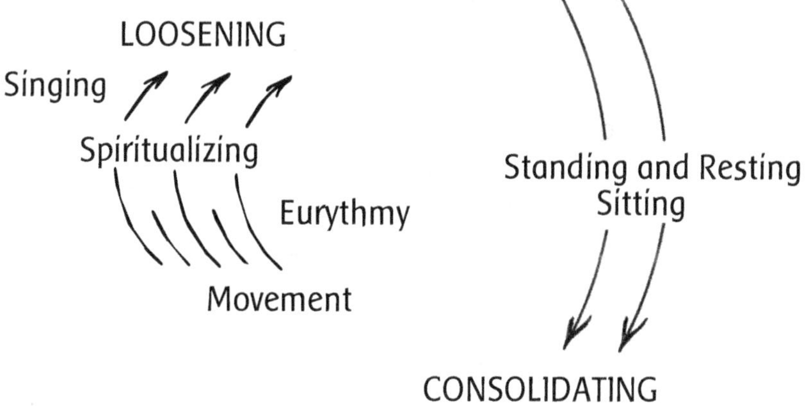

Figure 16: Activities that consolidate and loosen memory

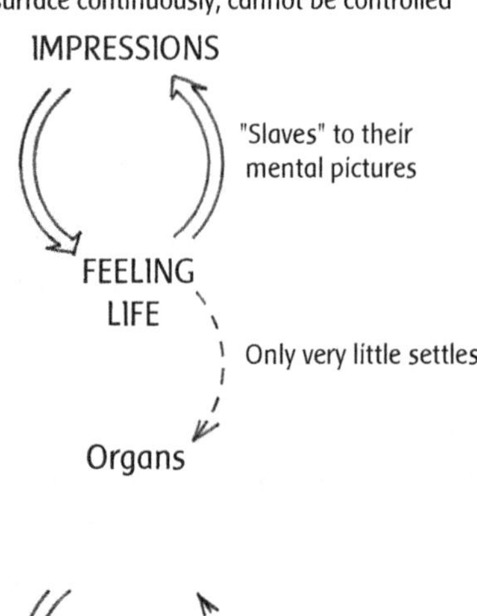

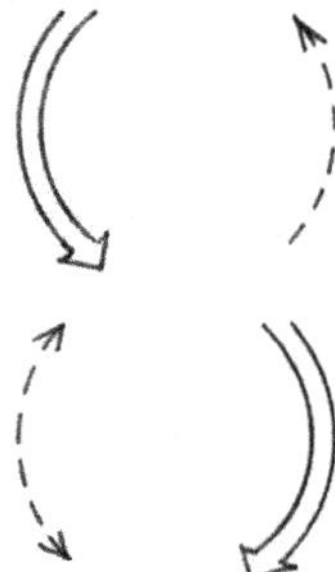

Figure 17: Imagination "rich"

Quickly forget what they have experienced

IMPRESSIONS

Mental Pictures Evaporate

Feeling Life

Everything Disappears

ORGANS

Figure 18: Imagination "poor"

Steiner then took this pedagogical process and extended it into a memory spectrum, in what is often described as the "fantasy rich" and "fantasy poor" or "imagination rich" and "imagination poor" polarities (Figs. 17 and 18):

> We shall now consider further uses for this knowledge. There are children in our school with a very vivid imagination, and there are children with very little imagination. We need not jump to the conclusion that half of our students are poets and half are not. We notice the difference not so much in the actual way the imagination shows itself but rather in the way memory develops. Memory is strongly related to imagination. We have some children—and we should notice them—who quickly forget what they have experienced and heard during a lesson, who cannot hold on to the pictures of what they have experienced, for whom the pictures disappear. And we have other children for whom the pictures remain, assume an independent life of their own, and surface continuously, cannot be controlled. We should be well aware of these two types of children. There is, of course, a whole range between these two extremes. For children with a vivid imagination, memory causes the pictures to surface in a changed form. Most frequently, however, the pictures surface unchanged, as reminiscences. The children are then slaves to what they have experienced during the lessons. And then there are the children for whom everything disappears, evaporates.[281]

Expanding the physiological polarity into therapeutic activity, with special emphasis for different aspects of reading and writing:

> It is now a matter of dealing with these two types of children appropriately. It is possible to occupy groups of children in the most diverse ways if we develop a routine in the best sense of the word—a routine in a spiritual sense. Children with poor memory, who have difficulty in getting the pictures to surface, should be made to observe better during reading. We should have them listen better. With children who are slaves to their mental pictures, we should see to it that they become more physically active,

> mobile; we should make them concentrate more on writing. We could have two groups in the class—giving the children who are poor in imagination the opportunity for cultivating their reading and observation, while for the other group, the children with vivid imagination, we should especially cultivate painting and writing. Naturally, it is a matter of degree, because everything is relative.
>
> We can take this distinction further. (But only the following observation is really important: We can only gradually learn these things; we cannot cover everything during the first year.) Children who are poor in imagination—that is, children who cannot easily remember—should be asked to do eurythmy standing up, mainly with their arms. Children with a vivid imagination who are tormented by their mental pictures will benefit by moving the whole body, be it by running or by walking. This we can encourage. It really is very important that we pay attention to such matters.[282]

Then Steiner indicated how both poles can be met through eurythmy:

> In addition, we ought to know the value of the consonants for phlegmatic children who find it difficult to recall mental pictures, whereas the children who are tormented by their ever-surfacing mental pictures will greatly benefit from eurythmy exercises that concentrate mainly on vowel sounds. It can indeed be observed that vowel exercises have a calming effect on the rising mental pictures, while consonant exercises engender them. Acting on this knowledge can help both groups.[283]

And through music:

> The same distinction applies to music lessons. Children poor in imagination and memory should be encouraged to play musical instruments; children with a vivid imagination should be occupied with singing. It would be ideal—if we had the necessary rooms—to teach both groups simultaneously, one in singing, the other in instrumental music. If we could practice a twofold method—listening to and making music—this would have

> a tremendous harmonizing effect on the children. It would be most valuable if we could make it possible to alternate between singing and listening: to let half the class sing and the other half listen, and then vice versa. This practice should really be cultivated, because listening to music has a hygienic, a healing effect on what the head is to do in the human organism; singing has a healing effect on what the body is to do in the head. If we carried out everything that we could in this way, we would have far healthier people about.[284]

The imagination-rich and imagination-poor polarity helps us understand the physiology of memory as it relates to the soul life, particularly to the feeling life. We are mostly still working in the realm of the "I" and astral body.

A second, related memory polarity was brought by Steiner in the curative course. This polarity of sulfur-rich and sulfur-poor allows us to see the continued settling of impressions as they meet the etheric and even the physical bodies. This description extends further down into the metabolism. We learn that the activity of the "I" and astral in the head organization engenders a reciprocal, but unconscious activity in the metabolism. The formation of a memory and the remembering of that memory live in the breathing activity between these two physiologic realms:

> Suppose we receive something through the medium of our head—as we do when, for instance, we listen to what another person is saying. Having been received by our head, it goes first into the "I" and into the astral body. But an interplay is always taking place in the human organism, and the moment something is caught and held fast, by means of an impression received in the one "I"-organization (here in the head), it immediately vibrates right through into the other "I"-organization (below). And then the same thing happens the moment something strikes home in the astral organization; that, too, vibrates right through into the other "I"-organization. If it were not so, we would not have memory. We owe our memory to the

> fact that all the impressions we receive from the external world have their reflections, their mirror images, in the metabolism-and-limbs organization. If I receive an impression from without, it disappears from the head organization.... For the "I" must maintain itself, it must hold its own. It cannot carry one single impression for hours on end; if it did, it would have to identify itself with the impression. No, it is down below that the impressions are preserved; and they have to make their way up again, for us to "remember" them.[285]

Steiner also gave a description of the process when it is weakened and memories are not able to settle:

> But now, it may well happen that the whole of the lower system, which, as we have seen, in direct polar contrast to the upper system, is constitutionally weak. In that case, when impressions occur, the impressions do not stamp themselves deeply enough into the lower system.... Then the impressions that fail to sink down into the "I"-organization of the lower system keep streaming back again into the head.
>
> We have with us a child who is constituted just in this way. One day I showed him, for the first time, a watch.... I sit down by this child, and begin to talk to him. All the time he is perpetually saying: "Lovely watch!" Hardly have I said a few more words than he says again: "A lovely watch!" The impression keeps coming back.... For if we do not succeed in strengthening the too-weak organization of metabolism and limbs, then this "streaming back" of impressions will go on happening with greater and greater intensity, and in later life the patient will suffer from the kind of paranoia that is associated with obsessive ideas. He will suffer from firmly fixed ideas. He will know that these ideas have no business to take up their abode, as it were, in his soul in this persistent way, but he will not be able to dismiss them. Why can he not dismiss them? Because while, up there above there is the conscious soul-life, the unconscious, down below, is out of control; it keeps pushing certain ideas back into consciousness, which then become obsessive ideas.[286]

And now the polarity extends all the way down to the physical level, as Steiner linked obsessive ideas with an inadequate substance activity, that of sulfur:

> When metabolism and limbs are too weakly developed, the protein substance in the human organism is prevented from containing the right amount of sulfur. We then have a metabolism-and-limbs system which produces proteins that are low in sulfur.[287]

Then, in contrast, is the opposite process, where there is too much sulfur:

> But now the opposite condition may arise. The system of metabolism and limbs may be so constituted that it is too strongly attracted to sulfur. The protein will then be too rich in sulfur.... In a metabolism-and-limbs system of this kind—for the system is influenced in its manifestations by the particular combination of the substances within it—there will not be, as before, the urge to push everything back. But, on the contrary, in consequence of the proteins being too rich in sulfur, the impressions will be absorbed too powerfully, they make themselves too much at home.
>
> Note that this is a different condition from the one I described in an earlier lecture, where there is a congestion at the surface of an organ [the epileptic process]. That condition gives rise, as we saw, to fits. It is not a congestion that we have now, but a kind of absorption of the impressions. The impressions are, as it were, sucked in—and consequently disappear. We bring it about that the child has impressions, but to no purpose; impressions of a particular nature simply disappear into the sulfur-rich proteins. And only if we can succeed in getting these impressions back, in drawing them out again from the sulfur-rich proteins—only then shall we be able to establish a certain balance in the whole organism of spirit, soul, and body. For the disappearance of the impressions in the sulfurousness of the metabolic–limb system induces a highly unsatisfactory condition of soul; it has a disturbing, exciting effect. The whole organism is a little agitated, a

> slight tremor runs through it.... Suppose I have a child to educate within whom I observe that impressions cause difficulties. This may, of course, be because of conditions described in the previous lectures. But if I am right in attributing it to the condition we have been describing today, then how am I to proceed?[288]

Rudolf Steiner next links qualities of the etheric body—relating to the sulfur content of proteins, which hold and store memories—with observable qualities of the physical body:

> To begin with, I look at the child. (The first thing is, of course, to know such children, to become thoroughly acquainted with them; this is the first essential.) I look at such children and notice one of the most superficial symptoms—namely, the hair color. If the child has black hair, I will not bother to investigate whether he is rich in sulfur, for those with black hair certainly cannot be rich in sulfur, though it is possible they are poor in sulfur. If, therefore, abnormal symptoms are present, I have to look for their cause in some other area. Even when recurring ideas show themselves, in the case of those with black hair, I will nevertheless have to look for the cause somewhere other than in the richness of sulfur. If, however, I am dealing with fair-haired or red-haired children, I look for signs of too much sulfur in the proteins. Fair hair is the result of excessive sulfur; black hair comes from iron in the human organism.[289]

Next we are given a psychological depiction of the child's inner state, where the metabolism stores all of these impressions. Such an excessive holding process leads to an agitation that is pervasive, though largely unconscious (as opposed to the very conscious, "slave"-like obsessional thinking of the sulfur-poor child):

> Now, let us take a little volcano of this kind—sulfurous children, who suck down impressions into the area of the will, where they stiffen and cannot get out. We are quickly able to detect this in such children. They will be subject to states of depression and melancholy. The hidden impressions they carry within

are a torment to them. We must raise them to the surface, and we must go about it not with psychoanalysis, as it is understood today, but with a true and right psychoanalysis. We must observe children and the kind of thing that is inclined to disappear in them. In the case of children who confront us, on the one hand, with inner excitement and outwardly, on the other hand, with a certain apathy, we have to watch them carefully until we can ascertain exactly what they easily remember and what they let disappear within them. We should repeatedly present things that do not come back to them again and again and, insofar as possible, in rhythmic sequence.[290]

Now a specific example:

A particularly odd little person. He was at once excited and apathetic.... His apathy showed itself in the fact that it was never easy to teach him anything; he never took anything in, he learned only very slowly and with difficulty. But scarcely had Herr K. turned away from him and begun to bend over another child in front, then up would jump this little spark and hit him smack on the backside! The boy was, you see, at one and the same time inwardly, in his will, like quicksilver and intellectually an apathetic child.

There are, in fact, quite a number of children who have this kind of disposition, in greater or lesser degree; and it is important to note that in such children the capacity for absorption of external impressions is as a rule limited to impressions of a particular kind and type. If we have the right inspiration—and it will come, once we have the right disposition of mind and soul—we shall find for the child a particular sentence, for example, and bring this very sentence to his attention. This can work wonders.[291]

Steiner built on this description. Having already linked a physical, "superficial" symptom (the color of the hair) to a functional imbalance (the simultaneous agitation and apathy), he went on to present a therapeutic intervention that addresses the thinking and feeling life of the child:

> As you live your way into this beholding of the world—not thinking about, but really beholding of the world—you will find that if you have children who is inwardly sulfurous, alert, and active but inwardly apathetic, then, through your ability to observe them, something will suggest itself to you in connection with them and their special constitution, which provides you with the right idea. Perhaps you will feel: Every morning I must say to them: *The sun is shining on the hill*—or it could be some other sentence, a very simple, ordinary statement. What matters is that it comes to rhythmically. When something of this kind is brought rhythmically to the children, approaching them from outside, as it were, then all the sulfurous element in them is unburdened; it becomes freer....
>
> Something quite wonderful can come out of letting the child repeat a verse that is in the nature of a prayer, even though there may be some among them who cannot say a word; you will find this repeating in chorus has a wonderful balancing influence. And particularly in the case of a child in whom impressions tend to disappear will it be important to induce certain impressions by means of such rhythmical impressions.... How can we explain this? The trouble is, as we have seen, that the internal parts of the child are not giving back the impressions; that is to say, the movement from below upward is too weak (and this is negative). If now we bring in a strong impulse from above, we rouse the movement from below (that is too weak) to a strong activity.[292]

Figure 19 brings together the different elements of Steiner's description of the sulfur-rich constitution and relates them to the four members.

After this first therapeutic picture, Steiner brought a contrasting indication for how we can soften thoughts for the sulfur-poor constitution, through murmuring:

> Suppose we have a child who already shows a tendency toward compulsive ideas. The raying back of impressions in these children is too strong; there is too little sulfur in the plasma. Here we shall have to do the contrary of what we did before. When we

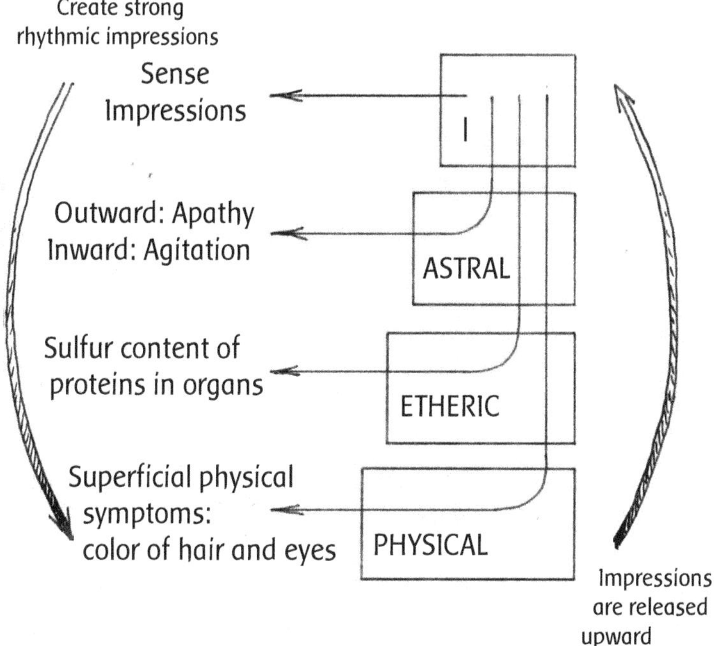

Figure 19: The relation of differentiated aspects of memory to the four members

observe that the same sentence, the same impression perpetually comes again and again to these children, it is helpful if we ourselves fabricate a new impression for them—one that our instinct tells us may be right for such children—and then bring it to them in a gentle whisper, murmuring softly in the ear.

The treatment could, for example, take the following form. The teacher says: "Look, that is red!" The child: "It's a lovely watch!" Teacher: "But you must look at the red." Child: "A lovely watch!" And now we try repeating, each time a little more softly, a new impression which has the effect of paralyzing the first. We say very softly: "Forget the watch!—Forget the watch!—Forget the watch!" Murmuring to the child in this way, you will find that you gradually murmur away the compulsive idea; as you murmur more and more softly, the compulsive idea begins to yield, it too grows fainter and fainter. The remarkable thing is that when the idea is spoken—when the child hears it spoken—it

> grows weaker; it gradually quiets down, and at length the child gets the better of it.[293]

This intentional murmuring—voicing a thought so that the child hears it spoken—helps to lift the impression up into more conscious "I"-activity so that it can then more fully move down to find a resting place in the etheric (and stop its bouncing in the astral body). It is very much the opposite of bringing a strongly repeated impression in order to stimulate an upward countermovement; it is a gentle stimulus so that the thought can fully settle.

Steiner rounded out his discussion by giving constitutional dietary recommendations. From pedagogical prayers and whispered murmurs, we now descend to the plant and mineral realms. For the sulfur-rich child we are instructed to give roots and salts:

> If we have children in whom impressions tend to disappear, it is good to begin with a definite resolve to combat a strong tendency in these children to develop sulfur in the protein. We can make good progress in this direction by seeing to it that they have the right kind of nourishment. If, for instance, we give them a great deal of fruit, or food prepared from fruit, we would be nurturing and fostering their sulfurous nature. If, on the other hand, we give them a diet derived from roots, containing substances that are rich not in sugar but in salts, then we will be able to heal such children. Naturally, this does not mean we are to sprinkle their food copiously with salt, but we should give them foods in which salts are present naturally.[294]

For the sulfur-poor child we should offer fruits and aromas:

> Take now the opposite case—children who fail to absorb impressions, children in whom the impressions stream back. These children are poor in sulfur, and the best treatment for them is to give them as much fruit as possible; they will soon acquire a taste for it and enjoy eating it. If their condition has become decidedly pathological, we should try also to bring fragrance and aroma to their food; they should have fruits that smell sweet. For aroma

contains a strong sulfurous element. And for a very serious case, we shall have to administer sulfur directly.[295]

These two memory polarities allow us to trace the interconnected but differentiated passing of impressions from the activity of the "I" of the head down to the receptive capacities of the etheric and physical bodies. Working with the two memory polarities in relation to each other brings several additional considerations:

- With these polarities we are given the possibility to offer therapeutic support on multiple levels: on the level of academic activity (emphasizing polar aspects of the reading and writing process); of artistic activity (through either making music and singing or the activity of listening); through eurythmy, running, or walking; by repeating a phrase or murmuring; through salty roots or aromatic fruits. The avenues for assistance are so generous that it is hard to imagine a situation where one (or even multiple) supports cannot be offered.
- The polarity of iron and sulfur is very helpful and striking when it is clinically encountered. It adds an additional, vital layer to the constitutional considerations described in the first three sections, as very sulfur-rich children with an epileptic constitution will likely struggle deeply to connect to the outside world (owing to disrupted consciousness) while also being less able to demonstrate that they are paying attention to what is happening around them (as their impressions disappear into their sulfurousness). Likewise, sulfur-poor (iron-rich) children with a hysteric constitution may well be both powerfully soul-sore (hysteric, sensing everything) and stuck (a slave to obsessively surfacing thoughts). In both cases, constitutional remedy treatments can be very powerful.
- Yet the sulfur-rich and sulfur-poor polarities are not universally applicable. For while variations in hair and eye color are present in some parts of the world, there are much larger populations and hereditary streams in

> which there are no children with blond hair and blue eyes (We may say, "If children have black hair, I will not take the trouble to investigate whether they are rich in sulfur, for those who have black hair certainly cannot be rich in sulfur, though it is possible they are poor in sulfur. If, therefore, abnormal symptoms are present, I shall have to look for their cause in some other sphere. Even if recurring ideas show themselves, I shall nevertheless, in the case of a child with black hair, have to look for the cause elsewhere than in the richness of sulfur.") This is important, as there are clearly great numbers of children in Japan, Egypt, or Guatemala whose impressions disappear, as well as in many other parts of the world where most every child has dark hair and eyes. We must then look for an imbalance more in the realm of soul activity (the astral body, imagination-rich / imagination-poor) than in qualities of the hereditary stream (etheric and physical, sulfur-rich / sulfur-poor), and consequently the appropriate therapeutic experiences will be brought through activities, not through diet.

It is also worth relating some of the specific pedagogical memory exercises Steiner brought before the teachers. Memory—much like another metabolic process, limb movement—is a pathway made smoother through practice. The exercises he suggested ask a child to move forward and then backward along a string of concepts or impressions. As an example:

> You can hardly strengthen memory other than by attempting to have the children imagine something backward, for instance, "the father reads in the book," turned around to, "book the in reads father the," so that they have a pictorial image of that. Or you can have them say the numbers 4, 6, 7, 3 in reverse order, 3, 7, 6, 4. Or perhaps the hardness scale back and forth.
>
> You also do not need to shy away from having the children repeat little poems that they have said word for word backward. That is a technique you can use when memory is so weak.[296]

When we carry out this kind of exercise we must lay down impressions (for there are too many items in the series to consciously hold in the "I" and astral activity of our sense organs at one time), but the impressions are soon liberated again as we come back to them when we work through the sequence in reverse order. With this kind of memory exercise the object spoken first (e.g., "the father") settles most deeply into the memory process (nearer to the etheric body) and then must correspondingly be mobilized the most when we get to the end of the phrase. This kind of memory work has a very long oral tradition and lives in the folk wisdom of many rhymes and songs ("This is the house that Jack built," "On the first day of Christmas my true love gave to me"). It is also the way that times tables and many other memory exercises are taught within the Waldorf curriculum.

In tracing these pathways, we become better and better able to understand a child's struggle and then bring healthy activities and experiences that will strengthen the child's capacity to know and learn from the outside world. Table 15 (pages 338–339) summarizes the main characteristics and variety of therapeutic support for both polarities: the imagination-rich / imagination-poor and sulfur-rich / sulfur-poor.

Table 15: Summary for memory polarities

Children who have trouble remembering	Children who have trouble forgetting
Imagination-poor	Imagination-rich
"[These] children quickly forget what they have...heard during a lesson [and] cannot hold on to the pictures of what they have experienced."	"Children for whom the pictures remain, assume an independent life of their own, and surface continuously" "Slaves to their mental pictures."
Therapeutic Pedagogical Activities	
Have them "listen better"; ask them to "observe better during reading."	"See to it that they become more physically active, mobile." "Make them concentrate more on writing."
Cultivate opportunities for "reading" and "observation."	"Especially cultivate painting and writing."
"[These] children...should be asked to do eurythmy standing up, mainly with their arms."	"Children with a vivid imagination who are tormented by their mental pictures will benefit by moving the whole body, be it by running or by walking."
"Children poor in imagination and memory should be encouraged to play musical instruments."	"Children with a vivid imagination should be occupied with singing."
Sulfur-rich	Sulfur-poor (iron rich)

Psychological Pattern

"They will be subject to states of depression and melancholy. The hidden impressions that they carry within them are a torment.... Up would jump this little spark and hit the boy smack on the backside! He was, you see, at one and the same time inwardly, in his will, like quicksilver and intellectually an apathetic child."

"If we do not succeed in strengthening the too weak metabolism-and-limbs organization, then this "streaming back" of impressions will go on happening with greater and greater intensity, and in later life the patient will suffer from the kind of paranoia that is associated with obsessive ideas."

Pedagogical Therapeutic Tools

"You will perhaps feel a need to say to them every morning: *The sun is shining on the hill*—or perhaps some other sentence; it can be quite a simple, ordinary statement. What matters is that it comes rhythmically. When something of this kind is brought to the children rhythmically, approaching them, as it were from outside, then all the sulfurous element in them is unburdened; it becomes freer."

"There is too little sulfur in the plasma. Here we shall have to do the contrary of what we did before. When we observe that the same sentence, the same impression is perpetually coming again and again to these children, it is helpful if we ourselves fabricate for them a new impression (one that our instinct tells us might be right for such children) and then bring it to them in a gentle whisper, murmuring softly in the ear."

"The trouble is, as we have seen, that the internal parts of the child are not giving back the impressions; that is to say, the movement from below upward is too weak (and this is negative). If now we bring in a strong impulse from above, we rouse the movement from below (that is too weak) to a strong activity."

"We say very softly: 'Forget the watch!—Forget the watch!—Forget the watch!' Murmuring to the child in this way, you will find that you gradually murmur away the compulsive idea; as you murmur more and more softly, the compulsive idea begins to yield, it too grows fainter and fainter. The remarkable thing is that when the idea is spoken—when the child hears it spoken—it grows weaker; it gradually quiets down, and at length the child gets the better of it."

Dietary Therapeutic Support

"These children are poor in sulfur, and the best treatment for them is to give them as much fruit as possible; they will soon acquire a taste for it and enjoy eating it. If their condition has become decidedly pathological, we should try also to bring fragrance and aroma to their food; they should have fruits that smell sweetly. For aroma contains a strong sulfurous element. And for a very serious case, we shall have to administer sulfur directly."	"If, for instance, we were to give them a great deal of fruit or food prepared from fruit, we would be nurturing and fostering their sulfurous nature. If, on the other hand, we give them a diet derived from roots, containing substances rich not in sugar but in salts, then we will be able to heal such children. Naturally, this does not mean we are to sprinkle the food copiously with salt, but we should give them foods in which salts are present naturally."

Chapter 29

Developmental Challenges, Opportunities, and Gifts

For Children Coming into the World Today

A question that often comes up in therapeutic circles is "Are the children coming into the world today different from the children of previous generations?" The answer is undoubtedly yes. Many teachers and doctors have observed that things are changing. The reasons for those changes are less certain, however, as they come from many different sides. It is clear, however, that there are an increasing number of incarnation challenges that make it more difficult to properly meet the physical body and then to come into healthy connection with the world around it.

A related comment, or concern, is that many of the steps of development that seemed to unfold more naturally, more instinctively in the past do not seem to unfold in the same way now. Many of today's children seem like a puzzle, needing extra attention and support. This means that we are being asked to look with new eyes. We are being asked to understand what underlies the most fundamental capacities of our humanity. Such knowledge informs the way we can nourish the life of all children. When anthroposophic medicine and Waldorf education were first being developed, there was perhaps a clearer distinction between the developmental supports needed for general education (pedagogy) and those needed for individualized (therapeutic) support. That distinction is blurred in many classrooms today.

The increasing prevalence of autism spectrum disorders is one expression of the challenges children meet in claiming and inhabiting the hereditary body. As a society, we have become quite aware of how the unfolding of higher social and moral capacities is hampered for these children. By learning about the different constitutions, we come to recognize that the ability to fully meet and sense another human being depends on how at home we are in the body. In the language of the polarities, the process of connection (through the nerve–sense system) builds upon a healthy process of integration (which builds the metabolic–limb system). So it is not unexpected to see, for example, that the formal diagnostic criteria for autism fall into categories of both challenged perceiving and reciprocating with the outside world and patterns of body-directed, self-stimulating behaviors. These closely mirror the outwardly directed and inwardly directed sensing pathway which make up the circle of the twelve senses (see fig. 20, page 346).

If we look, we can see how the developmental gestures of the polarities relate to autistic behaviors. It is necessary to look from several sides, because it is hard to identify one single pole or even one single polarity as being the main challenge in autistic behaviors. Nonetheless, we can find clues that give us very practical therapeutic orientation.

The diagnostic criteria begin by introducing the outer, more social expressions of autism (with additional commentary that relates to the constitutional polarities in italics):

> A. Persistent deficits in social communication and social interaction across multiple contexts, as manifested by the following, currently or by history (examples are illustrative, not exhaustive; see text):
>
> 1. Deficits in social-emotional reciprocity, ranging, for example, from abnormal social approach and failure of normal back-and-forth conversation; to reduced sharing of interests, emotions, or affect; to failure to initiate or respond to social interactions.[297]
>
> *These criteria show a spectrum of connection or, perhaps better said, lack of connection. We can think of this by asking, "How far out into the outer world can the child reach to sense the other?" Clearly part of the pathway through the outwardly directed senses is being blunted. The path from vision, to warmth,*

to hearing, to word, to thought, to sense of "I" is not easily traveled. We can gain insight by following this progression and asking, "Where is a step skipped, or where does the sensing stop?"

Generally, for children with autistic behaviors, the sense of vision is intact, but the next step, the sensing of warmth, may be underdeveloped. Bringing warmth into an interaction or responding to another person's warmth (social, emotional, or spiritual) may not routinely enter into social exchange. So we should look to see how the sense of warmth is present in any autistic behavior.

Next in the pathway comes hearing, and as we move further along, we may see another disruption, for although children with autistic behaviors may well be able to hear that another person is speaking (the hearing sense) and even understand the words (the word sense), they may not be able to reach further on to the ideas behind the words (the thought sense) or the nuances of experience and interpretation behind the thoughts (the "I" sense). Because sensing stops, communication is hampered. There is no easy flow through the higher senses, with the result that communication is sometimes puzzlingly concrete. To the child with an autistic experience, a word means a certain thing; interpretation is very literal, because sensing may stop with the word sense. Similarly, when information is shared by the child, it commonly comes without inflection or nuance. The more individual aspects of "thought" and "I" do not necessarily enter in, because they are not experienced. This necessarily affects the possibility for "normal back-and-forth conversation" and results in "reduced sharing" and even a full "failure to initiate or respond to social interactions." These children can really engage only with what they experience. They do not respond in the usual way because there are parts of the encounter that are not felt.

2. Deficits in nonverbal communicative behaviors used for social interaction, ranging, for example, from poorly integrated verbal and nonverbal communication; to abnormalities in eye contact and body language or deficits in understanding and use

of gestures; to a total lack of facial expressions and nonverbal communication.[298]

Here, again, there is a spectrum of connection—how much is felt? Now the sensing process depends not just on our sensing through the outer senses (see fig. 21, page 411) but also on how an outer perception resonates within our own bodies. Children's understanding of facial expression, body language, and gesture depends on the health of their own inner sense of movement, balance, and even the life sense. People know that a sad expression is sad because one imitatively reflect the other person's muscle movements (even if it is not outwardly visible), which then resonate into a child's own feeling life. If children have trouble sensing their own body, have trouble connecting their feeling life with their own physical movements and activities, then the ability to sense into the physical expression of another person will also be compromised. These challenges—though they express themselves as limited outer social interaction—are really grounded in an incomplete development of the lower senses. This second set of sensing activities, grounded in a sensing of self, remains opaque.

3. Deficits in developing, maintaining, and understanding relationships, ranging, for example, from difficulties adjusting behavior to suit various social contexts; to difficulties in sharing imaginative play or in making friends; to absence of interest in peers.[299]

These behaviors can be subtler and may be the only perceptible sensing imbalance with children who have Asperger's syndrome. Asperger's syndrome was discussed in the context of the kleptomaniacal pole (see chapter 8), where Steiner described how our capacity for moral perception is linked to the physiology of the limbs. This social challenge may relate not so much to a specific sense (like the sense of movement or the sense of thought) as to the whole physiology of the limbs.

Let us consider the capacity for social connection in yet another way. We are living in a world that overstimulates and prioritizes several of the middle senses—particularly smell, taste, and vision. Those sensory windows are bombarded continually, so that we are pulled to their activity over and over. Such a narrowed overemphasis distracts children from their inner sensing pathway and the development of the lower senses. It blunts their ability to self-soothe in very real ways (i.e., repeatedly offering a screen to a restless or bored child). This overemphasis on the middle senses also pulls attention away from the social/moral interaction that allows us to perceive beyond ourselves (as when a family is sitting at a table in a restaurant, all gazing independently at their smartphones). It is no wonder, then, that our ability to sense other human beings has stiffened and narrowed. We are all, as part of a modern, technological society less practiced in using all twelve of our senses. That change is pervasive. We should consider the possibility that autism spectrum disorders represent an accentuation of this process to the point of an illness, a karmic challenge to stimulate us to learn and remember what it means to truly perceive the other. We must work to stretch past the middle senses. This is emerging more and more as an urgent therapeutic, moral task.

The next set of diagnostic criteria relates to the ways children anchor themselves in their bodies. These patterns can give us very helpful clues about how to meet them therapeutically. While they are listed as "disorders," as part of a diagnosis, these patterns are more truthfully part of the innate wisdom that lives inside these children—they are sensory-seeking and orientation-seeking behaviors. When outer experiences or interactions are too difficult to navigate, returning to familiar patterns of self-stimulation helps a child feel safer and more grounded:

> B. Restricted, repetitive patterns of behavior, interests, or activities, as manifested by at least two of the following, currently or by history (examples are illustrative, not exhaustive...):

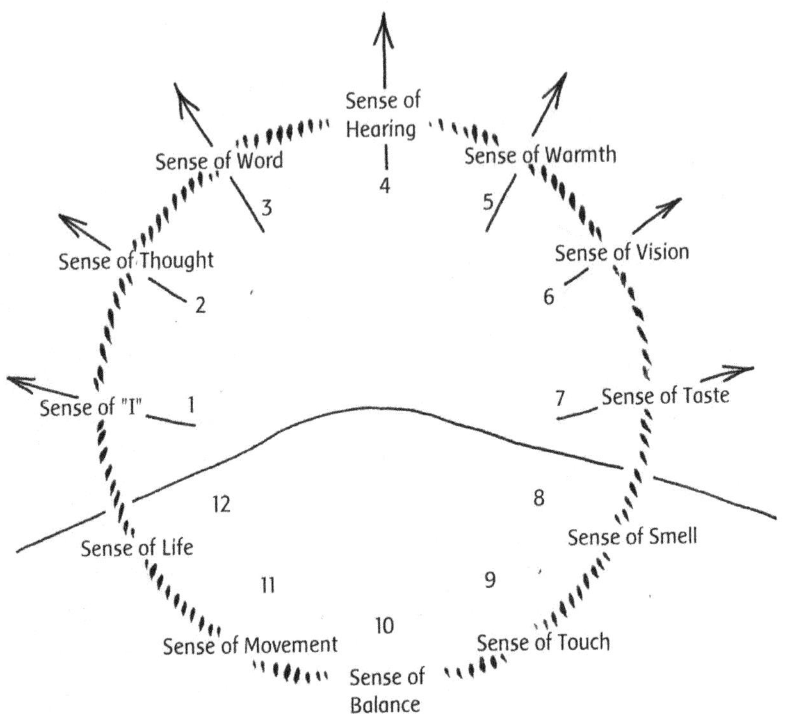

Figure 20: Inwardly and outwardly directed senses [300]

1. Stereotyped or repetitive motor movements, use of objects, or speech (e.g., simple motor stereotypies, lining up toys or flipping objects, echolalia, idiosyncratic phrases). [301]

Stereotyped or repetitive motor movements fall very much into the realm of anchoring through the lower senses. Hand flapping, rocking, or bouncing can be effective measures for following the inward pathway to the life sense, and if a child feels better inwardly, then outer experiences of disorientation are not so distressing. Even the examples of repetitive speech—"echolalia" (the repeating or parroting back of another's speech) or "idiosyncratic phrases" (repeating a stock phrase or set of words, which are often not in context)—are much more about inner anchoring and self-stimulation than an attempt to outwardly communicate. Many of the therapeutic indications for imbalanced movement (feeble/maniacal) and for strengthening the lower senses can be very helpful in these contexts.

2. Insistence on sameness, inflexible adherence to routines, or ritualized patterns of verbal or nonverbal behavior (e.g., extreme distress at small changes, difficulties with transitions, rigid thinking patterns, greeting rituals, need to take same route or eat same food every day).[302]

"Extreme distress at small changes" and consistent retreat to familiar patterns have been discussed as aspects of the hysteric constitution. Many children with autistic behaviors exhibit distinct pockets of soul-soreness, which are compounded by the challenge of not being able to rely on some of the usual sensing pathways (as discussed earlier). Some sense activities may be heightened to help compensate for others that are numbed. This is a little bit like the vulnerability that comes from being in complete darkness (unable to use the vision sense) and being surprised by an unexpected loud noise (a de facto hypersensitive). Steiner's therapeutic indications for bringing the astral body back into a more balanced relationship with the physical and etheric bodies are very helpful, especially the indications for consciously helping children to know that you are feeling with them and understanding their experience, that you help guide their hand (as with a paintbrush). Subtle "shocks," in the form of humor or distraction, can also help to ease some of this "insistence on sameness."

3. Highly restricted, fixated interests that are abnormal in intensity or focus (e.g., strong attachment to or preoccupation with unusual objects, excessively circumscribed or repetitive interests).[303]

These repetitive patterns can be part of a retreat to safe or known objects. Or they can speak to a rigidity of the body that extends into the soul life (see Appendix 2 for organ treatments, especially for the lung). Or they may be part of a repeated attempt to more fully penetrate the physical and etheric bodies, either via a more feeble pattern (repetitive gross motor) or an epileptic pushing through (working to connect over and over again with an outer element). It is good to look to see whether the perseverative pattern is more an expression of retreat (hysteric) or an attempt—however limited in its focus—to connect, connect, connect to what is outside (epileptic). Both this pulling back and pushing out can be seen.

4. Hyper- or hyporeactivity to sensory input or unusual interest in sensory aspects of the environment (e.g., apparent indifference to pain/temperature, adverse response to specific sounds or textures, excessive smelling or touching of objects, visual fascination with lights or movement).[304]

These behaviors speak to the fact that for an autistic child, constitution may need to be considered in pieces, that is, that it is very possible for a child to have an epileptic pattern with one sense (needing to smell over and over or touch and rub over and over) combined with a more hysteric pattern related to another sense activity (tremendous fear of loud or unexpected noise). The relationships of body and spirit are more complicated on this incarnation pathway, as the higher members may flow too far past the physical and etheric in one area yet be held back so strongly as to be nearly numbed in another. Therapeutic support, looking through the epileptic and hysteric lens, may need to be differentiated for specific sensory organs or sensory pathways.

The diagnostic criteria make clear that there can be a broad diversity of incarnation challenges in autism, but we can help the child find footholds through thoughtful observation and individualized therapeutic support.

An additional and sometimes challenging aspect of working with autism spectrum imbalances is that we may see incomplete development on both sides of a polarity, that is, that a child may have sluggish, heavy movement that alternates with quick, unpenetrated, and unguided movement. We may come to the conclusion that a child's body is both heavy from a dominant hereditary stream and unpenetrated because the "I" and astral body are only superficially engaged. In this way the child is both earthly and cosmic. This is an unusual situation, for most children truly do fall on one side or the other of the constitutional polarities, but when there are greater incarnation challenges, both sides of a child's physiology may need to be sculpted and guided.

We can see a similar paradoxical pattern with the other polarities as well, that a child with autism will sometimes show patterns of being both large-headed (challenged to really liberate forces away from the body in order to sense the outside world) and small-headed (challenged to fully meet and transform digestive substance taken into the body). Finding this constitutional duality in the sensing realm was just discussed (hyper- and hyposensitivity). Epileptic patterns (a thick-skinned numbness) and hysteric reactions (a true soul-soreness) may present in different sensory realms—like being numbed to self-movement but hypersensitive to sound—or both patterns may appear in the same sense organ, with a varying activity of the higher members flowing through (to be either thick-skinned or thin-skinned, depending on the specific stimulus and on the specific day).

Given all of these variations, it can be hard to know where to start. Here are a few observations that can help prioritize and organize therapeutic support. First, if we are faced with imbalances on both sides of a single polarity (say, both feeble and maniacal movement patterns), it is usually better to start with the more body-oriented side of the polarity—that is, start by making the density of the physical body more accessible and more comfortable. Then, once we have worked to warm and stir the body, we can invite the higher members in—loosening, then inviting, warming, then inviting, and so on. It does not work as well to ask the higher members to overcome their superficial engagement when the body is still hard to enter.

Similarly, if a child exhibits both a metabolic–limb system that is out of order (a small-headed tendency) and a nerve–sense system that is out of order (large-headed), we should work to strengthen digestion first. Many children with autism benefit from foundational digestive support. This should not seem unusual because it follows the archetypal patterning of childhood, that out of metabolic health and ripeness, thought and sensing activities emerge.

Within the epileptic-hysteric polarity, protecting hypersensitivity is often the best place to start. This does not mean that the child should be buffered to a place of constant retreat or isolation—no, there does need to be encounter. Firm, steady touch can feel very good for hysteric sensing too, it just needs to start from an experience of safety and security. Create opportunities for the child to initiate contact.

If support with anthroposophic medicines is being given, and there are imbalances on both sides of a polarity, supporting the rhythmic system can be very helpful. (We can think of medicines like Cardiodoron, Aurum, even Belladonna—see Appendix 2). Specifically supporting the middle can be helpful with other therapeutic modalities as well, such as eurythmy therapy, music therapy, and so forth.

Another important consideration is to respect the biographical age of the child, which may not necessarily be the same as the developmental age. In the first seven years, strengthening the integration process of the metabolism should be the priority for an autistic child. From seven to fourteen years, give special attention to the rhythmic realm, to the feeling life, and to how etheric forces are being liberated. From ages fourteen to twenty-one, work to foster deeper, fuller sensing connection with the outside world. Supporting the appropriate developmental process for a particular age speaks to the soul and spiritual development of the child. This is still coursing forward, even if the soul and spirit are not able to fully shine through the physical and etheric bodies.

All of these suggestions should, naturally, be considered with flexibility. When we really look with sincere interest and a devotion, answers are often whispered to us. If we are still totally without orientation, we can remember to look at the child's own (perhaps troubling) behaviors and ask what they are trying to accomplish. What experience are these children seeking, trying to create for themselves? They are being guided through an archetypal wisdom. We are, in fact, only humble partners in a seen and unseen developmental orchestration.

As a closing thought, we look at the gifts of the different constitutions. Most of our considerations have been devoted to understanding the challenges of leaning too far to one side or the other, but one should indeed ask what is gained by working through a process that does not archetypally unfold. The answer—gifts of greater consciousness and experience, which arise out of the will activity that is part of any constitutional rebalancing.

As described in part 1, children preparing for birth gather the substance of their astral body in relation to the knowledge they already carry (like iron filings responding to a passing magnet). How well the heart, sense of balance, or eye is formed depends on how deeply the activity of those organs has been known. When a hereditary body is chosen that does not have a healthy liver, it might be because the liver process has not yet been met in full consciousness. Constitutional imbalances ask us repeatedly to meet a specific part of our physiology. When that imbalance can be worked with and transformed, riches come. The fruits may not be immediately visible; they may not be evident for many years—or with a really significant imbalance, perhaps not even until a future incarnation—but they do come.

We can be reassured that there are indeed gifts associated with each constitution if we remember that a meditative activity has been presented in concert with each of the three major polarities. This points to the fact that there is indeed a relationship between the developmental work of coming into the body and higher spiritual or moral capacities.

What kinds of gifts are related to constitution? They come from two different sides. The first aspect is not hard to recognize, in that we are naturally good at doing what comes naturally, that is, when one aspect of our physiology naturally tends to lean to one side, we feel comfortable with it, and we know well how to live there. Such one-sidedness can be a challenge, but it can also act as a virtue. In other words, if one naturally connects to details (a small-headed inclination), then there will be lots of situations where that ability to analyze will be very helpful. Loving and living in details is then a great boon. Such innate gifts are granted to us as part of our constitutional tendencies—we receive them as part of our entry into life.

The secondary category of gifts is perhaps not quite so obvious and certainly not as easily won. They come out of the work we do with our own one-sidedness when we consciously strive to move past an inclination and to balance it. It might be very easy for a feeble child to sit all day and look at a well, to stay in the heaviness of the physical body, but for a maniacal child to learn to gaze in reverence—that has special potency. Children with a maniacal inclination have had to embrace their superficiality and move beyond it. We do not just happen into that activity—we help found it; we are a conscious participant in its creation. There is a will element involved, which lends a particularly moral quality to the new capacity.

The exact gifts revealed are, of course, as manifold as the individual variations of constitution. Here are some of the "fruits" that have been observed:

- A love of work, optimism for what can become. Children who have really worked through the earthly/feeble constitution have strengthened their own capacity for initiating and sustaining activity. The practice of stirring and loosening the physical body, over and over again, brings knowledge about how the earthly realm can be worked with in order to make it a good home for the spirit. Steadfastness, a love of real work and labor—those are some of the fruits of having wrestled repeatedly with the density and heaviness of the earthly body. The child has learned how stiff or unwieldy physicality can, in fact, be refined and transformed. Sculptors and builders, architects and engineers, gardeners and farmers all benefit from carrying this kind of special relationship to the earthly element. This gift also expresses itself as optimism, especially about what is possible and what can still come into being.

- A broad, impartial, but dedicated gaze. The child with a cosmic/maniacal constitution carries a certain natural freedom from earthly worries, a capacity for objectivity, and a skill for abstraction (as there is no burden of excessive sentimentality). Those qualities are innate, even as they are part of a certain superficiality. If that inherent tendency has really been worked with and transformed, inquisitiveness and a new reverence emerge—something along the lines of "I never realized how many different kinds of leaves there are in the world, until I started looking more closely." Learning to observe in this way brings powers of observation that are still flexible, not too enmeshed, yet quite astute. When this capacity for gazing with reverence ripens, many different ideas, topics, and interests can be pursued and investigated over the course of a lifetime. This could express itself in a love of invention, of inquiry into constitutional law, of anthropology or botany—all activities where a broad gaze needs to be combined with the power to penetrate very specific topics or activities and impartiality with a real reverence for ideas become manifest.
- Making archetypes practical and perceptible. The child with a large-headed constitution often carries a kind of emotional and social shielding from life and stays a little innocent. Awareness emerges more slowly, as it is first preceded by metabolic maturation. This means that there has been a stepwise, growing capacity to fully digest whatever is taken in, be it nutritional, social, or sensory. Inner preparation comes before outer activity. This is innate. When a child then learns to move past the amalgamation of large-headed thought (lumping it all into one) and instead finds connection to the details of the surrounding world, then a capacity emerges to make larger truths and archetypes approachable. The beauty or artistry of the whole is held, even as the details are being dealt with. A symphony conductor, grassroots organizer, novelist, or graphic designer all benefit from living in these larger realms of

harmony, idealism, narration, and proportion, while making sure the practical aspects are not neglected.

- Seeing nuance, with a potent sense for quality. The child with a small-headed constitution, who from early on has experienced an acute awareness of the world, is often very aware of the effect of outside influences on the body. This can be in the realm of substance, of food, of drink, of tone, or of form. When that sensing process evolves beyond distraction or brooding awareness, it can become a discerning sense for quality. Nuance, variation, freshness, and wholesomeness are evident and accessible. Most of the world's great chefs were probably not (large-headed) children who grew up content to eat anything. No, they knew right away what was good and what was not. Orienting toward the details of things but moving beyond that to a place of relation and comparison can make someone a wonderfully practical connoisseur. These are very healthy traits for an editor, a weaver, an accountant, a wine taster, or even an Olympic judge.
- Perseverance, pushing to find new skill and capacity. The child with an epileptic constitution has had to push and push from the inside in order to meet the outside. The physical and etheric bodies have not fit like a glove; they are not a natural vessel. Connecting to the outer world is always a task. This brings a certain sheltering for the child, since with thick-skinned sensing often only the strongest stimuli are felt. That can make one better able to bear physical hardship. The repeated practice of working to push into and through the substance of the body literally strengthens the process for resculpting the physical and etheric. In this way, the body can be pushed to do what might not usually be tolerated. Battling with an epileptic constitution brings a strong drive to make the body a more fitting vessel for the spirit and to connect that spirit with the outside world and its elements. Many great athletes, warriors, and explorers show this capacity. They carry this kind of conquering spirit. An additional quality of the epileptic constitution is that while outer connection is not easy, when it is made, it is often genuine and forthright.

- Finely tuned encounters with tremendous receptivity. The child with a hysteric constitution has always felt far out into the world, easily beyond the borders of the physical body. Outer mood and expectation have never been a mystery; in fact, the outer environment has been so well known that it often determines the state of the child's inner world. Knowing one's place in the world therefore comes quickly and naturally, as does swiftly perceiving one's influence on the surroundings. While this can make for vulnerability, it can also evolve into a gift for connection and communication. Sympathy is strong—an actor on the stage greatly benefits from noting and responding to the inflection of another performer while being able to simultaneously perceive the mood and attention of the audience. The artistry of encounter, whether through a finely tuned performance, a counseling session, a debate, or a nuanced negotiation, benefits from such strong sensing. Being able to feel and anticipate the other's reaction stands out as an important part of the process. Such receptivity makes for quick assessment and adjustment in all forms of interaction.

Each of these deeper gifts grows out of a process of self-knowledge. There are several archetypal steps.

- First comes the step of recognizing one's own inclination or a pattern. This can be great surprise, because up until now it was just natural—innate.
- Next, gather information about it. This allows us to step back from it a little, in order to begin to see it more objectively (perhaps even to begin to see it as an archetype or at least a pattern).
- Then we can take the additional step of actively engaging with that pattern in order to transform it or refine it. This third step is a will activity.

It is also what Steiner described as an essential aspect of personal development and which he related to the consciousness soul. Steiner characterized this modern phase of history we are in right now as the time of the consciousness soul, where we—as a whole social cohort of human beings—are being asked to move beyond mere sensing (which belongs to the "sentient," or sensing, soul) and beyond characterizing (which belongs to the "intellectual" or "mind" soul). We are being challenged—socially, emotionally, physiologically, morally—to recognize what belongs to our full humanity and then act in ways to claim and nurture those aspects. This third step is an important part of any illness and healing process, for we are generally not adequately aware of the importance of something until it falls far out of balance. When we then work to reclaim something, it becomes more truly ours than it ever was before, and we own it in a different way.

We learn to know things better through imbalance. One response to this is distress, to lament the loss of more instinctive, less complicated pathways into life. Indeed, when we focus on the immediate consequences of those challenges, there is reason to mourn, but if we can see the broader process and appreciate that something is also being learned, we find courage. By working through a process over and over—experiencing what it truly means to move, to feel, to sense, to connect—we know ourselves better.

The same process stands behind therapeutic work with children. We learn to observe, to know the patterns and pathways of growth and development, and then take a step to help someone who is struggling. Steiner brought a lovely imagination for this process with the image of a white rose:

> What is the difference among the sentient soul, intellectual (mind) soul, and consciousness soul? The sentient soul operates when we are merely gazing at the things of the external world. If we withdraw our attention for a while from the impressions of this outer world and work over them inwardly, then we are given over to the mind soul. But if we now take what has been worked over in thought, turn again to the outer world, and relate ourselves to it by passing over to deeds, then we are given over to the consciousness soul. For example, as long as I am simply looking

> at these flowers in front of me and my feelings are moved by the pure whiteness of the rose, I am given up to my sentient soul. If, however, I avert my gaze and no longer see the flowers but only think about them, then I am given over to my intellectual (mind) soul. In thought, I am working on the impressions I have received. If I say to myself now that—because the flowers have given me pleasure, I will gladden someone else by presenting them to that person and then pick them up to hand them over—I am performing a deed. I am passing from the realm of the mind soul into that of the consciousness soul and relating myself again to the outer world. Here is a third force that operates in human beings and enables us not only to work over the impressions of the outer world in thought, but also to relate ourselves to that world again.[305]

From this process we can see how working with the constitutional polarities contributes—one small step at a time, however humbly—toward the process of finding our true humanity. This is true when we work to help children find more balanced relationships with their bodies and with the world around and when we look toward the future fruits that will come out of their growth and experience and to the greater knowledge we all carry forward as fruits of our communal striving and spiritual work.

Appendices

Appendix 1

Constitutional Support through the Biographical Stages of Childhood

While we all carry overall constitutional leanings during our lifetime, each of us also experiences developmental swings as we work our way through the rhythms of biography. This means that at certain ages all of us, regardless of more individual inclinations, tend toward a specific experience of our body or of the world. Such rhythmic changes correspond to important nodal points of growth. These nodes often relate to the blossoming stages of growth we have already explored through the constitutional polarities. This means that a stage of growth that recapitulates the earthly heaviness of the physical body will be more challenging for a child with feeble movement and that a step of independent awareness will potentially be much more anxiety-provoking for a small-headed or hysteric child. All children work through these developmental changes. Some stages will be dramatic, some so natural they are hardly noticeable. If we look at the underlying developmental gestures of the first twenty-one years of life, we begin to discover links between constitution and biography.

These rhythms of biographical development unfold because of the differentiated and evolving activity of the four members of the human being. There are births not only of the physical body but also of the etheric, astral, and "I." Each member is present at birth but then makes significant steps in independent activity and conscious capacity over the first twenty-one years. That progression is very helpfully laid out by Dr. Edmond Schoorel in his book *The First Seven Years: Physiology of Childhood.*[306] He explains how the development of each member can be described in two different aspects: first, in terms of how its activity becomes individualized (relating to an activity within the body, an inner birth), which is followed by a corresponding later further step in which forces become independent from the body and move more into conscious activity (an outer birth, very much analogous to moving from a stage of building organs to using the organs). From Dr. Schoorel's description we can understand that the physical body becomes individualized with the process of conception, when a distinct physical structure is formed (the embryo, evolving into the fetus); then, about nine months later, the physical body becomes independent through the birthing process, when it physically separates from the mother's body. Parallel steps of maturation can also be traced for the etheric, astral, and "I":

- The shifts for the etheric body: first, the physical birth process (in which the etheric makes its first step, becoming individualized and etherically distinct from the mother's forces) and then the seventh year of life (when etheric forces are emancipated from their earlier task of organ development and freed for activities of abstract thought and memory)
- Shifts for the astral body: the first birth in the third year (ages two to three, "the terrible twos," when astral sensing and the emotional life awaken in a new way through the forces of sympathy and antipathy), and then outwardly through adolescence (ages twelve to fourteen, accompanied by physical changes of sexual maturation, when the feeling life opens to experience social cohesion and isolation, joy and sorrow, and artistic depth and sensitivity)
- Shifts for the "I"-being: the first birth in the ninth year (often referred to as the "Rubicon," when there a strong realization of individual identity, as a separateness from parents, teachers, siblings and friends comes to the fore) and then again in the twenty-first year (when the experience of true individual intention and morality dawns, often accompanied by a step out into independent adult life away from the family and community of origin).

We now take these nodal points (conception, birth, third year, seventh year, ninth year, fourteenth year, twenty-first year) and explore how the changing activity of the corresponding spiritual member relates to aspects of constitution and also how each phase can be supported therapeutically. Indications for select anthroposophic medicines are also included—this lays the first foundations for bridging the pedagogical and therapeutic pictures given in parts 1 to 4, and the medical work of a physician who is trained in prescribing these medicines (see Appendix 2 for more details).

Conception: With this step the physical body becomes distinct from the body of the mother and father, the very first step of individualization. Here begins the meeting of the hereditary and spiritual streams. All of the spiritual planning that has preceded this incarnation must now begin to reconcile itself to the physical body. The way in which the physical meeting of egg and sperm happens (the combining of two hereditary streams) can influence how accessible the hereditary body becomes for the incarnating individuality. Mechanically facilitated conception processes, such as in vitro fertilization or artificial insemination, remove the egg and sperm from the etheric sheaths of the mother's body, which can exaggerate the density and gravity of the hereditary body. Also, older ovum or sperm are known to increase the risk of birth defects and developmental challenges like autism, which we can similarly relate to an inherent physical density (and relatively weakened etheric) that limits or slows the healthy transformation of the physical body. It is therefore useful to consider the feeble/maniacal (earthly/cosmic) polarity for any situations where the meeting of the spiritual and hereditary streams has been "physicalized," either by older parents or by conception not being held in the etheric protection of the uterus. Preserving the possibility for strong childhood inflammations may also be particularly important for these children.

Birth and Infancy: With birth the physical body becomes independent and etheric forces individualized. The corresponding shifts of these two bodies (physical and etheric) are important, as the healthiest window for delivery comes when there has been enough organ growth that an infant can successfully switch from growing its organs to using them. When a child is born quite early, then on the physical level organs that should still be in the developing stage are suddenly forced to make functional use of them. This earlier-than-ideal transition accentuates a shift away from upbuilding, metabolic etheric activity to conscious, body-free etheric activity. (Think of building the eyes versus needing to use the eyes to see.) In that process some organs can become prematurely physicalized and fall into a hardened state, which will make it more difficult to really penetrate and claim the organs completely later on. Premature delivery can therefore predispose a child to more challenges with the polarity of integration in a way that is similar to the influence of artificially facilitated conception processes. In this way we can see how prematurity may accentuate the physicality of early life.

For children who then go on to experience very slowed development, particularly when there is a clear density and heaviness of the physical body, we can think of the remedies recommended for the feeble constitution (delayed gross motor milestones): for a heavy body with low tone, Arsenicum, Levico, or Scorodite, and, for limited mobility, Mercurius to the lower limbs

Prematurity also significantly impacts the etheric body, as physical independence comes before etheric forces are really ready to be fully individualized. This may leave an overall etheric depletion. That potential depletion is compounded by the required shift in etheric activity toward wakeful, sensing activity. We can therefore view prematurity as a kind of karmic, situational small-headedness (one that is already present at birth). For this reason, remedies that support and nurture the etheric are very helpful, especially where there is pronounced metabolic weakness and poor growth or a very low birth weight: Argentum, or Argentite (usually for children with darker hair and eyes), Bryophyllum, Oxalis.

Ages two to three years (the third year of life): This age marks an individualizing process for the astral body—with a newfound sense of self and not-self, sympathy and antipathy, that functions at a largely unconscious, nonvolitional level. These forces that work in the metabolism and feeling life are later liberated into conscious awareness (at puberty). The "terrible twos" can be recognized as a little adolescence and may bring forward a variety of excessively astral, cramp-like experiences and behaviors, such as temper tantrums; breath-holding spells; aggressive behaviors like hitting, biting, and yelling; mood swings; and newfound likes and dislikes. To help balance these newly strengthened astral forces with the established etheric forces, we can turn to the nightshades (Belladonna, Hyoscyamus) and Chamomile and Cuprum. Specific organ therapy may also be helpful, as the archetypes of independent organ activity are beginning to form. (For more on adolescent astral changes, see "Adolescence," page 367.)

Ages six to seven years (the seven-year change): This age marks when the etheric body becomes independent, with growth forces liberated into thinking activity. New capacities for abstract thought and memory develop. This signals the outward birth of the etheric and a step into a whole new way of understanding and remembering the world. At this time the large-headed and small-headed polarity—as an expression of being too young/too metabolic versus too aware/too soon—becomes particularly useful and pertinent. Before the age of seven, constitutional treatments with lead (Plumbum) should really be reserved for very specific conditions (such as *osteogenesis imperfecta*), because the child rightfully should not yet be coming into full wakeful sensing. It is obviously inappropriate to give a treatment for drawing forth a maturation process that has not yet rightfully appeared. By age seven, however, the shifting toward a stronger nerve–sense state should be happening, such that we can begin to critically judge a child's objectivity and awareness—that is, to ask the question whether this child is moving forward into the life of a grade school child, as we would expect.

At the same time, the dissolving of the etheric connections that have existed between child and mother can bring out separation fears and regressive behaviors on a very visceral level. Children recognize they are not held in the way they used to be. Bryophyllum helps anchor the child's own etheric in the metabolism (versus relying on the mother's etheric) and eases feelings of isolation, such as separation anxieties or newfound difficulty falling asleep. Etheric support of this kind is useful as a measured therapy (for weeks or for a few months). Regressive behaviors that persist beyond that period of time often instead benefit from iron (see nine-year change). For children who are old enough to go on to first grade but who do not show the expected physiologic changes of organ maturation, etheric support can also be given. Magnesium (for a younger child, in the form of Magnesite), which supports the eruption and progression of the adult teeth, can be administered. For children who seem to be having trouble liberating forces from the metabolism up into the thinking realm, etheric support with organ preparations containing Pulmo, Hepar, Renes, and Cor can be considered. This is an alternate kind of treatment for children who are staying "too young" and remain metabolically dominant but who perhaps are not etherically strong enough to do a Plumbum treatment or who show existing patterns of organ weakness.

Nine-year change: The "I" now becomes individualized (which will later unfold into the full step of "I" independence in the twenty-first year). There are several important aspects of this change. The child has a very strong growth experience of individuality, of truly being a single person, separate from parents, teachers, and siblings.[307] This often brings fears of death, of separation, and of loss. Etheric buffering (with a remedy like Bryophyllum) can sometimes be helpful, but only as a temporary measure, because this nine-year change does not bring a shift of etheric forces like that of the seven-year change. Remedies that support the "I" more directly are more helpful, such as Urtica (stinging nettle) when vitality is generally low or preparations of mineral iron, such as Meteoric Iron or Ferrum sidereum, a cosmic iron that is very supportive when there are fears or anxieties on a more spiritual level, or Ferrum carbonicum when the problems show up more in the realm of digestion and metabolism (such as early morning stomachaches that come while getting ready for school). The iron remedies generally help one to find the forces to meet and take on the new steps of individuation with more strength and courage. Aurum (gold) is also very helpful—balancing and bringing more inner light. It is often given at this age in a middle potency (10x). Aurum helps to bring reassurance. Stibium (antimony) provides more of an inner anchor, a remedy for the "I" that gives proper form and organization to metabolic processes.

Adolescence (twelve to fourteen years): This period is when the astral body becomes independent. This developmental milestone has become more complicated as physical, emotional, and spiritual changes separate from one another. It is increasingly common for the physical changes of sexual maturation to come much earlier, while true emotional and social maturation may come later (even if they are preceded by a kind of imitative precocious sexuality). In earlier times, when the astral aspect of social life and community was much more dominant, pubertal changes marked a true transition into adult life and readiness for marriage and children. With the current developmental emphasis on individualization, adult maturation depends more on the emancipation of forces connected to the "I" at ages twenty to twenty-one.

Metabolic forces and activities become more autonomous with puberty and separate from the models and patterns of adults or siblings in a child's life. Instinctive or intrinsic knowledge about when to sleep, when to eat, and what activities to prioritize seems to get lost. These patterns lose their previous consistency because the astral forces that regulate them have appropriately become independent. A certain chaos ensues because such children must now learn how to guide their own physiology. During this time the activity of the organs can easily become imbalanced, and so constitutional organ support can be very helpful, particularly through the "-doron" remedies. For example, Cardiodoron is used for challenges of circulatory regulation (syncope, hypotension) and also rhythmic disorders of many kinds, including disordered sleep/wake rhythms, aggressive behaviors, anger, or rage. Bidor (Biodoron) or Kalium phosphoricum comp. (Neurodoron) is indicated for sensory overload resulting in fatigue, worry, or a feeling of being overwhelmed, especially in the setting of too much stress with large academic workloads. The classic indication for Bidor, migraines, shows a clinical picture of excessive metabolism that comes up into the head when the sense pole has been worn down. Digestodoron is helpful for patterns of irregular eating and appetite, irregular digestive rhythms (resulting in either constipation or chronically loose stools) as well as eating disorders like anorexia or bulimia. Marjoram compound (Mendoron) is useful for disorders of menstrual timing, flow, severe cramping, or PMS.

In some cases the same kind of balancing or harmonizing of physiologic function can be achieved by combining complementary remedies in a rhythmic manner. Liver therapy involves giving Choleodoron, Chelidonium, or other bitters in the morning, when the adolescent has trouble waking and is slow to engage or initiate activity and may not really be hungry for a meal until midday. This remedy is complemented by Hepatodoron in the evening to support the absorptive, glucose-modulating activity of the liver in the late afternoon and into the night. Phosphorus, in a low potency (5x) in the morning helps to accentuate the waking process, matched with high potency phosphorus (20x or 30x) in the evening to help an adolescent child properly release when it is time to sleep (and not stay up all night). These kinds of organ or rhythm imbalances are common in adolescence and in some sense are developmentally normal and appropriate—though in the extreme, a child's inner world can become so chaotic that it leads to psychiatric imbalance.

A need to bring strong influences to that dysregulated inner world, to make the experience of the body and of the surrounding world more comfortable will commonly tempt an adolescent to find ways to self-medicate uncomfortable sensations away (really through manipulating one's own astral forces). This is done through very powerful sensory-seeking behaviors (extreme sports, video games, etc.) and/or substance-seeking behaviors (caffeine, nicotine, alcohol, drugs). Strong underlying constitutional imbalances may contribute to this—consider the impact of a heart or circulatory imbalance for someone who has a very hysterical constitution, which may then result in tremendous hypersensitivity combined with loss of equilibrium. Or think of a liver lethargy laid on top of a feeble/earthly constitution, resulting in a heavy, even numbed physicality that can really only be awakened through extreme physical encounter or aggression.

One addition—which is not actually part of this repeated birthing process for the four members but is very helpful to know and recognize—is the first moon node. This comes approximately every eighteen years and seven months (repeating at about thirty-seven, fifty-six, and seventy-four years), when the sun and moon cross paths in the same place in the heavens as when someone was first born. This repetition opens a window to a remembrance of the intention that first prompted one's incarnation. Questions emerge, like "How well does my life match what I am really supposed to be doing?" It brings both the possibility for significant introspection and depression as well as the emergence of new courage and enthusiasm. The first moon node acts as a prelude to the greater step of "I" independence that comes with age twenty-one.

Ages twenty to twenty-one (the twenty-first year): This age marks the time when the "I" becomes independent. A shift is now possible not just away from the characteristics of the hereditary body (physical body) but also from the family and sometimes the culture (etheric body) of origin and from the social and emotional turmoil of adolescence (astral body). The capacity for more independent and original thinking emerges, as an expression of one's unique viewpoint or style. Finer circulatory regulation is attained, particularly regarding the peripheral circulation and warmth regulation. The possible pathway for what one really wants to do in life becomes clearer (identifying a person's mission and vocation). Moral sensing becomes more refined, so that there can be a shift in relationships as one becomes better able to sense the "I" of another human being as well. Many of the remedies discussed for the nine-year change (Ferrum, Aurum, Stibium) can be helpful here as well, particularly if there is a strong experience of fear, depression, or disorientation. Experiences of the twenty-first year are different from the anxieties and insecurities of adolescence, as now the task relates to finding truth in one's inner orientation, rather than trying to find one's place in relation to the outside world and social environment.

Because of this newly deepening awareness of self, counseling concerning the archetypal rhythms of biography and self-development can have a powerful therapeutic effect all by itself at this twenty-first-year threshold. Being seen as an individual welcomes and supports the young adult's transition and places the changes in the context of growth of self, not loss of self, affirming the importance of shifting priorities and intentions.

Appendix 2

Medical Treatment Guide for Physicians

Remedy Pictures for Children with Feeble Movement and Feeble Moral Sensing

This consists of the astral body and ego acting too little on the physical body. Then one has to say to these members, "Please, gentlemen, get moving a bit more. You need to become more active in this person." In such a case you will have to use preparations of arsenic that are not too strongly diluted. They help the astral body enter into the physical organism.... If its effect is too weak, having become too lazy and thus allowing the etheric body to prevail since there are insufficient forces of resistance against what works from below, then we must resort to arsenic as a remedy.[308]

An important task for an anthroposophic physician is to carry these living pictures of constitution and the physiology of incarnation into the realm of substance. This makes possible the prescribing of a truly constitutional remedy treatment. In the same way that there is no fixed anthroposophic answer for the child who is "lazy" or who does not participate (because there are many reasons that may be happening), so too do we need to hold the individual child in our gaze when prescribing anthroposophic medicines. These special medicinal preparations are really therapeutic gestures. A selection of anthroposophic medicines are here presented for each constitutional polarity, with the wish to show how the realm of substance—as prepared through the anthroposophic pharmacy—can contribute to the spectrum of therapeutic support. There are surely other anthroposophic medicines that can also be used very effectively for addressing constitutional imbalances, but these have been selected because they present a solid foundation for understanding constitutional prescribing.

This section is intended for the use and reference of licensed prescribers who have been trained in anthroposophic medicine. The remedy pictures that follow are undoubtedly also helpful for the understanding of teachers and therapists who are working therapeutically, but this guide should not in any way be considered a substitute for a medical evaluation. The medicines described can have deep effects—that is why they are so useful—and so require proper dosing and monitoring.

We are fortunate that Steiner gave remedy indications relating to the constitutional polarities, particularly in the setting of the curative course. We also have the record of Steiner's indications for the many patients he saw in the first anthroposophic hospitals and curative homes, as documented by Dr. Hilma Walter and A. G. Degenaar.[309] Many of the following descriptions come from those sources. Table 16 provides summary points for a variety of anthroposophic preparations which have been found helpful in relation to the feeble and maniacal polarity.

We will begin with descriptions of several remedy pictures for the feeble constitution which allow us to learn about their rising, mobilizing activity (much like the therapeutic potency of the eurythmy sequence "R, L, S, I,") and also how these substances relate to the activity of the four ethers.

Arsenicum (Arsenic)

The remedy most directly indicated by Steiner for the feeble constitution is Arsenic, Arsenicum album. Arsenicum bears a special relationship to the astral body, such that Steiner equated "arsenizing" with "astralizing."[310] We can make sense of this connection if we return to Steiner's descriptions of a dominant hereditary body:

Table 16: Summary table of medical treatments to support the feeble and maniacal constitutions

Earthly constitution	**Cosmic constitution**
The child is helped through spiritualized activity: Music Eurythmy Painting and passing from minor to the major mood ***Feebleminded*** "R-L-S-I"	The child is helped by evoking strong feelings, ***Maniacal*** "M-N, B-P, A-U" ***Kleptomania*** Building memories and imagination of the past Having them hold their feet Vowels down into the legs Pedagogical stories, developed with real enthusiasm Learning practical tasks (making boots)
Primary remedy indication from Steiner: *Arsenicum*, often given in the form of Levico • For children, dosed as a drop per year of age (maximum 10 drops), 3x–6x, given 1–2 times daily; avoid evening dosing • Helps to astralize (stir and enliven) the metabolic-limb system • Also has an astral, sculpting activity for limbs that are very sculptable ("*plastisch*") **Additional remedy:** ***Mercurius*** • Indicated by Steiner for movement difficulties, as a powder by mouth • Give in a 3x–6x potency, or topically as an ointment applied to the lower legs and ankles	Primary remedy indication from Steiner: *Hypophysis* (Pituitary), given by mouth • Widely indicated by Steiner for many different kinds of developmental delays and formative weakness • Brings the stream of forces from the head down to the rest of the organism • The pituitary gland described as the highest metabolic organ in the body **Additional remedies:** ***Agaricus*** (often given in the form of *Mygale* compound, which contains *Agaricus* 6x, *Belladonna* 3x, *Stramonium* 6x) • formerly known as *Choreodoron #1* (traditionally given in alternation with Cuprum aceticum/Zincum valerianicum)

- Helps to bring mobility and levity to the limbs, to bring what is stuck into a freed state

Oxalis

- Applied as an ointment or essence, to the abdomen generally or to the liver specifically (the organ of the will)
- Strengthens the astral body in the limbs through the activity it engenders, converting oxalic acid to formic acid within the body
- Helps to lift what is too dense, what has become too mineralized

Hypericum

- Given in lower potency (1x–6x), can also be given as *Hypericum auro culta* (cultivated in gold-enriched soil)
- Addresses the melancholy and heaviness of the earthly constitution
- Brings light of consciousness to the moral process

Hepar magnesium (6x liquid)

- Magnesium has a special relationship to the plant world and to the etheric body.
- "Magnesium forces ray outward"
- Widely used remedy for depression, fibromyalgia, seasonal affective disorder
- Very helpful whenever there is an experience of excessive gravity

- Contains three poisonous plants—a strong picture of excessive astrality, held by the etheric body
- Very useful for stuck motor mannerisms—tics, or "choreiform" movements

Cuprum aceticum*/*Zincum valerianicum (both 4×)

- Formerly *Choreodoron #2* (traditionally given in alternation with *Mygale comp.*)
- Helps to relax both the astral body (*Cuprum*) and "I" (*Zincum*) out of the head and into a more metabolic activity
- Also useful for sleep onset difficulties or anxiety

Aurum (10x)/***Stibium*** (8x)/***Hyoscyamus*** (5x)

- Brings direction and balance to an unguided metabolic activity
- Helpful for motor impulsivity, for the toes and fingers that go everywhere
- Very commonly prescribed for ADHD, particularly the aspect of hyperactivity

Cardiodoron

- A balancing remedy, connecting inner processes and outer, above and below
- Archetypal remedy for the rhythmic system
- Particularly helpful for when motor patterns are perceived by others as aggressive or invasive

> The physical organization, let us say for example, is too dense. Such children will then be absolutely incapable of letting their astral body go down into this densified physical organization. They will receive an impression in the astral body, and the astral body can stimulate the corresponding astrality of the metabolic system, but the stimulation is not passed on to the etheric body, least of all to the physical.
>
> We can recognize this condition in children by noticing how they react if we say to them, "Take a few steps forward." They will be unable to do it. They correctly understand what they are supposed to do—that is, they well understand the words spoken, but they do not convey the meaning to their legs. It is as though the legs do not want to receive it. If we find this—that the child has difficulty when told to do something that involves using the legs—that the child hesitates to bring the legs into movement at all—then that is for us the first sign that the child's physical body has become too hardened and is unwilling to receive thoughts.[311]

Here is Steiner's description of the activity of Arsenicum as a remedy:

> Now, arsenic has a powerful effect on the mobility of the astral body, the mobility it requires for entering into the physical and etheric bodies—and, in fact, also on the form of the astral body. It can be observed in people who have undergone arsenic cures that their astral body just slips into the physical, glides smoothly into it. When therefore you have a child in whom you want to produce a right harmony between the astral and etheric and physical bodies, arsenic baths will be your obvious method. Prepare a certain quantity of Levico water of a particular percentage and let the child have a bath in it. This will work upon the nervous system and strengthen the astral body."[312]

Steiner very often recommended Arsenicum treatments—not in the form of Arsenic alone, but in the form of Levico water, which comes from a natural mineral spring in Roncegno, Italy:

> Let me remind you of how some good spirit seems to have formulated substances such as Roncegno water or Levico water,

> developed them in advance in outer, nonhuman nature under specific circumstances expressly in order to prepare a number of forces capable of playing a beneficial role in the human organism.... If we think about how wonderfully the two forces of copper and iron offset each other in this water and about how arsenic is also present to provide a broader basis for this interaction, we realize that something is being prepared in the outer world with specific regard to certain conditions in the human being."[313]

Iron and Copper also have a special relationship to the astral body—one stimulating the activity of incarnation into the physical body (Iron, Ferrum) the other making the body more receptive for that activity (Copper, Cuprum). They frame and harmonize the activity of Arsenic.

We can also connect the remedy picture for Arsenic to the sculptural pattern attributed to the earthly child—where the trunk and the limbs, hands, and feet are less formed (vital and doughy, without clear definition). Steiner indicated that "by driving the astral body further into the organs, we enhance the mineralizing process in the organs. If we notice that the organs are indicating a proliferative etheric, are too active vitally, and are developing life forces that are too strong, then the introduction of arsenic would have a healing effect."[314] He went on to describe Arsenicum as an important remedy for dysentery, a different, but related loss of form in the metabolic–limb system where etheric proliferation leads to watery diarrhea.[315]

Most of Steiner's references to Arsenic are for Levico baths (a form of treatment that is not widely available at this time), though he stated that while the usual treatment is to "use arsenic externally," it is also possible to "administer arsenic internally as well."

Arsenic works most strongly in the realm of the astral body and relates to the eurythmy "S," its activity a dynamic movement between fire and form. Arsenic guides the astral body to reach down and take hold of the etheric and physical bodies by enlivening the light ether.

As a constitutional treatment we can readily prescribe Arsenic (often in the form of Levico) when the most striking aspect of a child's constitution is the lack of any activity in the limbs, a kind of sleeping/lamed condition (a lack of astrality), and particularly when there is an accompanying proliferative lack of form in the trunk and limbs, expressing dominant and unguided physical and etheric activity. Arsenicum is prescribed at low potency to address the metabolic–limb system.

Specific pairings of Arsenicum with another metal can also be considered, such as:

- Scorodite (a naturally occurring form of Iron and Arsenic), for blond children, who carry a strong sulfur process[316] (see section on Sulfur and Iron for more information) or
- Olivenite (naturally occurring Copper and Arsenic) for dark-haired children who also carry a strong iron process.[317]

Levico holds both of these pairings, with its natural combination of Arsenic, Iron, Copper, and Sulfur. It is usually prescribed for children in the range of 3x–6x potencies, primarily in the morning because of its stimulating effect (though very feeble children may well be able to take additional doses in the afternoon or evening without significant change or disruption in their sleep patterns).

Two remedies discussed in more detail later are worth mentioning in relation to Levico: Sulfur and Phosphorus.

Sulfur

Another component of Levico mineral water is Sulfur. Its sulfurous component arises from a natural spring process, in which "mountain metal sulphide deposits are dissolved by spring water in a dynamic movement."[318] Sulfur contributes warmth and greater etheric activity, particularly at the level of protein formation. Steiner spoke about Sulfur's activity quite often, but he related it specifically to the use of

Arsenic, using the example of mustard or horseradish as an external application:

> Our chief concern must be to see that the astral body receives the right form and configuration that will enable it to fit itself into the ether and physical bodies in a harmonious manner.... Then, to ensure that the externally administered arsenic shall really strike home, we reinforce it by applying mustard juice compresses to the feet before and after the bath, using also grated horse-radish for this purpose. I should add that in the latter case, you must make sure that the horse-radish is not grated until immediately before use. It is most important that it should be freshly grated; if allowed to stand for some hours, it loses its efficacy.[319]

Sulfur has a transient activity—it brings loosening and warmth but does not linger. That is why the grated horseradish must be used promptly. In a similar way, a Sulfur crystal, exposed to air, will slowly sublimate into the air and eventually (over months to years) disappear. It always carries this loosening character, moving from the center out toward the periphery. Sulfur always leans toward a kind of combustion process. Steiner designated Sulfur as a light carrier, eager to release outward its inner light.

The application of a Sulfur process (such as horseradish juice or a mustard compress) stirs and loosens the physical and etheric bodies, so that the astralizing activity of Levico can really penetrate. Sulfur works most strongly at the level of the life ether.

Most of Steiner's therapeutic indications for the use of Sulfur relate to the epileptic constitution. It is discussed in more detail in the section of this appendix devoted to remedy pictures for the epileptic and hysteric polarity.

Phosphorus

Phosphorus is also a light carrier. While Steiner contrasted the opposing activity of Arsenic, on one hand (to bring the astral body in), and Phosphorus and Sulfur (in high potency, to help it release), on the other, he indicated that Phosphorus and Levico can work in a complementary way. In the chapter "Characteristic Illnesses" in *Extending Practical Medicine,* we are told that "phosphorus helps the ego to overcome the resistance of the physical body."[320] From this we can see how Phosphorus could be used as a remedy for the feeble constitution, working most strongly at the level of the warmth ether, and is an important consideration when feeble movement is accompanied by a lack of wakeful sensing activity.

Phosphorus is similarly discussed in more detail in the section of this appendix devoted to the epileptic and hysteric polarity.

It would perhaps suffice to limit our description to the activity of Arsenicum and its healing support for the feeble constitution. There is great therapeutic activity there, and Arsenic is indeed the remedy that Steiner indicated for its constitutional treatment. Just as there are many sides to having a dominant hereditary body—sculptability, movement, moral sensing—so too are there many other possible, related shades of remedy support. They are offered here because they help to enlarge the clinical spectrum of illnesses we might consider as falling under the feeble constitutional rubric and because they can also help expand our own imaginative considerations for how a dominant, untransformed physical body may manifest.

Mercurius (Mercury)

Whereas Arsenic astralizes an unwieldy hereditary body (through strengthening the activity of the light ether), other important therapeutic support can come by addressing the life and chemical ethers. One such remedy is the metal Mercury, Mercurius, which brings mobility and flexibility to the lower members so that we can really take hold of the solid constituents of our body:

> Let us take the Mercury forces. They are not concentrated exclusively in the planet Mercury but permeate the whole of space accessible to us, while the physical Mercury is merely a manifestation of the Mercury forces in a concentrated mineral form....

> Then we also acquire knowledge of what these Mercury forces signify for human beings and in the unconscious realms of life. Take a simple example: When we wish to walk, we must have certain forces by means of which, out of the spirit, we permeate our bones and muscles. With our spirit and soul we have to penetrate into the physical, or solid constituents of our body. That we are able to do this is due to the Mercury forces. It can therefore be said: The effect of the Mercury forces is that human beings can take hold of the solid constituents of the body. If there were no Mercury forces in the world, we would always remain outside the solid constituents of our body.[321]

From case studies, we know that Steiner recommended Mercury as a remedy for a nine-year-old girl with paralysis of the legs and lower body, in the form of Mercurius 3x, taken orally one time daily.[322] He also advised it for a twenty-one-year-old patient with cardiac dilatation and endocarditis (as Mercurius viv. 3x/Arsenicum met. 3x/Adrenal extract 2x, a pea-sized portion three times daily):

> "We have to work toward the restoration of the full functioning of the astral body. Adrenal hormone results in the activity of the astral body, directed toward the front. Arsenic gives rise to: the activity of the astral body from all sides, inwardly. Mercury gives: a certain affinity of the astral body for the etheric body, because it does not grasp it enough."[323]

Experience has consequently shown Mercury to be a helpful treatment for "motoric developmental delay with disturbance in flow of movement":

> The child falls into weight, movement appears inhibited, gravity dominates (to the point of spasticity).
>
> - Dosage: Apply thinly to lower leg ("where Mercury has his wings") and massage lightly.
>
> Overweight children with a pasty constitution: D5 ointment.
>
> Nervous and pale children: D14 ointment.

- Onset of action: Within 3–4 wks.
- Treatment duration: 6–8 wks.[324]

We can consider Mercurius an appropriate remedy for children whose feebleness extends beyond a simple slowness in initiating movement and manifests in motor delays where one senses that the limbs really cannot be taken hold of.

Oxalis

We will now consider Oxalis as a medicine to strengthen the life ether. Oxalis is most commonly used as an anthroposophic treatment for stone formation (such as gallstones or kidney stones), colicky pain, or constipation with dry stools—all conditions where substance has fallen out of healthy etheric activity and become too mineralized. *Oxalis* is additionally recommended by Steiner as a treatment for shock, as it helps to reconnect the etheric body, which has been displaced out of the lower abdominal and reproductive organs. We can consider Oxalis as a constitutional therapy for the feeble constitution, because of the enlivening activity it engenders in the etheric body, and then (through its conversion into formic acid) into a support for the astral body:

> Oxalic acid is found especially in clover, but it occurs in a certain quantity in the whole human being, particularly in the part that comprises the organs of digestion—spleen, liver, and so on. In the region of the digestive tract you have to reckon with processes under the influence of oxalic acid.... If human beings had never developed oxalic acid in the digestive tract we would simply be unable to live. That is, our etheric body would have no sort of basis in our organism. If we did not change the oxalic acid into formic acid, our astral body would have no basis in our organism. Human beings need oxalic acid for the ether body and formic acid for the astral body—or rather, we do not need the substances; we need the work, the inner activity that goes on in the oxalic acid process and in the formic acid process.[325]

From Steiner's description we can see that Oxalic Acid has a kind of stirring activity within the body, lifting congestions to etheric vigor (lifting mineral to etheric) while also pulling the forces of the "I"-organization down into astral activity:

> Oxalic acid production corresponds to the domain of the etheric.... Illness which comes to expression in gouty and rheumatic conditions can be ascribed to an inadequate activity of the astral body. Other conditions present in such a way that the causes, which stem from the astral organism in gout and rheumatism, lie further back in the etheric organism. Then not only force congestions toward the astral emerge, which inhibit the "I"-organization, but also inhibitory effects in the etheric which cannot be mastered by the astral organization. They manifest in sluggish, lower abdominal activity, in inhibited activity of liver and spleen, in stone-like deposits in the gallbladder and the like. If one gives oxalic acid in such cases, then the etheric organism is supported in its activity. Through oxalic acid the etheric body is strengthened since the force of the "I"-organization is converted by this acid to a force of the astral body which then works more strongly on the ether body.[326]

Steiner recommended Oxalis with specific reference to the astral body and the limbs for a thirty-six-year-old woman with amenorrhea and rheumatic complaints, commenting that "the astral body is not in the arms and legs."[327] Likewise, for another patient it was recommended that Oxalis salve be rubbed into the legs and Hypophysis injections be given for rheumatic complaints and delayed periods. In this case, "the astral body is not properly in the arms and legs."[328] Daily application of oxalic acid 5 percent to the upper chest and formic acid 5 percent daily to the lower chest was advised for a third patient "for strengthening the astral body."[329] With topical application in the form of compresses or being rubbed in, Steiner noted that "the best would be to rub it in. This will have an extraordinarily strong energizing effect on the etheric system in the digestive tract."[330] Other physicians have recommended rubbing Oxalis ointment over the liver (the main organ of the will).[331]

We can consider Oxalis as an additional constitutional treatment for a dominant physical heaviness and to help get the astral body into the limbs. It is particularly appropriate when where there are accompanying digestive congestions and as a way to quietly help re-seat the etheric body when there is a history of shock or trauma.

Two Additional Remedies: *Hypericum* and *Hepar Magnesium*

Both Hypericum and Hepar magnesium are included in this section, even though neither one was spoken about by Steiner in relationship to the earthly/feeble constitution. They do not address physical slowness or impeded movement. Instead, they speak to soul heaviness, to the melancholy that can accompany a dominant hereditary body.

Hypericum

Hypericum (St John's Wort) has long been known as a treatment for depression, an indication that is also true for anthroposophic medicine. Steiner, however, spoke most frequently about Hypericum as a remedy for bed-wetting (a symptom associated with the hysteric constitution), but we can mention it here because of its special relationship to the astral body and its comparison to Arsenic and Levico water:

> Bed-wetting in children arises out of a very characteristic weakness of the astral body. The astral body simply does not have the strength that it ought to have. If you were to use arsenic in just this situation, even when you use it in the healthy form of Levico water or Roncegno water, then as a general rule you would indeed see a strong, but extraordinarily short activity, that in these children who bed-wet the astral body comes into brief movement throughout the whole organism... [but] these children will remain bed-wetters. But you will achieve very good success, if for children who wet the bed you use the substance that can be pressed out of the leaves and flowers of St. John's wort, Hypericum performatum.... When you press this plant,

> then you obtain a juice...a bitter extract...a substance, which has a very powerful and lasting effect on the inner mobility of the astral body, and which makes the astral body stronger. Under certain circumstances it can really be healed if one works to influence children morally, even saying simply that they are obliged to pay attention to their own bodily functions. This moral influencing should actually take place exactly with these kinds of things, that lie on the border between misbehavior and illnesses. Please do not misunderstand me, I recognize, naturally, that this is an illness, but it stands on the border between impudence or misbehavior, and an illness.[332]

From this description we can perhaps see how Hypericum relates not so much to the child who is never able to penetrate the limbs and come into movement as to a child who feels uncomfortable or unsure about really descending into the body. On the soul level, we could almost speak of a kind of avoidance—that the physical body is heavy and does not feel good, and so there is a holding back of real engagement. Melancholy rules. This is different from the superficiality of the more cosmic/maniacal child, who bothers with the body so little that it is almost inconsequential.

Steiner added that Hypericum is helpful for conditions that "lie on the border between misbehavior and illnesses" and so speak to the moral aspect of making a healthy decision to enter more deeply into the body. This is somewhat different from not being at all able to enter the limbs and more an expression of a kind of incarnational "misbehavior." Although the language of Steiner's indication for Hypericum is certainly different from that for Arsenicum, we can see that it shares a gesture of mobilizing and strengthening the astral body.

Hypericum can be considered as a constitutional treatment for children who are melancholic and whose limb heaviness feels related to a reluctance to engage with the lower body (with a clear awareness of the burden of the physical body, which is different from the almost carelessness of the cosmic/maniacal process). Hypericum can also be helpful for biographical transitions, particularly when there is indecision about continuing to engage with the body and the physical world (such as the melancholy of the nine-year change—for more see Appendix 1).

Hepar magnesium

Steiner often made mention of the role of Magnesium in early childhood, particularly as it relates to the growth of adult teeth. Magnesium forces work into the teeth, helping them to grow up and erupt out of the gums. "The magnesium forces ray outward."[333] Magnesium is again a light carrier (like phosphorus and sulfur)—and so we can consider how this third light carrier helps to overcome the density and gravity of the hereditary body.

Magnesium has a special relationship to the plant world and to the slow, steady, radiating qualities of vegetative growth. Magnesium sits at the center of a chlorophyll molecule, which stands at the heart of the plant world's activity of light metabolism, as opposed to Iron, which takes the central place in hemoglobin in animal and human oxygen transport and metabolism.

Magnesium, combined in this remedy with a liver preparation, enhances this unrushed, gentle levity, which belongs to the etheric body. This makes it very helpful for balancing an exaggerated experience of lethargy and gravity in the limbs and for fatigue combined with melancholy or depression. In this way Hepar magnesium supports the healthy unfolding of will activity. Steiner designated the liver as the organ of will.[334]

Research studies have described the clinical use of Hepar magnesium for fibromyalgia[335] and for seasonal fatigue symptoms.[336] Fibromyalgia is characterized by the presence of pain and unusual trigger point tenderness in the muscles, with a sensing activity that has become too sharp and guarded. Seasonal fatigue, or seasonal affective disorder, is an experience of fatigue or melancholy related to longer nights and limited experience of the sun's light. *Hepar magnesium* can be helpful for both conditions, as its slow, gentle light helps to balance the sharpness and hardening of a fibromyalgia process as well as the loss of inner light that comes with winter seasonal disorders.

Hepar magnesium is useful as a constitutional remedy for experiences of the body becoming too hardened, yet too wakeful and for depressions with a strong experience of gravity and fatigue.

Remedy Pictures for Children with Maniacal Movement and Kleptomania

Hypophysis (Pituitary)

Steiner described as a primary treatment for kleptomania how glandular preparations of the Pituitary (Hypophysis) can be given when the forces of the head "are too feeble in their influence on the rest of the body."[337] He similarly recommended Hypophysis as a anthroposophic treatment for problems related to a range of developmental challenges (dwarfism, microcephaly, Down's syndrome, poor growth, and delays in soul and spiritual development). For one of the children discussed during the curative course he explained:

> We must come to the help of the stream of forces that goes from the head to the lower organism.... We can strengthen this stream of forces and so help to induce a right correspondence between metabolic system and nervous system, by making use of the secretion of Hypophysis. For this gives, as it were, a helping hand to the stream of forces, and exercises from the direction of the head a harmonizing influence upon the metabolic system. We shall therefore have, side-by-side, treatment with Hypophysis cerebri, arsenic baths, and curative eurythmy. With these three working together, we shall make progress with a body of this kind.[338]

It is striking that the treatment indicated for kleptomania (Hypophysis) is here combined with Arsenic baths, for as we shall see there is a certain overlap in the remedies between these two constitutional poles. This is true because both the feeble and the maniacal constitutions are healed by a meeting of the higher and the lower members in the middle.

Steiner elsewhere described the "centrifugal" activity of Hypophysis, which helps bring a child all the way to the periphery of the limbs:

> And now we must go on to speak of the child who is so restless and fidgety—a sleepy, backward little boy, still very young, who has not learned to speak and is behindhand with all the training he should have received in the first period of life.... Some medical treatment will be needed.... You must provide a dispersing influence that works centrifugally and drives the substantiality of the organism to the circumference. Hypophysis always works in this way.[339]

Hypophysis helps to bring the forces of the head down into the rest of the body. We can consider it as a foundational remedy for the maniacal or kleptomaniacal constitution, in which a child's whole incarnation gesture remains too peripheral and too much connected to the head. Hypophysis actually has broad application, especially when there are more global developmental or growth challenges. As an organ preparation, it works at the level of the etheric body and is usually used in a low potency (typically 6x).

Agaricus, as part of Mygale comp.

Mygale compound brings together three different poisonous substances, from plants in which the astral forces (which usually only touch into the brightly colored and highly sculptural aspects of the flowering process) enter more deeply into the rest of a plant's activity. This unusual penetration of the astral body into the plants gives rise to poisonous compounds, which very often contain a high level of alkaloids.

If we consider the spiritual activity of the maniacal or kleptomaniacal constitution, the higher members (astral body and "I") stay too much in the head and are too superficial in their engagement, precisely because they do not engage in this kind of bridging activity between the astral body and etheric body. The maniacal child's physiology shows a kind of hole in the middle, while the poisonous mushroom Agaricus and the other two nightshade plants included in the preparation show an excessive interpenetration:

> What takes place when a plant develops properly—the blossom unfolding always a little above the earth's surface—can develop right on the earth's surface. Then fungi arise; this is the basis for fungus formation.... Fungi arise from such a special astralizing process.[340]

We hear that the therapeutic potency of the fungi arise out of a "special astralizing process." This activity is more specific than the general astralizing of arsenic (which was recommended for the dominant hereditary body). The indication for Agaricus is different than for Arsenicum, because the challenge in bridging the upper and lower members in a maniacal child lies not so much with an inaccessible or overly dense physical body as a kind of self-limiting activity of the "I" and astral body. The Agaricus mushroom helps to shift the direction and activity of the astral body, from the head down:

> The golden agaric substance, with its particular content of organized nitrogen, acts in such a way that an effect coming from the head makes the ether body more lively through the ego organization and increases its affinity with the astral body.[341]

This nuance is further elucidated by Steiner when he contrasted it with Algae (which speaks more to the feeble constitution):

> In cases where we perceive a disorder due to the "I"-organization making too great a demand upon the astral body and not allowing it to enter into the etheric body, we must have recourse rather to the fungi [to Agaricus]. The algae [in contrast], which come nearer to the ordinary plant, are to be used when the physical

> body and the etheric body refuse to allow the astral body to enter—that is to say, when the disharmony is due not to an excessive attraction exerted by the "I"-organization, but to a special relationship put up by the ether body.[342]

The nightshade plants (Belladonna and Stramonium) present a similar picture, with related excessive astral penetration. The nightshades are described in more detail as part of Steiner's indications for Hyoscyamus, described later in this listing.

The clinical picture for this remedy would be excessive movement, but with the rigidity of an astral body that stays too much in the activity of the head pole. This can be recognized as largely unconscious repetitive or spasming movement. As a constitutional remedy, we can therefore consider Agaricus (as a single remedy or as an ingredient in Mygale compound) as a helpful treatment for motor tics or unguided, stereotyped movement patterns.

Cuprum aceticum / Zincum valerianicum

Any time there is dominant activity of the astral body working out of the head pole, it can result in a kind of cramp. This cramping process happens when the astral body works directly on the physical body, without the etheric body acting as a bridge. Sometimes this manifests clearly in the realm of movement, other times more prominently in the realm of feeling or thought. Cuprum aceticum/Zincum valerianicum is helpful in this second situation, when a cramping process relates more to consciousness than to bodily activity. Cuprum aceticum/Zincum valerianicum is often prescribed as a complement to Mygale compound for tics or spastic movement. It, too, helps to release the "I" and astral body out of the head but with a somewhat different gesture. Agaricus guides the "I" and astral down into connection with the etheric (a kind of inhalation down into the body). Cuprum aceticum/Zincum valerianicum work more to breathe the higher members out of the head (an outbreathing gesture away from the consciousness pole, but that can nonetheless have an effect complementary to that of *Agaricus*).

Steiner described how Cuprum directs the astral body away from the centripetal activity of the head to a more centrifugal, radiating, and relaxing activity, which is seated in the kidneys. The use of copper in an acid form (Cuprum aceticum) directs copper's activity more specifically to the astral body.[343] Cuprum aceticum alone is commonly prescribed for cramping illnesses of the respiratory system (like asthma or the spasmodic coughing seen with pertussis). In that illness picture a rhythmic process—respiration—gets stuck because of a dominant forming, hardening activity coming from the head pole. Cuprum aceticum helps to relax the breathing cramp in the lungs and upper airways.

Zincum valerianicum combines a plant remedy, Valerian, with a mineral, Zinc. Zinc also has a relaxing effect, but one that is directed not to the astral body but to the "I"-organization.[344] The Valerian plant is well known as an aid for sleep difficulties because of the way it models the process of release of the higher members from the sensing pole.

The combination Cuprum aceticum/Zincum valerianicum works also as a sleep remedy—best prescribed for those children who have trouble falling asleep because they are too wakeful, too busily sensing. As a constitutional treatment it helps address a rhythmic activity of sleeping and waking that has become stuck owing to a dominant head pole. Cuprum aceticum/Zincum valerianicum is included in this description, however, because of the way it can be used constitutionally to help soften and release a stuck, cramping process in the realm of limb movement—such as motor tics or cool intellectuality that is anxious and without much moral warmth.

Aurum / Stibium / Hyoscyamus

Aurum (Gold)

The first three remedies just described give different pictures of therapeutic balancing for the cosmic process, as all three work to help the "I" and astral body to move down, out of an isolated head activity to instead work cooperatively with the etheric body. A different, but nonetheless related therapeutic possibility comes not by bringing the head forces down but by supporting a healthy meeting place in the middle, by strengthening and balancing the rhythmic system. The meeting of head and limbs physiology in the rhythmic system is a microcosm of the much larger meeting of the spiritual world and the physical world. Steiner consistently related this kind of mediating activity to the sun, as a planet, and to the metal Gold, as a material substance:

> The Sun holds the balance between the spiritual and the material in the cosmos. For this reason the Sun, you might say, is a cosmic body that both maintains order in the solar system and brings order into the forces pervading our material system.... There is a connection between the Sun and gold. In this instance, too, the ancients valued gold for its connection to the balance between spirit and matter rather than for its ahrimanic value.[345]

Steiner also related that balancing quality to the organization of the human being:

> This is naturally the case in a normal person, where everything that works downward from the upper human being is counterbalanced by the effect of the lower human being on the upper.... When this balance is disturbed, however, the metal that can bring equilibrium is gold, aurum. This restores the balance between this enveloping process and what lies in the middle.[346]

The "enveloping process" mentioned relates to the activity of the head. We have seen how the head forces are not properly mediated in both maniacal movement and kleptomaniacal behaviors. Aurum's therapeutic effect comes through connecting the upper members (which work independently in the realm of thought) down to the etheric, which can then work upon the physical (making healthy limb activity possible):

> Gold is an impulse for the quickening of human thought, so that human thought can work down as far as into the etheric body.... "I"-organization, astral body, etheric body and physical body are members of the human organism, and we may say that through gold the "I"-organization becomes capable of working down into the etheric body. The etheric body can then go further and work upon the physical body, but gold brings it about that one can actually hold the thoughts in all their power as far as the etheric body.[347]

Aurum (Gold) is given as part of this compound remedy in a 10x potency—considered anthroposophically to be a "middle" potency—which addresses the rhythmic system.

Stibium (Antimony)

Steiner spoke many times about *Stibium* (Antimony), not just as a mineral but as an actual dynamic activity. In much the same way that he described the activity of arsenic as astralizing, he also referred to an "antimonizing" activity. Where arsenic strengthens the astral body, Stibium works more with the "I" to bring proper form to the metabolic–limb pole—examples of this include Stibium's ability to help bring form to the blood (as a treatment for clotting problems in a hemophiliac) and its use as a treatment for loose stools or diarrhea. As a constitutional remedy, we can think about Stibium as a helper for bringing proper form to the will pole:

> Antimonizing forces are the sculptors, as it were, that work inward from the outside to give shape to the substances that build up our organs. Thus, the forces of antimony have a certain relationship to our organs' internal organizing forces.[348]

Most of the remedies that bring an organizing activity are related to the head and the nerve–sense system (like Silica or Plumbum), but accentuating a head activity would only reinforce the imbalance already seen in a maniacal or kleptomaniacal constitution. In contrast, Stibium's organizing forces are directed to the limbs and metabolism and belong not to the formative activities of the upper pole (Saturn, Jupiter, and Mars) but to those of the lower pole (Venus, Mercury, and Moon):

> The obvious question is, what is this antimonizing force in the supra-earthly domain? From the planetary perspective, it is the interaction of Mercury, Venus, and the Moon. When these planets work together rather than separately, their effects are not mercurial, silvery, or coppery. Instead, they work just as antimony works in the Earth.... The force that works out of the Earth from all of its antimony is the same as the force that works down on the Earth from these three planetary bodies above the Earth."[349]

Stibium is given in this compound is a liquid, part of a tincture taken by mouth. Steiner pointed out that Stibium has different effects relating to its specific route of administration:

> You will have to restrict the internal use of antimony to patients who are very strong-willed and external applications to individuals who tend to be very weak-willed. You will have to make this distinction. As you see, the antimony in the mineral kingdom manifests as something that has an inner relationship to human will, in that the more conscious human will becomes, the more it feels the need to bring about an effect opposite to that of antimony. Human will has a destructive effect on all the forces that I described earlier as constituting the characteristic action of antimony. Human will has a destructive effect on all forces, especially the subconscious thought forces that are still active in children. Antimony's forces work together with these particular forces.[350]

Oral Stibium (included as an 8x liquid in this compound remedy) therefore works to address the child who is strong-willed and who needs to be stimulated to make the activities of the will more conscious.

Hyoscyamus (Henbane)

As a complement to the two mineral remedies described comes Hyoscyamus (henbane), a plant remedy that has a special relationship to the astral body.[351] Hyoscyamus is a nightshade plant, part of a plant family that can be very helpful therapeutically when there is an imbalanced interaction between the astral and etheric bodies. Steiner made reference to Hyoscyamus multiple times, but usually in combination with Belladonna. He did make an important distinction between the two, however, indicating that Belladonna should be used when an illness process is related more to the rhythmic system or the head, while the activity of Hyoscyamus speaks much more to the metabolism. In the course of his medical lectures Steiner described the contrasting qualities of a "cross spider" (*Araneus diadematus*)—which he characterized as strongly linked to cosmic, planetary activities—and Hyoscyamus, which is more earthly. From this description we see that Hyoscyamus has a special relationship to the earth and therefore a therapeutic relationship to the limb pole:

> Blackbirds—which are not, after all, totally ascetic animals—occasionally eat cross spiders. But when a blackbird eats a cross spider and begins to feel very uncomfortable... it heads straight for a henbane plant. If there is a henbane plant nearby, the blackbird will go straight to it to get the appropriate remedy. If no henbane is available, the blackbird develops convulsions and dies a terrible death. Its own healing instinct, however, protects it from this fate; it immediately begins pecking away at henbane, the appropriate remedy.... What is actually going on when a blackbird eats a cross spider? The cross spider's entire organization is closely linked to certain cosmic relationships in supra-earthly nature, and this connection gives rise to its

> overall limb development as well as its markings. If I may put it in this way, the cross spider has a lot of planetary life in it.... As soon as the bird has consumed the garden spider, its inner will becomes a copy of supra-earthly life, and it goes straight to a specific plant. This plant has become similar to earthly factors, the opposite of the planetary factors, because of the very way it grows out of the Earth—specifically, because of its inability to fully process a substance influenced by the planets, which it retains as a poison instead.[352]

If we paraphrase Steiner's picture, using slightly different vocabulary, then we can say that the blackbird that has eaten a cross spider becomes suddenly poisoned by too much cosmos and is rescued, healed, by a plant that has brought that astrality right down to the earth. As a remedy, Hyoscyamus brings the cosmic constitution down to the earth. Steiner separately indicated that Hyoscyamus stimulates the solar plexus, such that "if the solar plexus was stimulated by means of henbane, it was permeated with spirit; in such a case, astral body and ego organization take firm hold of the solar plexus."[353] In this way the disengaged "I" and astral body are stimulated to find an anchor in the metabolic–limb pole. Hyoscyamus is usually given in a 5x potency as part of the mixture with Gold and Stibium.

In summary: Aurum 10x/Stibium 8x/Hyoscyamus 5x can be seen as a constitutional treatment for helping a child unite the spirit with the limbs. It is directed toward strong-willed but unguided limb activity. It is a helpful remedy for maniacal hyperactivity and restless limbs.

Cardiodoron

Cardiodoron is one of the original "*-doron*" ("gift") remedies that came from Steiner. *Cardiodoron*—a gift for the heart—is composed of three different plants: *Hyoscyamus, Primula* (the Pasque flower), and *Onopordon* (Scotch thistle), which balance each other to present a complete and balanced rhythmic process. *Hyoscyamus* has already been described—it helps balance too cosmic a gesture by bringing the

"I"-organization and astral body down to the solar plexus and into a healthier relationship with the limb pole. The flower of *Hyoscyamus,* with crude, unusual, yellow-green petals, stays close to the ground as the whole plant twists and snakes horizontally.

Primula, a delicate, tender, yellow alpine flower, brings a striking contrast, as the flower rises high above the rosette of leaves that crowns the base of the plant. Its flowering process leaves the earthly realm so that the astral activity reaches far up into the realm of air and light.

Onopordon draws a strong contrast, bringing a very strong form principle. It is a large and grand member of the thistle family, rising as tall as a human being, with many sequences of spiraling, thorny leaves. It also carries a strong rhythmic process, growing gradually but consistently over the course of the first year and only in a second year of growth coming into a flowering process. Its longevity and resiliency (it likes dry areas) contrast with the delicate transience of the Primula flower, and whereas Hyoscyamus shows its strongly astral process inwardly, through the production of poisons, Onopordon holds its strong astral process at the periphery through the contracted thorns of a strong boundary.

The many varied sides of this Onopordon/Primula/Hyoscyamus composition have been described by many authors in nuanced ways.[354] What is remarkable about the triad of these plants is that if one takes almost any physiologic process, then looks to find its exaggeration and its polar opposite, one can find that pairing represented in the contrasts of these three plants. In this way Cardiodoron helps to model an inherent balance and flexibility between extremes. It holds the gesture of contrasting activities for growth and form, rigidity and flexibility, inner world and outer boundary.

Precisely because it presents such a balanced picture, Cardiodoron can support an imbalance on either pole and has proved helpful for regulating both the excessive, invasive physicality of the maniacal pole and the crude, often too strong movement of the feeble pole. It can similarly help a child navigate the balancing of inner and outer world when there are challenging social encounters, for as we have seen, the extremes of limb movement and moral sensing share a certain disconnection in the middle. Cardiodoron models and strengthens the bridging activity in that middle, rhythmic, heart space.

Cardiodoron is given as a fixed combination, so there is no specific variation in potency. It is also called Onopordon comp.—working out of the same principles but in a different pharmaceutical preparation.[355]

Archetypal Remedy Pictures for Working with the Large-headed Constitution

Table 17: Summary table of medical treatments to support the large-headed and small-headed constitutions

Nerve-sense System Is out of Order *Large-headed Constitution*	**Metabolic-limb System Is out of Order** *Small-headed Constitution*
Primary remedy *Plumbum* (Lead) • Lower potency (6x) is administered if there are marked physical signs of delayed maturation (like open fontanels, difficulty moving, very young appearing face).[1] • Higher potency is more commonly given (20x), generally once in the morning over the course of a month (five weeks). Follow with a shorter course of Cuprum (6x), in the evening for two weeks. • Plumbum helps bring sensory maturation and the capacity for antipathy so that a child can find proper distance from sensory impressions.	**Primary remedy** *Argentum* (Silver) • Lower potency (3x–6x) is given several times daily. It can be given for a longer period of time, but a usual course is 4–8 weeks. It has broad application for both digestive and sensory signs of weakened metabolism. • It can be used both for overactive digestion (diarrhea) and slowed excretion (like dry constipation). • Argentite (Silver and Sulfur) more specifically supports the loosening and vitalizing of the physical body, mobilizing the digestion into greater activity. It is particularly useful for a more iron-rich coloring (dark hair and dark eyes).

• It can also be used for sensory-seeking behaviors related to "perverted instincts," especially to smell (such as a desire to smell gasoline fumes). • Plumbum silicicum, a related remedy, brings particular definition to boundaries (as 20x, in situations like autism).[2] • Cichorium plumbo culta helps to bring that distancing more into the digestive and metabolic spheres. • Stannum (Tin) addresses formative weakness when the child is present in the world but not yet able to fully organize the body. Often given in combination with Hypophysis (Pituitary). • Bidor (as a Silica remedy) is used for the child whose nerve-sense pole becomes quickly worn down through too much stimulation or intellectual work.	• Ferrum (8x) can follow a Silver treatment for several weeks, especially for those with more "sulfurous" coloring (blond or red hair and blue eyes). • Bryophyllum argento culta works to anchor the etheric in the metabolism. It is good for the restless aspects of the small-headed constitution, especially when there are sleep disturbances. 1 Medical Section of the School of Spiritual Science, Dornach, Switzerland, et al., "Plumbum," Vademecum of Anthroposophic Medicines. 2 Henning Schramm, "Plumbum," Heilmittel-Fibel zur anthroposophischen Medizin.
• Application of cool water to the forehead in the morning • Need for salt in the diet	• Application of hot water bottle to the abdomen in the evening and even through the night • Need for proper sugars in the diet

Steiner linked the balance between blood and nerve activities directly with substance and the use of remedies. His indications for the feeble and maniacal processes of the will pole were different—movement (eurythmy sequences) and curricular activities (pedagogical experiences)—with substances mentioned only in relation to specific cases. In his description of a nerve–sense system that is not in order (large-headed constitution), however, he promptly spoke to the teachers about the use of lead and silver for a child whose metabolic–limb system is not in order (small-headed). He made reference to these two substances in other medical lectures as well, emphasizing the activities they embody and placing them at the center of medical meditative work. Between the activity of lead and the activity of silver, we find the full unfolding of life—connecting on one end with our journey out of the spiritual world and on the other with our earthly encounter and digestion of substance and experience. The therapeutic uses of lead and silver create important reference points for many aspects of anthroposophic medical therapy (see Table 17).

Plumbum (Lead)

Let us begin with lead. Lead (Plumbum) is the metal that most powerfully stimulates the formative activities of the head, which makes possible the sensing activity of our nerves:

> In lead, for instance, you have a substance that acts with extraordinary strength on the nerve–sense activity.... In patients suffering from weaknesses in the head region—i.e., in which the upper human being develops neither a proper nerve–sense activity nor a proper breathing activity—we will be able to achieve a great deal with such lead cures, provided we do not go too far and cause lead-poisoning.... Those substances tending more toward silver have a polar relationship to those tending more toward lead.[358]

Lead has a very bad reputation, and it is, of course, poisonous when it is taken in a substantial, material way into the body. We should not have lead in us, but Steiner indicated that we are, in fact, continuously bathed in very finely dispersed amounts of it. The therapeutic activity of a constitutional (homeopathic) lead treatment comes not from the substance itself but from what is stimulated as we clear lead out of our bodies:

> The organism begins to fight against the process that is contained in the lead substance—substances are always processes.

> Lead spreads out within the organic process, and the organism, exerting its opposition, tries to drive out the lead.... It cannot tolerate the formative forces of lead. If we now try to learn what it means to human beings that we will not put up with having lead in our organism, we are led to the following: The human is a being of sense. We perceive things around us and then think about them. We need both forms of activity. We must perceive things so that we can be connected with the world; we must also think about them. We must repress the act of actual perception and then unfold our own, independent activity. If we were only to perceive, we would lose ourselves all the time in acts of external seeing. But by retreating from the things themselves, by thinking about them—thereby one becomes a personality, an individuality. We do not lose ourselves in the things. When we study the human etheric body, we find that it has within it a center for the forces that throw out lead. This center, approximately, lies where the hairs grow in a kind of vortex at the back of the crown of the head.... The forces that the body has developed for overcoming lead have great significance; they are the same forces that enable me, when I am looking, for example, at this piece of chalk, not to be entirely caught up in the simple act of looking at the chalk.... It is because of these forces that human beings can be self-contained personalities; these forces enable a person to separate from the world.[359]

That capacity for separation, which is necessary for objective sense activity, is stimulated and strengthened through a constitutional treatment with lead. Lead also helps to bring the possibility for memory:

> You must therefore imagine the Earth and, in the distance, Saturn filling the whole planetary system with finely distributed lead; and then imagine this fine lead substance working in on humankind. You can still find evidence that this was taught to those to be initiated in ancient Greece, and that they came to understand how this lead worked. They knew that without it the sense organs, especially the eye, would claim the whole human being and not allow us to reach self-independence. Humanity

would be able only to see and not to think about what one had seen. We would be unable to detach ourselves from what we saw and say: I see. We would, as it were, be overpowered by seeing, unless this lead influence were present in the cosmos. It is this activity of lead that makes it possible for us to be independent in ourselves, placing us as "I"-beings in the face of this sensitivity to the outer world that is in us. It is these lead forces that, entering the human ether body first, and then from the ether body also, in a sense, impregnating the physical body, bestowing on us the faculty and power of memory.... We are human beings only because we can recollect today what we knew ten or twenty years ago. Consider how the human part of us would suffer if we did not carry within us what we experienced ten or twenty years ago. Our "I"-force would be shattered unless this power of memory were fully present. The power of memory is the result of what streams to us from distant Saturn...and then we were told that another force must be placed over against the Saturn force—that of the Moon. Let us suppose that these two forces act in such a way that the Saturn force and the Moon force approach from opposite sides and, flowing into each other, descend to the Earth and to humanity on Earth. Then what Saturn takes from us the Moon gives to us. And what Saturn gives to us, the Moon takes from us.... It was a deeply solemn moment when the Greek pupil was led to see this opposition of Saturn and the Moon. In the holy solemnity of night, one was told: Look up to Saturn surrounded by his rings. To him you owe the fact that you are an independent human being. Look to the other side, to the Moon streaming out her rays of silver. To her you owe the fact that you are able to bear the Saturn forces without being cut off from the rest of the cosmos."[360]

Clear sensing, objective perception, and memory all express how the "I" is able to make a home in the physical body. Steiner took his description of the Lead process further and also related it to morality. This aspect of morality is different from the imbalances that we have seen with the feebleminded and kleptomaniacal polarities (in which the challenge lies in incomplete moral perception, in an inability to properly sense the other, owing to a weakened limb activity). Lead, in contrast, speaks more to an inner corruption or imbalance of the feeling life:

> In that, as human beings, we have this process of [lead] elimination within us, we are able to receive independent moral forces into ourselves. We can imagine that the human organism as presently constituted may be unable to make use of lead but contains certain forces that compensate for lead; we can imagine the organism containing lead in the same way that it now contains iron. If this were so, human beings would bring themselves into semi-moral qualities—for so it is with lead. We would then have a morbid affinity (we should call it a "morbid" or "pathological affinity") to the impurities in the outside world. Such individuals would always be on the lookout for evil-smelling substances and like to smell them. If we notice that some child has perverted instincts of this kind—and there are children who are partial to everything that smells—they will sniff petroleum, for instance—then we may be sure that the quality of the blood that rejects lead, is not present. And it is then a matter of calling up this lead-rejecting power by clinical methods or even by medications. It is possible to do this.[361]

We can summarize several main points on the use of constitutional Lead treatments in the following way:

- Lead (Plumbum) brings definition and maturity to the nerve–sense system. In this way it is the main treatment for the large-headed constitution. For very specific circumstances it can be given in a low potency (6x), such as if there are clear physical signs of a delayed maturation process (like persistently open fontanels, difficulty with movement, or a face that looks very young for the chronological age), but it is much more commonly prescribed in a higher potency (20x). This higher potency is generally appropriate for the school-age child,[362] for in this situation the therapeutic goal is usually to address the cognitive, sensory weakness of the large-headed pole, and a higher potency (20x–30x) addresses the head pole. Once-daily dosing, in the morning, is sufficient. It is important to give lead preparations for only a limited period of time (typically five weeks, a full etheric cycle), then to heal it over with a course of low-potency copper (Cuprum 6x), given in the evening for a couple weeks to balance the lead.[363] The cycle can be repeated, if necessary, but it is important to treat once and then leave some time to see what changes have taken place before initiating a second cycle. The impact of a lead treatment is deep and therefore must be prescribed only very judiciously.

- Lead also supports powers of memory when there is a loss of oneself in the stream of time. Lack of memory results in a very real loss of orientation as we are not able to remember what we have already done or learned or said. This leaves little memory foundation to build upon. This situation can be observed in certain children, particularly those who are experiencing more profound developmental delay. It is an imbalance on the incarnation pathway that in some ways parallels the dementia and loss of orientation more commonly experienced as part of the excarnation pathway toward the end of life. (Indeed, lead—combined with sugar and honey—is a remedy indicated by Steiner and Dr. Ita Wegman for memory loss and sclerosis in old age, in the form of Scleron.[364]) When children seem unable to build upon their experience and perpetually need to start anew (with learning, with language) we sense that a weakened capacity for memory is part of their developmental delay and consider a Lead treatment.
- There has also been experience with Lead to treat cruel behaviors, including the mistreatment of animals and other sensory-seeking behaviors related to perverse instincts. The potency should be based on the larger constitutional picture—that is, based on clear physical markers of imbalance (low potency), more in feeling life (middle potency), or in the thinking life (higher potency), though again a higher potency is most commonly indicated.

In considering constitutional treatments for strengthening and shaping the head pole, we can include several other related remedies, even though Steiner did not specifically reference them for treatment of the large-headed constitution. Their activities can help us to better recognize and define the character of a lead process. On one side we can look at the relationship between lead and silica and, on the other, the metamorphosis of activity from lead to tin and from tin to iron.

Lead, tin, and iron stand within the range of planetary metals, moving us from the outmost planet (Saturn) in toward the sun. One step in from the sobering activity of lead we find tin (and the planetary activity of Jupiter) and then, a step further, iron (related to the activity of Mars).

Lead process	Saturn activity
Tin process	Jupiter activity
Iron process	Mars activity

For each of these three planetary activities there is natural kinship with silica, for although it does not fall into this sequence of planetary metals, silica bears a relationship to the head and to the whole nerve–sense system:

> If we look first at the siliceous quality that gives form to human beings, we must not forget that the particular areas within the human organization that resemble this siliceous quality, for reasons I have already explained in part on previous days, have a relationship to the metallic qualities of lead, tin, and iron. Thus we can say that when we look at the area above the heart, we must look at what works within the human being on the basis of silicic acid on the one hand and on the basis of the qualities of lead, tin, and iron on the other. The iron quality has more to do with the lung's formative process, the tin quality with the head's general formative principle, and the lead quality with the formative force that is located in the bones, because bone structure and bone growth essentially originate from the upper part of the human being, not the lower part.[365]

Steiner here connected the metals to organs and built a spectrum of activity: from bones (which are most inward and hidden), to the general formative activity (which works downward from the head and can be outwardly observed as it is visible from the outside), to the lungs (the organ system, which even more directly continually engages with the outside world through a continual exchange of air). Similarly, we can build that progression on a larger developmental spectrum—including Lead, which works to bring children from the spiritual world and works to draw them into real relationship with the physical world; Tin, which addresses children more on the level of the bodily form; and Iron, which strengthens the capacity to be in the organs and make good use of them (but no longer carries such a formative activity). An analogy might be helping children decide to plan and build a house (Plumbum), bringing in workers to construct the house with proper form (Stannum), and then moving all the furniture in and actually starting to live in one's new home (Ferrum).

Plumbum	bone structure and growth	leaving the spiritual
Stannum	head's formative principle	forming the body
Ferrum	lung's formative process	inhabiting the body

This formative spectrum of activity helps when considering variations of nerve–sense imbalance. We can also now look at the spectrum of activity of each of these metals and the ways in which silica may be used with them in therapeutic combination.

Silica

When we speak of Silica, we are really describing a silica process. The silica process underlies all sensing and nerve organ activities. Silica does this by opening a space between two fields of action in which "consciousness must unfold."[366] Consciousness, mirroring, is allowed to arise in this inwardly and outwardly bordered space: "Silica has a twofold task. Inwardly, it sets a border to processes such as growth, nutrition, and so on. To the outside it closes the mere effects of nature off from the inner organism, so that it does not continue the workings of nature within its own sphere, but is able to unfold its own."[367] This "own" space defines sensory maturation. From this, we can see how silica (which commonly occurs in natural combination with lead) can be used for the treatment of a child with excessive growth and nutrition processes, creating a sensing space between inner metabolism and outer world. Silica sets a border to processes of growth and nutrition (like the dominant metabolism of the large-headed constitution), and Plumbum crystallizes the sense organs into their proper form. A constitutional treatment with both Plumbum and *Silicicum* can therefore be used as a successful treatment when there is an incomplete formation, a delayed maturation of the nerve–sense pole. As a therapeutic example, *Plumbum silicicum*, 20x, can meet the very young sensing and thinking capacities seen in conditions like autism.

Cichorium (Chicory)

A similar therapeutic process can be invoked when the closing off of the inner organism from the outer world needs to happen more in the realm of digestion, though in this case we need to find a way to bring boundary activity, in a lower potency, but without too strong a devitalizing effect. Lack of proper boundary in the metabolic realm means that we are too immediately affected by the substances of the world and are not able to create the proper antipathy to fully meet and transform them (an imbalance that frequently happens with food allergies). For this situation a lead and silica process can be brought in a different form, through Chicory. *Cichorium plumbo culta* (a vegetabilized lead remedy, given in a low potency, 2x or 3x) helps to bring form and boundary to the digestion, without deadening the metabolic process. Chicory, well known for its powerfully bitter taste, invokes strong digestive activity. The associated digestive sensing is made possible because of the plant's special relationship to silica: "*Cichorium intybus*...in addition, a considerable amount of silicic acid is present."[368] Further, "we find that *Cichorium intybus* is not only an antidote to digestive weakness but also to weakness in the organs immediately exposed to the external world."[369] We are even told that Chicory prevents us "from admitting disturbances in the composition of the blood fluid itself." Chicory is more than a digestive remedy. It exerts a broader effect; its protective activity guards against the outside world and can even "reach to the periphery and under certain conditions may affect the organs of the head but especially of the throat and chest, and the lungs."[370] Chicory plant that has been cultivated in lead-enriched soil stimulates better digestive activity at the organ level but also carries that digestive strength over into other boundary organs like the intestines, throat, chest, lungs, and head. Indications include "psychological boundary disorder...[with characteristics such as] sensitivity to smells; easily influenced and irritated by external sense experiences; sleep disturbance; addictive patterns (smoking, computer, internet, television, gambling); digestive weakness coupled with weak will forces."[371]

Stannum (Tin)

A step in from lead we encounter the formative activity of tin, *Stannum.* Whereas lead and silica work to build strong boundaries—a delimiting of one activity from another—tin works a little more gently, acting to bring form to life without totally stopping life. It works in a refining way, guiding and forming a process without deadening it. *Stannum* is commonly prescribed for formative weakness—such as dysplastic conditions, in which the formative forces of the head are not yet able to fully descend into and meet the physical body. This is true with almost any kind of anomalous or incomplete organ formation (cleft palate, horseshoe kidney, undescended testes) or a loss of form evidenced on a general, structural level through conditions like low muscle tone, exceptionally loose joints, or flat feet. *Stannum* is usually given as a high potency to support organ formation (20x), frequently in combination with *Hypophysis* (which was discussed for the klepto-maniacal pole for helping bring the activity of the head down into the body). *Stannum* can also be prescribed in a higher potency for weakened thinking. Tin can be helpful when the architecture or formality of thoughts remains elusive (like grasping the lawfulness of mathematical concepts). *Stannum* can also be given in combination with silica (*Stannum silicicum*), a remedy that directs the formative activity of tin more toward the organs of the head, as opposed to the more metabolic activity of combining *Stannum* with *Hypophysis* (Pituitary).

Bidor

We can also consider the combination of Iron and Silica. There are still other situations in which a child remains weak in thought, but the weakness is mostly related to the fatigue that comes with too much thinking, reading, listening, or watching. This is another variation of a weakened nerve–sense system that is not in order, but it is different from the lead picture because the head pole loses its proper function through being worn down. For these children the nerve–sense organs have already reached a certain completeness and maturity (which the classically large-headed child has not yet achieved), but the child cannot sustain proper nerve–sense activity in the face of too much sensory work. Once the nerve–sense system is worn down, metabolic forces rise, which cloud clear sensing activity. This imbalance results in headache (a migraine). The picture, then, is of a child whose thinking quickly fatigues and who loses orientation and cannot make intellectual connections. The remedy *Bidor* helps to balance this weakness of the nerve–sense system. It was indicated by Steiner as a treatment for migraine but also as a remedy for too much "civilization." In this way we can see that *Bidor*, a silica and iron remedy (sulfur too), helps protect and balance a child when the nerve–sense system loses its order from being overwhelmed:

> A diagnosis-specific dose of correctly formulated silica supports the forces of the sensory–nervous system as they are meant to develop in the organism. A remedy prepared from quartz or silica supports what the senses are meant to do. Depending on the

> patient's secondary symptoms, other substances will need to be included in the preparation, but the most important factor in this case is the effect of the silica formative process. When introduced into the human organism, the activity of silica supports weakened sensory–nervous activity and brings it up to the appropriate level of intensity. When sensory–nervous activity becomes too weak, digestive activity extends forcefully into the head, and migraine-like conditions ensue. If we reinforce sensory–nervous functions in the right way with a remedy that has been correctly prepared from quartz or silica, the migraine sufferer's sensory–nervous system will become strong enough to force back the digestive process that has invaded the head.[372]

Bidor works strongly as a Silica remedy, but its balanced threefold composition—of silica for the nerve–sense system, iron for the rhythmic, and sulfur for the metabolic system—finds wide application for support of a child who is overwhelmed by the demands of academic work. *Bidor* can help balance the proper allocation of life forces after the seven-year change, reflected in the fact that Steiner's original name for the remedy was *Biodoron*—a "gift" to "life."

Archetypal Remedy Pictures for Working with the Small-headed Constitution

Argentum (Silver)

Silver stands at the opposite pole from lead. Lead breaks things down, brings distance, matures; silver builds things up and makes them more cohesive. If we imagine the filling up, the rejuvenation of the sclerotic, hollow old man described in *Understanding Healing*, we come into the activity of silver:

> The forces that split up the physical organism so that the spiritual could find a place are also present in lead. Forces of disintegration have brought lead into existence. If we introduce lead into the human organism, splitting takes place. If there is too

> little destruction within human beings and they need certain processes of disintegration, we must give them lead in some form. Vice versa; if the condition is such that the formative power is lacking to the degree that the human organism is becoming too "spongy," so to speak, ancient knowledge teaches that the forces of the Moon (which in ancient times streamed the substance of silver into form) must be brought into play. The forces of silver can bring a spongy quality to form; they support the Moon forces. The whole planetary system is connected with substances that are remedial:
>
> | | | |
> |---|---|---|
> | Saturn | = | Lead |
> | Jupiter | = | Tin |
> | Mars | = | Iron |
> | Sun | = | Gold |
> | Venus | = | Copper |
> | Mercury | = | Quicksilver |
> | Moon | = | Silver |
>
> These correspondences are treated with unbelievable superficiality nowadays, whereas in reality they are based upon most minute investigations which were carried on in the ancient mysteries.[373]

The spongy quality described is another picture of the hollowness of age, when things have been split too far and there is no longer cohesiveness. *Argentum* balances excessive formative activity, excessive catabolism:

> Silver is connected, in a certain respect, with the building forces, so that when we notice in human beings that the building forces are being overpowered by the forces of demolition, we can genrally correct this by means of some medication derived from silver.[374]

In this way *Argentum* is a broadly applicable remedy, because today so many children are bombarded with such overpowering sensory input, which by its very nature overemphasizes the catabolic activity of the head pole. Today there are generally more children who will benefit from a constitutional treatment with silver than children who need lead (though lead is a very helpful remedy when it is applied in the correct developmental situations). The external forces that make us aware too soon far outnumber those that keep us young too long.

Like the spectrum of nerve–sense activity seen with lead, tin, and iron, different aspects of metabolic–limb activity are supported through the metals of silver, mercury, and copper. All three of these remedies were indicated by Dr. Ita Wegman as a combination (Argentum/Mercurius/Cuprum 15x trituration) for "insufficient digestion and uptake of what has been taken in as nourishment: for people who are weakened and have little vitality, and who, in spite of sufficient nourishment stay thin."[375] Silver's activity within this spectrum is to build the foundation upon which all other metabolic activity can take place. It helps shift activity away from an independent astral activity to one that is united with the etheric. Returning to Steiner's faculty discussion of the small-headed polarity in a first-grade girl:

> First try to get the parents to give her a warm stomach wrap, perhaps even a little damp, for a longer period, so that the astral body becomes more firmly seated in the metabolic–limb being. Silver would be the right remedy for her. For her, much depends upon getting the metabolic–limb system to take over the activities of the astral body. Give her silver and stomach wraps. She is a child who does not live in herself and is not in her metabolism at all.[376]

Silver constitutional treatment is directed primarily toward the etheric. It bears a strong relationship to the reproductive organs (which have exceptional etheric forces) and supports the nutritive activity and growth forces for the whole body. Supporting etheric forces encourages the higher members to find their way down into the metabolism, into fourfold interweaving. The etheric acts as an essential bridge. When the etheric body is weakened, metabolic activity will necessarily be compromised, because the "I" and astral body cannot find their way into this cooperative activity. They will be active, but working more from the head pole (nerve and respiratory pathway). Through silver the lower pathways for pulse and blood are opened and encouraged (see fig. 21).

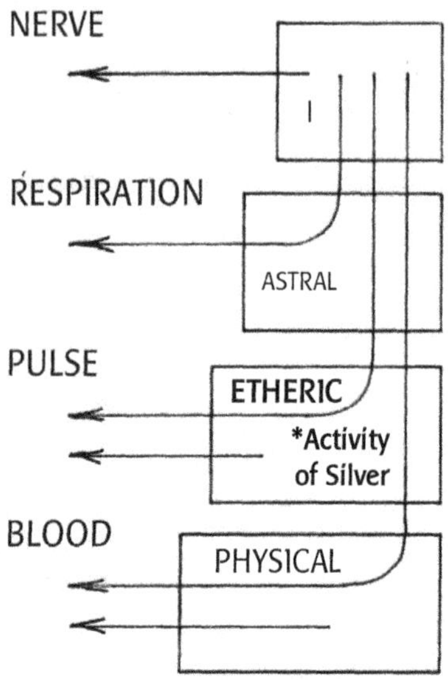

Figure 21: Activity of silver within the fourfold metabolic stream

Silver thereby has a supportive and harmonizing effect on all metabolic activity. Even seemingly contradictory imbalances (such as diarrhea and constipation) can both find support through a silver treatment. On the one side we can think of prescribing *Argentum* when the digestion is too active, or stimulated. Silver acts to free the higher members when they are penetrating too deeply into the metabolism and causing excessive digestive activity. The resulting increased etheric activity buffers the astral and "I":

> But suppose the astral body and "I" are working too actively in the digestive organs. These two organizations are the active motors as it were of the digestive organization in the metabolic–limb

> system. If they work too strongly, penetrate too deeply, then there is excessive digestive activity. Too much is digested, too strongly and too fast. There is a tendency to diarrhea and other kindred symptoms, which are the result of too rapid and thus too superficial digestion.... If we know that the astral body and the "I"-organization are driven out of the metabolic–limb system by the administration of a certain dosage of silver, we are further aware that if the astral organism and the "I"-organization are too deeply embedded in the metabolic–limb system, we can raise them out of the latter by giving a remedy consisting of silver or silver combined with some other substance.[377]

Silver, as a treatment for a metabolic–limb system that is "not in order" includes this clinical picture of too superficial, too quick digestive activity with associated diarrhea. This is a pattern frequently seen in children with food allergies. These children do indeed greatly benefit from an Argentum treatment—though they bring quite a different constitutional picture from the lack of sufficient boundary when one is overcome by foreign food substance (see the preceding description of *Chicory* as a lead remedy). As with attention problems, where it is helpful to differentiate between inattention and distraction, parallel distinctions can be observed in a child's engagement with food substances. Working between the poles of lead and silver we can ask, "Is the child too open and overcome by nourishment or so metabolically weakened as to be able to engage only superficially with it?"

Silver also supports underactive, slowed digestion (like constipation). The enlivened etheric activity stimulated by *Argentum* can bring greater mobility, which then allows more complete excretion to take place:

> As paradoxical as it may sound, we discover in silver an activity that can be enhanced to the point of the excretion that occurs when an egg cell is released in the human organism. In silver's functional aspect, we find an external, natural manifestation of the excretion forces at work in the human being. The pronounced excretion effects of silver reveal its tremendous significance (in the appropriate dosage) for the human abdomen in general. Thus

> when we introduce silver, in combination with the appropriate finders and additions, into the digestive system, it affects elimination. Silver remedies can have an extremely significant effect on blocked elimination processes.[378]

Silver (*Argentum*) is generally given in a low potency (6x) several times daily for a period of four to eight weeks.[379] Silver can also be given in the form of *Argentite* 6x (natural silver sulfide). This combination with sulfur brings the activity of silver more specifically to the metabolism (just as combining Plumbum with silica brings the lead activity more directly to the nerve–sense system). Sulfur also has a special relationship with protein synthesis and therefore the whole upbuilding, nutritive aspect of metabolism. It is most indicated when the physical body needs to be opened up to greater etheric activity[380]—like the slowed digestive picture mentioned previously. It is also helpful for the child with a small-headed constitution who also carries a denser, iron-rich process (with dark hair and dark eyes). A child with blond hair and blue eyes (more sulfurous constitution) usually benefits more from a course of just the metal (Argentum). Sulfurous children often benefit from a healing over of silver with a short course of iron (Ferrum 8x).[381] The etheric bounty engendered by a silver treatment, especially if it seems to lead to too much expansion (even euphoria), can then be properly spurred into activity with a little iron. In this way, the outermost metabolic metal, silver, is balanced with the innermost nerve–sense metal, iron (just as lead, the outermost nerve–sense metal, is balanced with the innermost metabolic metal, copper).

We find related expressions of the silver process in the plant world. Bryophyllum, the "mother of thousands," can also be considered as a treatment for the small-headed constitution. It is a remarkable plant, prolific in its reproductive process as it repeatedly moves from the growth process of the leaves right into the formation of hundreds and indeed sometimes thousands of new plants. Light and warmth ether intervene just enough to separate the young new plants from the mother leaf but not to unfold a true flower or fruit process. The etheric is too strong. Bryophyllum helps create greater etheric shielding from the surrounding world and is particularly helpful with sleep disturbances. The remedy *Bryophyllum argento cultum* (2x or 3x) quiets restless behaviors and allows the child to let go of overwhelming sensory impressions that have become somatized. It works best on the sensory side (less so the digestive side) of the small-headed constitution. (It is discussed in more detail as a remedy for the hysteric constitution.)

Just as Steiner indicated a relationship between the upper planetary metals (lead, tin, and iron) with silica, so did he link the lower planetary metals (silver, mercury, and copper) with the carbonates.[382] One can also consider calcium carbonate as a treatment for a metabolic–limb system not in order, particularly when excretion is imbalanced. It is described in more depth in the next section in relation to the epileptic and hysteric constitutions.

Archetypal Remedy Pictures for Working with the Epileptic Constitution

> For we shall not get to the heart of the trouble, when epileptic phenomena are present, without employing medicines, nor should we shrink from doing so.... Anyone who has observed many epileptic children, or many children with a tendency to epilepsy, will have noticed two conditions which differ very considerably from one another. There is, first, the condition where the child does not defy moral judgment; he adapts himself to the moral and ethical standards that one would desire to impart to every child. When we have to do with epileptic or epileptoid children who readily adapt themselves in this way to the moral order, then the indications that have already been given will perhaps suffice. But if we have to do with children who are not accessible to moral influence—who, for example, readily become violent

Table 18: Summary table of medical treatments to support the epileptic and hysteric constitutions

<table>
<tr><th>Epileptic Constitution</th><th>Hysteric Constitution</th></tr>
<tr><td>

Belladonna

- Balances activity between the astral and etheric bodies
- Mirrors the "waking process" in the human being
- Can be used in a wide range of potencies (2x–30x), lower potencies used for an epileptic process that is more physically manifest; middle or higher potencies for when the imbalance shows itself more in feeling life or thought and consciousness
- Often recommended by Steiner in combination with other nightshades (*Hyoscyamus* or *Stramonium*)

Sulfur

- Increases the disposition of physical substance for intervention of the organism's etheric activity
- Works in the realm of the etheric and physical bodies (does not address the astral directly)
- Generally used in low potencies

Algae (Vaucheria)

- For obtuseness, when "the physical body and the etheric body refuse to allow the astral body to enter... due not to an excessive attraction exerted by the "I"-organization but to a special resistance from the ether body"
- To support the process of finding greater capacity, such as for inflammations in which the child is working to overcome the hereditary body (scarlet fever)

Chamomile

- An example of an organ-specific treatment for disturbance of the "nerves" in the digestive organs

</td><td>

Bryophyllum

- Anchors the etheric in the metabolism, working to balance a hysteric process by strengthening etheric activity
- Helpful for bringing an etheric "buffer" to create more protection from the outside
- Used in low potency (50 % titration to 6x), also in the vegetabilized form *Bryophyllum argento culta*

Conchae (Calcium carbonicum)

- Directs excessive activity of spirit and soul out from the metabolism (the lower human being); helps to release too much intelligence from what should be a restful, sleeping metabolism
- Stimulates processes of excretion

Berberis

- Brings vitalized astral activity to the bladder and kidney
- An organ-specific treatment for the hysteric constitution (compare with the picture of *Chamomile*)

~

Phosphorus—important as a *contrast* to the other remedies for the hysteric child

- Drives inhalation
- Has a wakening effect
- Excess creates a state where we "vehemently desire that sense impressions come quickly"

A remedy polar to *Conchae, Argentum, Silica,* and *Arsenicum*

</td></tr>
</table>

> during their attacks, since epileptic attacks might disguise themselves as outbursts of violence, of which such children later have no memory—if, in short, defects present at a moral level, then it is important to intervene in early childhood with actual medicines. In these cases, we shall quite definitely try to fight the epilepsy with the medicines that are in general use for the purpose, or with remedies prescribed by us under certain conditions, medicines like Sulfur or Belladonna—thus entering upon a regular medical treatment.[383]

Belladonna

Belladonna can be understood as an archetypal plant remedy for the epileptic process. *Belladonna* is important because it embodies an intense interaction between the astral and etheric bodies, one that is unusual for the plant world. Steiner mentioned it (in the previous quotation) as part of a "regular medical treatment" for the epileptic constitution. He also recommended *Belladonna* for many other illness processes where the same kind of excessive or blocked astral activity is present.

We can know that *Belladonna* carries an unusually strong astral process because it is a poisonous plant. The presence of a poison in the plant world means that an astral impulse has penetrated into the plant itself (which usually has only physical and etheric activity). Cosmic astrality usually meets a plant only at its periphery—through the sculpting of the edges of the leaves, the coloring of flowers, the forming of petals—but in some plants that astrality goes beyond the flower realm and is pulled more deeply into the living activity of the plant. This astrality does not enter harmoniously into the etheric; it retains a strong, independent astral quality. That same kind of strong, penetrating astrality is present in the other plants of the nightshade family, including *Hyoscyamus* (Henbane) and *Stramonium* (Jimson weed), both of which Steiner similarly recommended for the treatment of seizures. He described the nightshade plant family in this way:

> Poisonous substances have the peculiarity that they do not make use of the etheric as do the normal green substances in the plant; instead they turn directly to the astral, so that the astral enters into this substance. With Belladonna, the fruit becomes especially greedy and is not satiated by absorbing the etheric element alone; instead the fruit absorbs the astral element directly, before this astral element has absorbed on its path downward the life forces through the etheric.... Such drops of the astral being, which have not gone through the ether atmosphere in the right way, can, for example, be found in the poison of the deadly nightshade. We also have this cosmic astral element dripping down into the plant in the poison of the Jimsonweed, or thornapple (Stramonium), fruit, in henbane (Hyoscyamus), and so on.
>
> What therefore lives in this plant substance, for example in the deadly nightshade, is related to the activity that enters the human nerves and circulation of oxygen directly from the "I" or the astral body. Thus, by taking in the poison of the deadly nightshade, we get a significant strengthening of the breakdown processes in us, those processes that otherwise enter the physical body directly from the "I."[384]

Such breakdown processes make possible the conscious activity of the nerve–sense pole. Belladonna treatment strengthens those pathways that the "I" and astral body take when they enter the physical body directly (as opposed to the fully interpenetrating, fourfold weaving that creates limb and metabolic activity). In this way, Belladonna is related to the waking process, which is held back in the epileptic process:

> Deadly nightshade (Atropa belladonna)... is related to everything in the human organism that moves in the direction of the type of form of development that can happen only in the domain of the senses, to something that lifts human beings out of the domain of their internal organization and into the domain of the senses. The process that takes place when tiny potentized amounts of deadly nightshade are ingested is

> extremely interesting, because it is very similar to the normal version of this same process—namely, the waking-up process that is mingled with dreaming. Waking up (the state when we are still not quite perceiving with our senses and sensory perception is still directed inward, pervading our consciousness with dreams) is a type of deadly nightshade process within the human being."[385]

Steiner generally recommended Belladonna for patients with epilepsy in a lower potency (6x),[386] though for a fifteen-year-old boy presented during the curative course lectures, Steiner recommended Belladonna in ascending potencies: 4x, 10x, 15x, 20x, 30x. For a different, twenty-one-year-old patient, he advised ascending potencies of 15x, 30x, 60x.[387] Steiner also sometimes recommended *Belladonna* in ointment form, to be rubbed into the calves.[388] This route of administration is interesting, because elsewhere Steiner described how the use of topical applications (like creams, ointments, oils, and metal foils) more specifically address the nerve–sense system.[389] We have heard how the waking process, via the entry of the "I" and astral body, begins at the periphery of the body, at the fingers and toes, and slowly works its way in. With the application of *Belladonna* ointment, we are then appealing to a nerve–sense activity in the metabolic–limb system—a therapeutic gesture that addresses a child who still seems very dull and asleep in the limbs. The process of applying an ointment or cream brings better consciousness and connection with the limbs in of itself, through both the activity of application as well as the sensation of having something rubbed into the skin and muscles.

When we use *Belladonna* as an oral medication, we are directing therapy more to the metabolic system. A low-potency *Belladonna* tincture (2x–6x) addresses an epileptic constitution in which the initial stages of the waking process are really imbalanced, as with manifest seizures (the early morning hours are a common time for people with generalized epilepsy to have a seizure), or, alternately, those who are very deep sleepers and have difficulty awakening. Here we are supporting the waking process when it is still very close to the metabolic state of deep sleep. As we move up in potency to address the rhythmic system (8x–15x) or the nerve–sense system (20x–30x, even 60x), we are working to balance the epileptic process more on a feeling and then on a thinking level. Steiner's recommendations for a rising sequence of potencies can be understood as working through an astral/etheric imbalance from the metabolism through to full waking consciousness (as with the 4x to 30x sequence for the fifteen-year-old boy).

The nightshade plants (Belladonna, Hyoscyamus, and Stramonium) were also recommended by Steiner for epilepsy, often in combination and usually in lower potency, though Steiner did differentiate the activities of Belladonna and Hyoscyamus in the following way (even when he sometimes recommended both Belladonna and Hyoscyamus at the same time):

> Belladonna will then work especially well if you know that there are abnormalities in the brain, or at the least, in organs that have a relationship to the nerve–sense system. But as soon as one has something in the lower tract, one must see that *Hyoscyamus* works.[390]

Hyoscyamus was previously considered as part of a compound remedy for the maniacal constitution (Aurum/Stibium/Hyoscyamus) for calming excessive, unguided activity of the metabolic–limb system. In the treatment of the epileptic constitution it is a helpful addition, particularly when the fit process involves violent or aggressive limb activity (hitting, kicking).

Sulfur

Sulfur is the other remedy that was specifically indicated by Steiner for the epileptic constitution during the curative course. Belladonna's activity lies at the interface of the astral and etheric, supporting the wakening activity of the astral body in order to support a fuller sensing activity. Sulfur similarly works to bring harmony between the etheric and astral, but it does so by loosening the physical body so that it is better able to take up the etheric. Sulfur is also connected with the excretory processes of digestion, thereby relieving the body of unneeded substance—another kind of mobilization of physical material. Steiner recommended sulfur for such diverse conditions as lumps in the breast, gouty arthritis, and a "tendency to consolidation,"[391] all of which are aided by sulfur's work to help make physical substance more accessible:

> It is essential to bring harmony between etheric and astral activity. The etheric body must be strengthened, the astral toned down. This can be made to happen by bringing the physical substances, which the etheric body is processing, into a condition in which they accommodate activity more easily than when a state of disease is present.... [Sulfur] functions in the sphere of the physical and ether body. This is also apparent from the fact that an increased supply of sulfur evokes feelings of dizziness, suppression of consciousness in the organism. Sleep, the state of the body in which the astral body and "I"-organization are not at work as soul beings, also becomes more intensive when the sulfur supply is increased.... One can learn from this that sulfur, introduced as a medication, will increase the disposition of the physical activities for intervention of the organism's etheric activities."[392]

This loosening aspect speaks—with regard to the epileptic constitution—to the very fine organ infiltrates Steiner described. *Sulfur* can make an organ more pliable and accessible for the entering astral and "I."

Sulfur is elsewhere indicated as being important for the shifting interplay between circulation and respiration. Sulfur's role on that threshold is emphasized for both Pyrite and Cinnabar remedies, which Steiner and Wegman included as "Typical Medicines":

> [Pyrite, the natural combination of iron and sulfur] embodies that process by which rhythm inclined to the digestive system is transformed to one that inclines to breathing.... Sulfur mediates the connection between blood circulation and breathing.[393]

They went on to say:

> The characteristic property of sulfur, which has been mentioned before, is that sulfur proves its efficacy in the area of the organism where circulation and breathing border on each other [in relation to cinnabar, a natural combination of mercury and sulfur].[394]

Sulfur's activity helps to mediate this shifting from "I" and astral alone (related to breathing) to "I" and astral working in concert with the etheric (related to pulse), another interface between the etheric and astral bodies.

We can therefore characterize sulfur's contribution to therapy for the epileptic constitution as an aid to opening the physical body for the etheric (especially if we have the sense that the body is too consolidated) and as a balancing influence for the shifting physiology between circulation and breath.

The Algae (Vaucheria)

The fifteen-year-old epileptic boy mentioned in the quotation at the opening of this section is one of the children Steiner examined during the curative course. The boy is described as having "a certain obtuseness to external impressions," with an accompanying recommendation that the boy should paint with color. Steiner then brought a remedy picture:

> There can be no question but that we must intervene here also with medical treatment. We have not, I think up to now, prescribed any medicaments? The boy should have Algae and Belladonna. Treatment will consist of these two medicines.... Why do we propose for this boy Algae injections? In the algae we have plants that have neither strong root development nor strongly developed flower development. It is indeed almost as though flower and root had been telescoped. The leaf organization is the main thing; everything else is produced from it. In algae therefore, since foliage preponderates, we find no intensive relationship to the earth. Nor, on the other hand, is there an intensive relationship to the outer cosmos. There is, however, a relationship to the watery and airy elements that are active immediately over the surface of the earth. Algae—and the same applies also to fungi—are plants that are, as it were, completely steeped in the interplay of air and water. And these two kinds of plants have in addition this characteristic in common, that they are strongly attracted to the minute quantity of sulfur which is to be found everywhere today in water as well as in air. Consequently, when these plants are introduced into the human rhythmic organism, they are peculiarly adapted to restore harmony between astral body and ether body.... In cases where we perceive a disorder due to the "I"-organization making too great a demand upon the astral body and not allowing it to enter into the etheric body, we must have recourse rather to the fungi. The algae, which come nearer to the ordinary plant, are to be used when the physical body and etheric body refuse to allow the astral body to enter—that is to say, when the disharmony is due not to an excessive attraction exerted by the "I"-organization, but to a special resistance put up by the ether body.[395]

This overcoming of the physical and etheric body is also very much the picture of the young child's overcoming the hereditary body. Steiner recommended the use of Algae in low potency both for epilepsy (5x) and for scarlet fever (3x, 5x),[396] the childhood illness that comes when the "I" and astral body are excessive in their activity.[397]

Steiner elsewhere spoke of algae, lichens, and mushrooms as being related to our earliest developmental stages[398] and gave instruction to the teachers about how the plant world can be connected directly with the temperaments and how particular kinds of plants could be described to the children:

> Now we will go out into nature and look for something there that is asleep just like you when you were tiny little mites. Naturally you could not think of this yourselves, but there are those who know, and they can tell you that all the fungi and mushrooms which you find in the woods are fast asleep just as you were when you were tiny babies. Fungi and mushrooms are the sleeping souls of childhood.
>
> Then you came to the time when you learned to walk and to speak. You know from watching your little brothers and sisters that little children have first of all to learn speaking and walking, or you can say walking and then speaking. That was something new for you, which you could not do when your life began: you learned something fresh and you could do many more things when you learned to walk and speak.
>
> Now we will go out into nature again and search for something that can do more than mushrooms and fungi. These are the algae. (I must show the children some examples of algae), and the mosses (I must show them some mosses). There is something in algae and mosses which can do much more than what is in the fungi.[399]

We can see from this pedagogical picture how the Algae (such as Vaucheria) help a child to come into greater capacity by overcoming an obtuseness, lifting the child from predominantly vegetative (etheric) to mobile and wakeful (astral) activity.

Chamomile

Steiner's description of the epileptic constitution includes symptoms associated with different outside elements (like gravity, water, light, and warmth) as well as relationships to specific organs (e.g., nausea and the circulatory system). The chamomile plant is introduced here as an example of an organ-specific epileptic therapy. Chamomile has a strong relationship to the astral airy element—with thin, long stems; lacy, fine leaves; and delicate, aromatic, hollow flowers—as well as a strong sulfur component. It can be understood as another remedy that helps to balance a blocked or cramped astrality and has long been used as a natural aid for cramping pain, anxiety, and sleep problems. Steiner spoke of its special relationship to the digestion, as a remedy for "nerve" illnesses:

> Now it is very interesting how, if one localizes a disorder of the nerves to the digestive tract or right in the stomach, and it does not continue on out of the digestive organs, one can achieve the same thing—this is really extraordinarily interesting—if one uses Chamomile instead of Arnica, especially as injections.[400]

Chamomile therefore stands as a treatment for the epileptic constitution when symptoms are primarily below the diaphragm (as opposed to Arnica, whose activity relates much more to the central nervous system).

Chamomile can be used in the form of a vegetabilized metal preparation, where Chamomile and Cuprum (copper) are combined. Cuprum has a similar and closely related remedy picture to that of Chamomile: "With a [copper] process, which dampens down the oversensitivity of the astral body in the digestive tract, we were able to divert this astral activity to the ether body, where it normally belongs."[401] Cuprum was recommended by Steiner as an epilepsy remedy distinct from Chamomile for a five-year-old girl with spastic paresis and epilepsy (in a 4x potency) as well as an ointment rubbed into the soles of the feet in a twenty-six-year-old woman.[402]

In terms of other organ pictures, an indication for Mucilago levistici (the gumlike substance that can be extracted from Levisticum, lovage) is given for epileptiform conditions associated with palpitations and an irregular activity of the astral body in the blood circulation.[403]

Nicotiana tabacum could also be considered in this realm, as it was recommended by Steiner for conditions such as asthma, stuttering, dysmenorrhea, and obstipation—all illnesses marked by a disordered interaction between the astral and etheric bodies.[404]

Archetypal Remedy Pictures for Working with the Hysteric Constitution

Bryophyllum

Remedy support for the hysteric constitution can be considered from several different sides. A first and often most immediate goal is to help soothe the child's soul-soreness by bringing greater etheric buffering to the metabolic limb system. In this way the independent, exposed astrality ("I" into astral alone, a pathway belonging to the upper human being) can be shifted if it is better housed and held by the etheric body ("I" into astral into etheric, an activity that belongs to the lower human being). Any therapy that supports the etheric body, especially in the metabolism, can help to calm and redirect an overactive sensing process.

Bryophyllum (also known as "mother of thousands") was described by Steiner as a plant that helps to anchor the etheric in the metabolism.[405] A vital, succulent plant, Bryophyllum is remarkable for the way it moves from a rich leafing process directly into a reproductive process, as small astral serrations at the edges of the succulent leaves become the birthplace of hundreds, if not thousands, of baby plants—complete miniature plants—with formed leaves and even roots. The new baby plants grow and mature at the edge of the leaves for several weeks, then fall to the ground, ready to anchor themselves and start growing. The Bryophyllum plant routinely skips the usual growth processes of blossoming and fruiting. In fact, the main kind of astral sculptural activity seen in the plant—the scalloped indentations at the edge of the juicy, smooth, flat leaves—quickly shifts into a new growth process.

As a remedy, Bryophyllum helps bring protection from the surrounding world and softens problems like difficulties falling asleep, anxiety, and irritability related to exhaustion or overwork. It is used in both herbal and lower-potency preparations (50 percent powder to 6x liquid). Its pronounced etheric, metabolic activity as a plant corresponds to the etheric, metabolic activity of silver as a metal. Thus, the vegetabilized form, Bryophyllum argento culta, also works well for the hysteric constitution, particularly if there is a wish to also address the "I"-organization (which is more specifically addressed through metal preparations).

Bryophyllum helps to heal shock and trauma, experiences that excarnate the etheric forces from the reproductive organs. Bryophyllum reseats the etheric back into those organs. Such disturbing experiences, especially if they come in the early years of development, are particularly disruptive for the child who already tends toward a hysteric constitution. Traumatic experiences may also push someone who is normally well protected into a thin-skinned experience of the world, by inducing a defensive, anticipatory hypervigilance. Bryophyllum as an oral remedy is often combined with Oxalis ointment (over the solar plexus) as a treatment for shock.

Conchae

Whenever there is an imbalanced relationship between two of the spiritual members, the disturbance can be addressed therapeutically from at least two different sides. One approach for healing soul-soreness and its unrestrained astral activity is to strengthen and anchor a weakened etheric, so that it can better contain and cushion the astral (as is done with Bryophyllum). A second pathway is to direct activity toward the astral body itself. This can be accomplished with Conchae, a form of calcium carbonate harvested from the oyster shell that helps a child to breathe out the higher members when they bring excessive sensory activity to the metabolic pole:

> Studying the oyster may be a revelation to you with regard to certain methods of treatment that apply to the lower parts of the human body in their relationship to the upper areas. Shell formation in the oyster is an extremely interesting subject because, you see, the oyster produces its calcium carbonate shell from the inside out. If you study the oyster from a spiritual-scientific perspective—and it is indeed necessary for Spiritual Science to assist us somewhat in this investigation—you will realize that although the oyster occupies a very low position in the evolution of animals, its standing in the cosmos as a whole is quite elevated because it secretes what human beings carry within them in the form of thinking. In a certain way, the forces that shape the oyster's shell, working from the inside out, show how the oyster extrudes a substance that would make it very intelligent if it were linked to its organic growth, a substance that would shape the oyster into a very highly evolved animal being. Instead, this factor is channeled to the outside. You can positively see the work of calcium carbonite, Calcarea carbonica, in the development of an oyster shell. This work guides excessive activity of spirit and soul out of the organism.
>
> If you find evidence of excessive activity of soul and spirit in the lower part of the body—and this does indeed appear in certain forms of illness that we will describe further—you will need to turn to the remedies we owe to oyster shells or similar substances that work from the inside out through the mysterious forces of calcium carbonate. Thus, an essential component of our therapeutic repertoire will depend on our understanding of the specific healing forces present in this outward-directed impulse.[406]

Conchae was recommended by Steiner for a three-year-old girl who was "very nervous" and also for "sleeplessness" in a thirty-seven-year-old, "conditions of agitation" in a thirty-five-year-old, and "depressions" in a sixty-six-year-old patient.[407] In all of these situations the forces of calcium carbonate help to release excessive activity of soul and spirit from the lower part of the body, which then soften a person's sensory relationship to the outside world.

Other manifestations of a hysteric imbalance between astral and etheric forces include excessive excretion—like sweating or bed-wetting. For these kinds of physiologic secretions Conchae helps to better balance the way substance is released from the body. Oyster shell calcium carbonate was recommended by Steiner to balance excretion processes like acute diarrhea, eczema, and urticaria (hives).[408] It is broadly related to processes of release:

> In the lowest part of the body, calcium carbonate competes with silver, but even there it has an eliminating effect. Throughout the body, calcium carbonate eliminates both fluids and gases. The calcium forces in the human organism also include the forces that underlie exhalation and those that drive warmth out of the nerve–sense system in a cooling process of sorts. Thus calcium carbonate eliminates fluids from the lower parts of the human body, or the metabolic–limb system; gases from the rhythmic system; and the warmth ether—or simply warmth, if you prefer—from the sensory–nervous system.[409]

Additionally, Steiner pointed out:

> When administered as a remedy, this substance also has the peculiar tendency to encourage elimination. Calcium carbonate is the external, natural counterpart of the radiating, centrifugal forces in the human being. Consequently, calcium carbonate preparations can be used to alleviate diseases that develop when these radiating forces become too strong."[410]

Because they address the hysteric constitution from two complementary sides, Bryophyllum and Conchae are often used together: Bryophyllum anchors the etheric body while Conchae guides excessive astral and "I" activity (excessive radiating, centrifugal activity) out of the body. They are both used in a low potency (usually 4x or 5x).

Berberis vulgaris (Barberry)

An alternate way to work with an overflowing secretion, such as bed-wetting, is to strengthen and thereby restrain the astral body in itself. This is a somewhat different therapeutic gesture than that of either Bryophyllum or Conchae, but it is included here, as there are a whole group of children who do indeed wet the bed but exhibit a kind of sleepiness in the lower body, as opposed to the soul-soreness of a classically hysteric sensing process. These children also experience an astral/etheric imbalance but without such pronounced anxiety or hypervigilance. Berberis (Barberry) is therefore included as another way to approach an astral–etheric imbalance, though it addresses more of a sleepy boundary experience than an overly wakeful one.

Berberis can also be considered as another example of an organ-specific therapy. Where Chamomile helps release a cramped or stuck nerve process in the digestion, Berberis pulls in, consolidates astral activity in the bladder and kidney system. Steiner described a ten-year-old girl during the eleventh lecture of the curative course who suffered "from a loss of memory" and "adenoids." He attributed this to "an excess of etheric powers of growth in the region of the bladder, which condition is then reflected in the head... clear evidence of the fact that the ether body is not properly at home in the organism—the reason being that its cooperation with the astral body is not able to come about as it should."[411] Steiner recommended that "strong impressions must be brought to bear on the child" in three different forms:

- Take with the child little poems where a refrain is repeated—say, after every three lines. She will in this way receive a powerful impression of rhythm; and then later on, the moment will come when we can approach her with impressions that are without rhythm. Do not imagine that any substantial success can be looked for in under three or four years—that is, up until puberty [the age that marks a certain physiologic maturation of the astral body].

- The medical treatment we have already indicated: the girl should have compresses with *Berberis vulgaris* 10 percent,
- and therapeutic eurythmy: L, M : S–U.[412]

Rhythm and repetition through poetry help to "induce strong impressions,"[413] passing from the nerve–sense pole through the rhythmic system and then into the lower part of the body where memories are imprinted (see part 4 for a more detailed discussion of the physiology of memory). Through this kind of pedagogical activity, an astral impulse from the senses works down, over and over, to progressively take hold of a largely unbounded etheric activity. Such rhythmic memory practice brings an astralizing activity, reminiscent of the therapeutic pictures discussed earlier for uniting the spiritual and hereditary streams.

Steiner did not give specifics about the therapeutic use of *Berberis* for this girl, but we can build additional insight by working through his indications for the individual elements of the eurythmy sequence:

> Note that an inner perception underlies the giving of these particular sounds in therapeutic eurythmy. The formative, molding influence will enter right into the mobile astral body. Then the M, as I have told you, is the sound that places the whole organization into the out-breathing, and so the astral organization will there meet the etheric. With S, the aim is to bring the astral body into powerful and living activity—but it must be an activity that is restrained, held in check; and for this purpose the *U* is added.[414]

These steps—of guiding the astral body to encounter the etheric, of bringing the astral body into living activity and then helping to contain it, to give it healthy boundary—also belong to the therapeutic activity of Berberis. Berberis brings healthy form and boundary by uniting the astral body with an overflowing etheric (when there is too much growth) and/or renewing and vitalizing what has become too dried out or sclerotic (for organs of both the lower body—bladder and uterus—and the upper body—nose and sinuses).[415]

From this picture we can see how fortifying the astral body can also bring a stronger experience of boundary. We can appreciate why Steiner recommended Berberis as treatment for a nine-year-old girl with enuresis and swollen glands (excessive etheric) as well as for an older patient with exhaustion and nervousness (more the devitalizing, or drying out).[416] In both cases an enlivened astral activity helps to bring an experience of proper boundary and a proper seating of the astral and etheric body.

The therapeutic application of Berberis for bed-wetting relates in some ways to the astralizing described for the feeble constitution, and there is indeed sometimes some symptomatic overlap between the feeble and hysteric constitutions, although the former does not feel a boundary because the body has not yet been adequately penetrated, while the latter has lost the boundary by flowing out too far beyond the body. Levico and Hypericum actually offer additional treatment options for the child who wets the bed and who still needs to awaken more in the lower body.

Bringing all of these different considerations into view, we can see that there are at least three differentiated (though often complementary) approaches to support a child in whom there is an imbalanced interaction of the etheric and astral bodies:

- **Bryophyllum**, which works to anchor and support the etheric body in the metabolism, thereby bringing a more vital etheric buffer to the outside world as it creates a better housing for the astral body.
- **Conchae** (calcium carbonate), which helps relieve anxiety and sensitivity by driving out excessive activity of the higher members (spirit and soul) in the metabolism.
- **Berberis vulgaris**, which helps to bring more vitalized and better boundaried astral activity to the organs of the bladder and kidney system.

All three remedies were, with various patients, recommended by Steiner as a therapy for “nervousness.”

If we look at these three remedies from a slightly different angle, we recognize that they speak to a kind of therapeutic sequence, which is helpful to have in mind when treating a hysteric constitution (or the hypervigilance after a trauma). Early in a therapeutic process, the thing a child usually needs most is to be shielded, to have the etheric body supported and anchored with a remedy like Bryophyllum. This is particularly true when the idea of going to a quiet, safe space sounds ideal. The child needs to be protected from the world, and sometimes this is enough. But then, at a certain point—even if the immediate environment has become quiet, predictable, and safe—the child may still not feel restful. An imbalanced astral sensitivity continues, is carried around within the child and cannot quite be let go of. *Conchae* can then help breathe out such excessive astral and "I" activity from the metabolic pole. But then, perhaps after a still longer period of time, we may see that an additional step needs to be taken, because the process is no longer helped simply through providing protection (Bryophyllum) and because outbreathing (Conchae) proves to be only a temporary help. The boundary instead needs to be taken hold of in a new way. It is much like following the "L" of the eurythmy sequence (bringing mobility to the formative, molding activity, a strengthening of the etheric) and the "outbreathing" of *M* with the ending sounds of *S* and *U*. To make the therapeutic process our own, we must eventually step into that consolidating process. *Berberis* lends us an option for helping to do that for the astral body in the bladder, kidney, and adenoid organs and to bring a stronger experience of boundary.

Phosphorus

Phosphorus is included here not because it is a classical treatment for hysteria—it is not; in fact, it brings a very polar kind of activity. But it can work in a complementary way to the remedies so far described, especially for stimulating the kind of consolidation that may be needed at a certain point in the therapeutic process, though now not in the realm of the astral body but of the "I." Phosphorus as a remedy belongs to the "I"-organization. In various lecture cycles, Steiner described Phosphorus as having an opposite activity to that of calcium carbonicum (Conchae), to silver, and also to arsenic and to silica.[417] With such varied activity, it is perhaps difficult to assign phosphorus to a particular constitution or even to a single polarity, but we can gain important insight by focusing on it in relation to calcium carbonicum.

We have already seen how calcium carbonicum (Conchae) has "the peculiar tendency to eliminate fluids from the lower part of the human body, gases from the rhythmic system, and warmth ether from the sensory–nervous system."[418] Steiner continued that sequence:

> In each of these contexts, the effects of calcium carbonate are diametrically opposed to those of phosphorus.... Phosphorus drives inhalation, or all inward-directed respiratory processes. It pulls the gaseous element into the organism in a way that warms the sensory–nervous system.[419]

This inbreathing of warmth increases the activity of the astral and "I" so that phosphorus helps when:

> a pathological condition appears that is characterized outwardly by an additional symptom—a too strong tendency to sleep. Thus if one has to deal with an illness complex including, among other symptoms, a tendency to fall into states of dulled consciousness, one must work with phosphorus.[420]

Phosphorus has a wakening effect; it opposes the breathing out and releasing of Conchae.

An additional description brings us to an even clearer understanding of the phosphorus remedy picture, one related to phosphorus excess:

> Imagine for yourself, that you are in a terribly anticipating mood. This means for your senses system that you vehemently desire that sense impressions come quickly. You come into a soul fever.

> Think that this process progresses even further, then you have the activity of phosphorus. An inflammatory process comes into being when the effect of phosphorus is too strong in the organism. The will process comes about through burning through of organic substance. If you have an excessive, internal inflammatory process, then you will be brought into the state, as if the external impressions must come as quickly as possible. If your normal temperature were to become much higher, then the world must proceed much more rapidly.[421]

This phosphorus picture, of waking dulled consciousness and desiring that impressions should come more and more "quickly," is precisely what the hysteric child is fighting to escape. Such a treatment would, in fact, most certainly exacerbate the underlying soul-soreness of a hysteric constitution. Learning to feel into that strong contrast is another way to help us identify when a hysteric process is present. Sometimes a child's lack of engagement can be difficult to identify: Is it restraint, a constant pulling back, that keeps the child from engaging, or is it a dulled consciousness that needs to be inflamed into more interest?

It is also good to include phosphorus as a remedy in this section because there are certain points when, even if the primary therapy has been to support the working together of the etheric and astral bodies, the "I"-organization then needs to be called in. This can be true even when it feels contrary to the original constitutional picture of needing to protect a soul-soreness and becomes more of a therapeutic consideration with an older child or a young adult. As astral forces are liberated into consciousness with puberty—having reached a certain metabolic ripeness and completion—support for the developing "I"-organization now fits the underlying developmental activity. One can shield and buffer for only so long; then (perhaps after months or years) a treatment with phosphorus can be very helpful.

This use of phosphorus can also be considered as a kind of healing over, as when, after a course of homeopathic lead treatment, a shorter treatment with copper is given (for the large-headed child) or, after a course of silver, a few of weeks of iron (for the small-headed child) is administered. Working in time with polar remedies can yield a certain consolidation for the therapy overall. Steiner recommended just such an alternating therapy, in relation to the shifting phases of the moon for a thirteen-year-old boy who sleepwalked and wet the bed (Argentum 5x during the waxing moon, Phosphorus 5x during the waning moon)[422]—silver helping to strengthen and buffer the etheric, phosphorus to penetrate and guide the activity.

Finally, we can consider phosphorus any time we are working with a hypertrophy of astral activity. This is worth considering when there are repeated improvements and then relapses. A physiologic change is stimulated, but it cannot be held or sustained. Then a step of self-consciousness, of self-determination, needs to be taken. This relates to the polarity of Arsenicum (and its astralizing activity) and phosphorus. Phosphorus in this context then works to stimulate "the conscious activity of the human being.... Phosphorus will therefore act as a medication when the pathological condition consists of a hypertrophy of the astral region over the "I"-organization and the latter needs to be strengthened so that the astral is pushed back."[423]

Archetypal Remedy Pictures for Working with Organ Imbalances

An additional section on organ imbalances is included as an extension of the remedy pictures given for the epileptic and hysteric polarity. These are offered, partly as an elaboration of the organ-specific remedies already introduced (i.e., Chamomile for the epileptic constitution, Berberis for the hysteric) but more so because organ imbalances strongly influence the quality and development of liberated thought and conscious connection. When, during puberty, astral forces are freed up into conscious awareness, many organ pictures present themselves. These kinds of pathologic inclinations, interestingly enough, may also emerge around other developmental shifts when other steps of new awareness are similarly burgeoning forth.

Knowledge of the functional processes of the four main organs underlies much of anthroposophic psychiatry (see next page, table 19). Steiner stressed that these are real medical problems and need to be treated as such. For this reason, too, they are included only here in the remedy section, not as part of the broader pedagogical discussions in the main part of the book.

> The primary factor in psychiatric disorders, even if it is sometimes more difficult to observe, always lies in the lower organ systems. This accounts for the often dishearteningly low rate of success of psychotherapy.... We will have to get used to treating psychiatric disorders with remedies. [424]

Steiner's description of epilepsy includes mention that a specific organ system is often involved: "Nothing of any real value can be said about fits if we do not know that, at the surface of some organ, astral body and "I"-organization are being terribly squeezed and crushed."[425] Steiner used the example of a fine infiltrate in the lung as blocking proper connection between the astral body and "I" with the outside world and urged consideration of an organ imbalance as part of any treatment for seizures. A series of symptoms are then given, relating to barriers between the higher members and outside elements, as well as different kinds of activity that can help to restore a proper connection: for example, gravity and balance, water and tasting, air and breathing exercises, warmth and sweating. Aside from those general indications, specific organ therapies are not examined in any detail in the curative course lectures.

In other settings Steiner did elaborate on often unrecognized aspects of organ imbalance. He designated four cardinal, or meteorologic, organs (because of their relationship to the elements of earth, water, air, and fire): "These four organ systems play a crucial role in the human being's relationship to meteorology, to what is outside."[426]

Table 19: Summary table of medical treatments to support the characteristic organ imbalances

Organ	**Characteristics of Imbalance**	**Remedies for Organ Treatment**
Lungs	Disturbed sense of hunger	*Pulmo*
Earth	Frequent repetitions	*Ferrum*
	Compulsive thoughts or illusions	Ash preparations: *Cinis urtica*
		Mercurius, Mercurius auratus
Liver	Disturbed sense of thirst	*Hepar, Hepar magnesium*
Water	Obstinacy and self-righteousness	*Taraxacum*
	Immobility or rigidity in thinking	*Chelidonium*
	Calm hallucinations	*Phosphorus*
Kidney	Shortness of breath	*Renes*
Air	Inner, or "soul" overexcitement	*Equisetum* (also *Cum sulfure tosta*)
	Hypochondriasis	*Cuprum*
	Excited, emotional hallucinations	*Carbo vegetabilis* (*Carbo betulae*)
Heart	Pangs of conscience	*Cor*
warmth	Raving madness (anger)	*Cardiodoron*
		Hypericum
		Aurum

He also noted the ways in which they influence our thought, feeling, and behavior. Those descriptions differ some from the epileptic process, because instead of an outward-reaching process of the higher members being blocked in an organ, psychiatric symptoms instead arise when an impression that has already come into the body and been stored is released inappropriately, too early. The timetable for proper release is perhaps not what we might expect—Steiner indicated that the activity of such impressions should really carry over, as formative activity, into the next incarnation. Through a process of proper metamorphosis, what is gathered through experience in one incarnation becomes formative activity for creating the body of the next incarnation. When those formative forces are released in the present incarnation, they rise up and unduly influence our thinking and feeling.

Consideration of an organ imbalance helps deepen medical constitutional assessment, although organ imbalances are not an inherent part of the shifting developmental gestures experienced in childhood in the same way that the constitutional polarities are. When organ patterns are present in a predictable and observable way, they warrant early support with remedies.

An organ imbalance will sometimes magnify—or perhaps a better term is exacerbate—an underlying constitutional leaning. For example, a hysteric child with a lung imbalance will usually be exceptionally anxious and also tend toward obsessive thinking; an epileptic child with a heart imbalance may have a pattern of truly explosive anger. Organ imbalances do not necessarily correlate with other constitutional patterns, however, so that organ pictures should be considered as an independent aspect of the child's inner life. This is similar to when Steiner indicated that with an earthly child "even when the child does not appear to be melancholic, there is, nonetheless, alongside the apparent temperament a nuance of melancholy." [427]

Constitution does not necessarily determine temperament, and temperament does not dictate constitution; temperament likewise does not dictate organ imbalance. There may be some instances when a melancholic child has an earthly constitution and a liver imbalance, but we should not expect for there to be such correlations.

The normal anatomy and physiology of these four cardinal organs as well as their potential imbalances and supportive treatments have been explored in depth by other authors. The reader is directed to those discussions as very helpful additional resources.[428]

The Lung

In his lectures on the four cardinal organs, Steiner placed the lungs first (before going on to describe the liver, kidney, and heart). There is a certain primacy about the lungs; they make possible our most immediate interface and encounter with the outside environment. We meet the physical environment, directly and continuously, through our breath. Steiner linked the lungs to the element of earth. He described how the health of the lungs is dependent on the conditions of our physical environment and the work we do in that environment:

> In pointing out the lung's dependency on the environment, I am not referring to respiration. I mean the internal structure of the lungs themselves. Of course, respiration in turn is dependent on good or poor functioning, which in turn is determined by the lungs' internal structure. But with regard to this dependency, I am referring to the actual internal structure of the lungs. Whether a tendency toward incrustation or excessive mucus or the like is present essentially depends on the environment. But then the lungs are also very sensitive to physical labor and will certainly be damaged if a person has to do physical work to the point of excessive fatigue.[429]

The first part of this description is medically not such a foreign concept, as the influence of environment factors on the lung are well known, like pollen, dust mites, animal dander, asbestos, chemicals, and smog. In many ways we are more immediately affected by our surroundings through our lungs than through our skin or even through our digestion. The digestive system's task is to meet and transform the substances we take in. The lungs instead meet and exchange substances (oxygen, carbon dioxide, nitrogen) without necessarily altering them. The lungs must be capable of meeting and interfacing with the world as it is (without trying to transform it).

We can see the lungs' relationship to the earthly element in its structure and architecture. The hard, cartilaginous structures of the larynx and the rings of the trachea are almost bony. Just as the mineralized enamel of the teeth first meets the food that enters into our digestive system, the hard cartilage structures of the upper airway meet the air element that enters into our respiratory system.

That hardening process belongs to the structure of the lungs. The lungs embody this kind of mineralizing activity, but this activity can also metamorphose into a sculptural force. Steiner shared that these hardening, formative forces will, in the next incarnation, give rise to the shape, the morphologic characteristics of the head. When those formative forces are released prematurely, in this lifetime, they make our thinking hard as well. Thought loses its flexibility for meeting new outside impressions:

> We will have to look carefully at any abnormalities in the process of lung formation—not in the respiratory process, but the lungs' formative process, in pulmonary metabolism.... In the case of someone who is losing interest in outer life and beginning to brood and act out delusions, the most important concern is always to get an idea of the constitution of the person's pulmonary process. This is extremely important.... The person who suffers from frequent repetitions always has a potential for illness that is related to a formative lung process that is not in order.[430]

Additionally, Steiner noted:

> Certain organs instead absorb something that becomes latent within them and constitutes an inner force. For example, all thoughts that we absorb in this way are connected mainly

> with outer objects. The forces developed in these thoughts are stored, as it were, in the inner aspect of the lungs.... If what has been stored in the lungs is not controlled in the right way, it is pressed out, as I said yesterday as water in a sponge is pressed out, and then, from what actually should only form the head in the next incarnation there arise abnormal phenomena that are usually designated as compulsive thoughts or illusions.... You see, the thoughts that are pressed out are compulsive thoughts, because they already contain the forming forces. The thoughts that now we ought normally to have in consciousness must be only forces; they must not have in themselves a forming force; they must not compel us.[431]

Support for an organ imbalance must therefore focus on medical treatment and work to heal a problem that is coming from the inside out. It is not really possible to transform these imbalances just with pedagogical experiences (like telling the child to relax, to stop thinking the repetitive thoughts), which work more formatively from the outside in.

If we now move to specific remedy indications: the inner structure and activity of an organ can be supported in a foundational way through the use of a corresponding potentized animal organ preparation. This works to support the etheric activity of that organ. So in the case of a child with repetitive, compulsive thoughts or behaviors, an organ lung preparation can be prescribed: Pulmo, usually given as a 6x preparation. It is possible and often useful to bring in a corresponding organ preparation for any of the cardinal organs. In fact, a broad-based treatment for psychiatric imbalance is the combination of Pulmo (lung), Hepar (liver), Renes (kidney), and Cor (heart).

We can look to the lungs' relationship with the earthly element as a way to identify additional kinds of lung remedies. The prescribing of an earthly substance for an "earthly" organ may initially seem like a simple "like treats like," but what is really being stimulated is the overcoming of earthly substance. Strengthening that capacity for transforming or transcending what has become too earthly, that is the therapeutic goal. Such overcoming creates more vital spiritual activity within the organ, with a resulting improvement of lung function. In this way, Ferrum (iron) is a very helpful lung remedy:

> Upon examination in the blood, iron reveals itself as the only metal which, within the human organism, has the tendency toward crystallization. Thus it maintains forces which are in fact external, physical, mineral forces of nature. Within the human organism they form a system of forces, oriented in terms of outer physical nature. This, however, is continually being overcome by the "I"-organization.[432]

More specifically addressing the relationship between the metal iron and the pulmonary system:

> Iron plays the mediating role between the sphere within the boundary of human skin and the sphere outside that boundary. We may therefore maintain that the whole pulmonary system—the "pulmonary human," possessing the urge to become a whole human being—is linked strongly with the whole human relationship to the universal life of nature.[433]

Furthermore,

> All that opens outward from lungs to larynx, with its starting point in the lungs, is akin to iron.[434]

The strengthening effect of an iron remedy can be intensified through a pharmaceutical process:

> If you examine the earthly qualities of plants you will find in them the remedies for everything connected with diseases that have their origin in the lungs.[435]

The most earthly parts of a plant, the most mineralized components, are identified and gathered by burning a plant to ash:

> The specific chemistry of the earth is revealed in the ashes; it is represented in the refuse, the dross of the living sphere. This dross and ash is subject to gravity, whereas the upward urge and growth of the plant is a continual conquest of gravity, and of other earth-bound forces, so that we may properly speak of a polar opposition between gravity and light. Light is that which continually overcomes gravity. And the plant is, so to speak, set into the tension of this combat between light and weight, between that which strives toward ashes and that which strives toward fire. And this polar contrast between what becomes ashes and what is revealed in flame, is the opposition of ponderable and imponderable elements.[436]

Ash preparations are indicated for the lungs and particularly for the overcoming of excessively fixed or obsessive thought patterns arising out of a pathologic lung condition. Cinis urtica, the ash of stinging nettle (an iron-rich plant) is commonly used for obsessive-compulsive disorder and given in a low potency, 3x–6x. We are able to give an ash of an iron-rich plant.

A quite different, but often complementary way to work with an overly formed thought process is to try to bring a loosening, mobilizing remedy. This can be done with Mercurius (mercury) or the combination of mercury and gold (Mercurius auratus). Both forms are generally given in a middle potency, corresponding to the rhythmic system, such as 12x, 15x, or 20x.

Another consideration, which may be helpful as a confirmatory symptom, is that a lung imbalance may also manifest in a disturbed sense of hunger: "The manifestations of hunger and all of its accessory symptoms are intimately connected with the internal condition of the lungs."[437] Our lung physiology underlies our longing and our sensing for when we need to take in as substance from the earthy world. This connection can prompt us to inquire about hunger whenever we are considering a lung imbalance and vice versa (such as obsessive thoughts and anorexia nervosa).

The Liver

After the earthly element comes the watery realm, and this is the sphere of activity for the liver. The liver rules the fluid processes within the human being. In the watery element we become freer from the conditions and substances of the outside world and work to begin to incorporate them into our own activity. While the lungs meet and exchange substance with the earthly environment, liver activity takes place more internally, in the process of digestion as we work to transform and then to incorporate new substance into ourselves. The lungs underlie our sense of hunger (for solid food); the liver stimulates our sense of thirst.[438] The liver is open to and influenced by the water we take in:

> To properly consider the liver health of the people living in a particular place, we would always have to study the composition of the local water. Tasting promotes liver development, but when it occurs in excess it promotes liver degeneration. In human beings, liver degeneration is the same as excessive indulgence. Finding food pleasant or unpleasant, sympathetic or unsympathetic, ought to be restricted to the tongue and the palate, and extending this sympathy and antipathy to the interior leads to liver degeneration. We need to pay attention to this and try to persuade people with any type of liver damage (which is often difficult to notice) to investigate taste and to discover something essential in taste.[439]

This relationship has already been alluded to in Steiner's indication that children with an epileptic constitution should "specially taste" their food in order to strengthen the astral body and "I"s relation to the watery element. The liver is not only a digestive organ but also a sense organ, and a specific sensing activity—taste—can strengthen its inherent activity.

When there is an imbalance in the liver we find corresponding imbalances in the realm of thinking—namely, a difficulty assimilating new thoughts (though this has more the quality of stagnation than the obsessive repetition of a lung imbalance):

> If we observe someone in whom obstinacy, pigheadedness, and self-righteousness appear, indicating a certain immobility or rigidity in thinking, this should lead us to investigate the status of the liver function in the person in question.... The one who suffers from omission of thoughts always has an inherent predisposition to a liver process that is not functioning properly.[440]

A liver imbalance can result in omission of thoughts. It can also result in excessively active thoughts that are not a result of assimilation. These thoughts we can categorize as hallucinations:

> Within the liver are concentrated all the forces that in the next incarnation determine the inner disposition of the brain.... Whether or not some are to be acute thinkers in the next incarnation depends upon behavior in the present incarnation. Thus by through the metabolism certain forces may appear within the liver; if those forces are pressed out during the present incarnation, however, they lead to hallucinations or to powerful visions...calm hallucinations, that merely appear, are liver hallucinations, as it were.[441]

Liver pathologic conditions fall on two poles in the influence of thought: those that are the result of a stagnation of thought (leading to omission or obstinacy) and those related to an excessive, inwardly engendered activity of thought (hallucination).

These liver processes can be met with their own corresponding set of remedies. We have already looked at one liver remedy in relation to the earthly or feeble constitution, Hepar magnesium. It is based on an organ preparation (Hepar) and helps the child overcome the heaviness and melancholy of an untransformed hereditary body through stimulating liver activity. That lifting, levity-filling process belongs to other liver treatments as well. Where for the lungs we are directed to turn to the earthly qualities of the plants, for liver treatment we are directed to the watery, dynamic elements:

> If you take what circulates in the plant, the circulation of the plant's juices, you will have therein the remedy for all disturbances connected with the liver organization.[442]

Several classic liver remedies show this inner circulation: both Taraxacum (dandelion) and Chelidonium (the greater celandine). They contain a characteristic milky fluid (which even finds its way into the name of another traditional liver remedy, Carduus marianus, or "milk" thistle).

Steiner spoke with great admiration about dandelion in the lectures on biodynamic agriculture. The dandelion's bitter greens have long been valued as a liver tonic. Steiner spoke about the much broader role of dandelion within an environment's whole living activity in describing the biodynamic preparations:

> The innocent, yellow dandelion is a tremendous asset because it mediates between the fine homeopathic distribution of silicic acid in the cosmos, and the silicic acid that is actually used over the whole region. The dandelion is really a kind of messenger from heaven.... It will give the soil the ability to attract as much silicic acid from the atmosphere and from the cosmos as is needed by the plants. In this way the plants will become sensitive to everything at work in their environment and then be able themselves to draw in whatever else they need.[443]

In this way Taraxacum can help to overcome "obstinacy, pigheadedness, and self-righteousness," for the dandelion not only has an enlivening effect (which is very helpful for moving liver lethargy) but also supports the liver's sensing—and thereby the whole life of thinking—to be open and to better recognize what should be accepted and incorporated. It speaks to obstinate narrow-mindedness (which again is different from the stuck, repetitive inflexibility of a lung pathologic condition) and is usually given in a low potency.

The stimulatory effect of Chelidonium is different; it works not so much to lift up, like Taraxacum (levity) as to release out. Chelidonium stimulates gall secretion, a physiologic pathway for healthy detoxification and excretion. Gall secretion is also associated in many ancient healing traditions with the release of emotion. It mediates between stagnation and lethargy on one side and sudden anger or activity (even mania) on the other. The liver influences not only how we take up and assimilate thought but also how our thoughts then move into deeds:

> For you must know that the liver is not merely the organ modern physiologists describe; it is pre-eminently the organ that gives the human being the courage to transform a deed which has been thought of into an accomplished deed.... The liver is the mediator which enables an idea that has been resolved upon to be transformed into an action carried out by the limbs. In point of fact, every organ is there in the body for the purpose of acting as mediator for something to come about.[444]

As a remedy, Chelidonium was most often discussed by Steiner as one of the components in Choleodoron (in which it is combined with Curcuma, or turmeric). Chelidonium helps to balance just that movement from thought to deed. It serves as an important remedy for aggressive behaviors, particularly if they show a pattern of alternating, irritably "toxic" congestion and then an excessive release and anger. Chelidonium opens the pathway for more regular connection between thought and deed (making it easier for something to be promptly released, an aspect that is worth mentioning, as there is sometimes a surprising, but healthy release of emotion that appears when an existing liver congestion is overcome). Chelidonium is usually given in very low potency, low enough that it can actually be tasted (2x or 3x), alone or in the form of Choleodoron.

Phosphorus can also have a place in liver treatment. It brings the "I"-organization into better connection with the limbs and metabolism and, through them, with the world around. Phosphorus has already been mentioned as a remedy that stimulates a child to "vehemently desire that sense impressions come quickly," which in the context of a liver imbalance can be considered a healthy counterbalance to a strong liver obstinacy. Phosphorus—in low potency—brings greater wakefulness and engagement through the limbs, sparking more interest for tasting the surrounding world. A 5x or 6x preparation addresses the metabolic–limb system and is usually indicated for an organ treatment.

The Kidney

The kidney, ureters, and bladder are united in their activity as a third organ system. They relate to the element of air: "Air activity corresponds to everything that is associated with the renal system in the broadest sense, and especially to all urinary functions."[445] This is not an obvious connection, because we usually think of the lungs as being most connected with air; the lungs are indeed very connected to air, but to the movement of air. To better understand the connection between the kidneys and the air organism, it is necessary to draw a distinction between the structure of an organ and the process of an organ. Steiner's indications about the lungs and the earthly element relate to the physical structure of the lungs, and the lungs are certainly the most solid of the cardinal organs, particularly when we look at the uppermost structures of the larynx and trachea. That is structure, and, as was already described, the lungs as a whole organ system hold strong formative forces. The very fine process of exchange, however, that happens as oxygen is absorbed and carbon dioxide released is related to lung process. That kind of nuanced, bidirectional exchange is a signature of the astral body—choosing between more or less, inside and outside, concentrating or diluting. The alternation of inhalation and exhalation is similarly an astral process, so there are clearly astral processes in the lung, but the lungs are not the primary astral organ. The primary seat of astral differentiation in the body is the kidneys.

The very fine sensing process that occurs in the kidney—which begins with the excretion process of the glomeruli (a tremendous push outward) that is balanced with a very conscious reabsorption (almost all of the filtered fluid being reabsorbed) and ends with a strong concentration and final excretion of waste products in the urine—this is an astral activity of sympathy and antipathy par excellence. Kidney activity relates to sorting and sifting, filling, then emptying, and this is happening continuously on a grand scale.

The etheric body alone knows only how to grow, to stream, and to expand. It is the activity of astral body that makes it possible for us to reduce, shape, refine, and take away. A related signature of strongly astral organs is that they are hollow. Something is first created (through physical and etheric activity) and then sculpturally hollowed out by the astral body. For example, the sinus spaces of the skull are sculpted out of what is initially more solid bone; the lungs and kidney systems arise embryologically from invaginations out of the endoderm and into the mesoderm. The bladder, as a hollow, astral organ, creates a pulling movement toward the outside. That process of pulling and hollowing makes excretion possible. The kidney guides and balances all of these, finely differentiated, simultaneous, and sometimes contrary movements. These fine, internal movements underlie kidney and bladder activity:

> Essentially, the bladder is a suction device. It is dependent on the fact that the human organism is hollowed out at this particular location.... With regard to all the bladder's intended functions, we create disturbances if we have little opportunity to complete internal movements in the right way. One example of this is failing to pay careful attention to the act of eating, disrupting the entire digestive process by gulping down our food instead of chewing. Another is not maintaining the right balance between rest and movement during the digestive process, and so on. Everything that disrupts inner mobility from within also disrupts what we might call the life of the bladder.[446]

This description of "internal movements," of the "right balance between rest and movement," and of "internal mobility" helps build a picture of how imbalanced kidney activity can influence our thinking and feeling life—either as lack of awareness or as exaggerated inner awareness.

An important symptom of pathologic kidney function relates to the element of air, specifically to the feeling of not being able to get enough air: "Shortness of breath and its regulation are associated with the kidneys."[447] A standard medical response for someone feeling short of breath is to check to see if the person is getting enough oxygen, and that is, of course, an important acute concern. There may not be enough oxygen in the body. Shortness of breath, however, is also a classic symptom of an anxiety attack, where the person is hyperventilating and symptoms come not from a deficit of oxygen but from a loss of carbon dioxide. Both processes can be understood as kidney symptoms, because they really are an expression of dysregulation, of having lost the proper sense of what air should be inside and what should be out. That kind of dysregulation, on many different levels, brings anxiety. Kidney anxiety is different from the anxiety of the hysteric constitution, which comes from loss of boundary and then creates hesitation and withdrawal as a means of protection. Kidney anxiety is more restless and agitated:

> If we study in the same way everything that is connected with the kidney-excretory organs, we will see that they concentrate within themselves the forces that in the next incarnation influence the head organization more from the emotional side...that which has to do with the temperamental tendencies in the broadest sense.... If these forces are pressed out during the present incarnation, they display all the nervous conditions, all the conditions connected with over-excitement of the human being, inner or soul over-excitement specifically, hypochondriacal conditions, depression, and so forth, in short all the conditions connected particularly with this side of the metabolism.... In fact, everything that is memorable more from the feeling or emotional side is also connected with what is reflected from the kidneys.... Hallucinations that appear as though crawling on a person so

> that the victim wants to brush them off come from the kidney system. These are excitatory hallucinations, which have to do with the emotional system, with the system of temperament.[448]

Kidney therapy is not based on stimulating greater encounter (like iron for the lungs) or on enlivening and lifting fluids (like the "milky" plants for liver therapy), but rather on enhancing inward sensing and orientation:

> In a certain sense, all organs are sense organs. The kidney is a particularly important abdominal organ in this respect. Using silica as it occurs in Equisetum...increase[s] the kidney's sensitivity and positively affects processes in the human organism that stem from a deadening of the kidney's inner sensing ability.[449]

Moreover, Steiner told us,

> Suppose the symptoms suggest that a disease originates in the kidneys. Applying Spiritual Science to diagnosis reveals that the kidneys are not functioning adequately as sense organs for the neighboring digestive and excretory processes.... The metabolic function of the kidneys has become excessive.... We must make sure to supply the kidneys with the silica they.[450]

Equisetum (Horsetail) was a favorite plant for Steiner, and he often described its special relationship to both silica and sulfur. These are, in many ways, polar substances, but sulfur was indicated by Steiner as the proper treatment for an accumulation of silica in one part of the body, which usually means there is a resultant deficit somewhere else. Sulfur works to effect a proper distribution of silica in the body and a more balanced inner sensing process.[451] The balancing of these two activities stands behind Equisetum's role as a kidney treatment. Equisetum can be further developed as a remedy, slowly roasting it with sulfur, into a treatment for inner restlessness, Equisetum cum sulfure tosta. Both the Equisetum and the preparation with sulfur are usually given in a low potency (6x).

The organ preparation for the kidney, Renes, is also useful. It is often combined with Cuprum (copper), the metal that mirrors kidney activity. Cuprum was repeatedly recommended by Steiner as a treatment for anxiety as well as related symptoms because of how it "dampens down the oversensitivity of the astral body in the digestive tract" and can lead to "a diminution of abnormal heart activity and dissipation of the anxiety"; it also works "to support the influence of the astral forces on the circulatory system."[452] Copper helps not so much by increasing sensitivity as by rebalancing or redirecting sensing activity. Cuprum is frequently given as an anthroposophic medicine in the form of an ointment application rubbed over the kidneys (0.4 percent ointment in a sideways lemniscate) or orally as a low potency, often 6x.

A different treatment for the kidney system relates back to the symptom of shortness of breath. Burning and combustion bear a strong relationship to the air element, and Steiner linked this process to the formation of a coal, Carbo:

> The earth's coal or carbon content regulates the oxygen content of the Earth's environment.... The Earth as such, if understood as an organism—as indeed it must be—is subject to a breathing process and that its coal or carbon content has to do with this process.[453]

Notice how he emphasized that this is a coal or carbon process, as it regulates the breathing process of the earth's environment. Steiner went further in his description of Carbo and connected it to the kidney:

> Air activity corresponds to everything that is associated with the renal system in the broadest sense, and especially to all urinary functions. Under certain circumstances, this system, of which the kidney is the part that lies deepest in the interior, can provoke shortness of breath, as can ingesting Carbo vegetabilis.[454]

The ingestion of Carbo vegetabilis, which is produced through the burning of plant matter—not to the point of ash, but burned under conditions of limited air (oxygen) access—brings an excessive and thereby imbalanced astrality:

> We are introducing nothing less than the principle that strives to become animal. All the symptoms that appear, from belching to bloating to foul-smelling diarrhea to hemorrhoid formation on the one hand and burning pain of all sorts on the other, stem from the fact that animal nature, which has been externalized by humankind in its process of becoming human, has been taken back into the individual human being.... If you manage to enhance or heighten the kidney process by administering higher potencies of Carbo vegetabilis—then you are working to counteract this disease process in the human being that resembles the allopathic effects of Carbo vegetabilis.[455]

The most commonly used form of Carbo vegetabilis is Carbo betulae (Birch carbon), prescribed in a broad range of preparations, ranging from 1 percent up to the higher potencies mentioned here by Steiner (such as 20x). The cruder, lower potencies address more of the physical symptoms, the higher potencies more constitutional imbalances. Clinical symptoms indicating its use include, on one hand, an imbalanced air process (such as shortness of breath but also "belching" and "bloating") and an imbalanced sensitivity, on the other ("burning pain" of all sorts).

The Heart

The heart is the organ related to the element of warmth. The heart, too, is a sensing organ—not so much for the substance we ingest, the water we drink, or the air we breathe as for the integrating and harmonizing of all of those processes together. That is what makes the heart different from the kidney. Through the kidney the astral body creates contrasts and polarities as well as the sensing of those contrasts, to switch between in and out, sympathy and antipathy, waking and sleeping. The astral body can move between one pole and the other, but it cannot be in both at the same time. Heart activity goes a step further. The heart establishes a meeting place, a middle space of active engagement and balancing where both poles can be held at the same time (not just to push in or push out, to receive or reject, but to consider both possibilities at the same time). It is a sensing process on a higher order:

> Ultimately, what is the heart? It is a sense organ. And ultimately, even if we are not directly conscious of the heart's sensory function, even though this is one of our subconscious sensory activities, the heart nonetheless exists so that our upper activities may sense and perceive our lower activities. Just as you perceive color processes in the environment with your eyes, you also perceive with your heart, although in the dimness of the subconscious. You perceive what is taking place in the lower part of your body. Ultimately, the heart is an organ of inner perception, and it must be addressed as such.[456]

We could say the heart is our greatest sensing pathway to connect our inner world to our conscious sensing.

The activity of the heart and circulation is anything but a fixed machine. To focus on the anatomic shape and structure of the heart is to miss its essence, for the heart is fully dynamic. To see its function during surgery is a marvel, for the moment we think we have captured its shape or activity in our mind it has already changed and then changed again and then changed once again. It is able to be so nuanced and responsive because it lives in full engagement and adjustment all the time:

> Physicians today reach a diagnosis in such a way that they prefer to delineate the contours of the heart as though it were a finished organ. The important thing is not to look at what the finished organ is, for actually it is an organ that is always flowing away and reappearing. In this going away and reappearing there is something inwardly mobile; if I were to try to sketch the process,

> it would basically be as if I were to try to sketch lightning; it is in continuous movement.[457]

It is continuously creating and adapting its activity anew.

Steiner linked heart problems with modern modes of transportation, which move us without our active involvement. In that process we create a chasm between what we are sensing and what we are doing—and that connecting place is where the heart lives. When it is absent, the heart is affected, as is our experience of warmth:

> You will find that the tendency to cardiac disease is essentially dependent on whether or not people sit still when they are being transported by some outer vehicle, as is the case with a car or a train. Passive submission to being moved "deforms" all the processes that are held back by the heart. Everything that plays into the human world in this way is related to how human beings maintain bodily warmth. Here you see how cardiac function relates to the impulse of warmth in the outer world to which we are connected. You can see that if individuals engender enough warmth through their own activity, this adequate measure of self-engendered warmth in their vital processes is also the measure of their heart. With cardiac patients, we would always have to make sure to induce thoroughly enlivened self-movement.[458]

The heart lives in and also engenders the element of warmth.

When the heart becomes unhealthy, it affects our sense of health, not so much on the level of an individual organ or physiologic process but for our sense of self as a whole. Our ability to sense and measure proper activity in the world is similarly hampered, and we can become either unduly preoccupied with what we should have done (guilt) or let everything fly without due consideration (rage):

> Something is reflected from the surface of the heart that is no longer merely a matter of habit or memory but is life that is already spiritualized when it reaches the outer surface of the

> heart. For what is thrown back from the heart are the pangs of conscience. This is to be considered, I would like to say, entirely from the physical aspect: the pangs of conscience that radiate into our consciousness are what is reflected by the heart from our experiences.... If the heart presses out its contents, however, this is really a system of forces, pushed out and brought into consciousness, that call forth in the next incarnation that strange inclination to live out one's karma.... This living out of karma can only be described as a kind of hunger and its satisfaction.... The forces that manifest themselves as such a hunger, leading to karmic fulfillment, living themselves out in this way, are concentrated in the heart; and when they are pressed out and thereby come into consciousness in the present incarnation, they create pictures that form a stimulus, and then raving madness results. Raving madness is basically a premature living out in this incarnation of a force of karma intended for the following incarnation.[459]

We can perhaps best frame these two symptoms as a diminution of self-worth and security (through guilt and "pangs of conscience") and an exaggeration of self-interest and the need to satisfy it ("raving madness").

As an introduction to remedy support, we can again mention an animal organ preparation, this time Cor as an etheric support for healthy organ function. Cor is particularly helpful when there are basic functional or structural imbalances with heart activity (such as congenital malformations).

For balancing the polarities of the upper and lower human being, of expansion and contraction, of inside and outside, Cardiodoron is a foundational medicine. It was discussed previously in relation to the cosmic and maniacal constitutions. The pedagogical indication for the cosmic child is to engender strong feeling and for the maniacal child is to bring experiences of self in the context of the world (through activities like body geography). The middle realm is very often weakened for these children, as the incomplete feeling connection between thinking that does not engage with the body (cosmic) and limbs that are not guided (maniacal) leaves a void in the middle. Cardiodoron is a plant remedy, with each component plant holding a very striking relationship to the astral body (Hyoscyamus, almost ugly and animal-like, with yellow-green flowers; Onopordon, a giant thistle filled with points and thorns but strong seasonal and architectural rhythms; and Primula, a delicate, yellow flower on a long stem that lifts high above the rosette of flowers down on the ground).[460] Through a threefold composition of such strikingly different plants, Cardiodoron brings a physiologic modeling for simultaneously holding such disparate gestures. Balancing those kinds of very different gestures belongs to the heart. Whenever children lose their balance between polarities and swing recklessly between engagement and disengagement, anger and guilt, we can turn to Cardiodoron.

Another remedy used to support the heart is Hypericum, St John's wort. It was previously discussed in relationship to the earthly or feeble constitution. Hypericum was also recommended by Steiner as a heart remedy, specifically as a treatment for palpitations with fear,[461] and has a long and well-known history as a treatment for melancholy and depression. We can find its broader application as a heart remedy if we revisit the process of bed-wetting and Steiner's recommendation for Hypericum as a treatment to bring better self-awareness:

> Under certain circumstances it [enuresis] can really be healed, if one works to influence children morally, even saying simply that the children are obliged to pay attention to their own bodily functions. Such moral influence should actually take place exactly with these kinds of things lying on the border between misbehavior and illnesses. Please do not misunderstand me; I recognize, naturally, that this is an illness, but it stands on the border between impudence, or misbehavior, and an illness.[462]

Hypericum assists the heart by allowing children to deepen their experience of self, to bring more light and warmth into themselves.

Hypericum exemplifies these processes of inwardly held light and warmth. In this way it relates to the activity of the heart as an inwardly directed sense organ.

A very good companion to Cardiodoron and Hypericum, is Aurum (gold). As a metal remedy it addresses the "I"-being. This makes it helpful in all questions of destiny and the decision to fully incarnate or a wish to excarnate. Aurum helps a child find balance and clarity with respect to these questions of whether to be in the world. Aurum does not force or push a particular decision or reaction but presents the healthy archetype so that proper insight can be attained. Aurum holds within it the archetypal threefold balance of thinking, feeling, and willing, of sal (the salt process), mercury, and phosphorus (as a fire process):

> In our thoughts, we separate what is subject to gravity (and therefore tends toward salt formation) from both the bearers of light, which tend toward the effect of light, and from what forms the basis of the balance between the two. There is no such separation, however, in the natural world. In nature, these ways of working are united with one another and interpenetrate, forming very intricate structural systems. These intricate edifices are present in the gleam of gold, because through gold, in a certain way, the spiritual element in its pure form looks into the outer world.... *Facilius est aurum facere quam destruere* ["It is easier to make gold than to destroy it"]. This is really one of the examples that makes us revere ancient knowledge, because people thought that the three essential principles of nature—the saltlike, the mercurial, and the phosphoric—were so strongly connected to each other in gold that it would be more difficult to extract them from that substance than from any other.[463]

Aurum is particularly helpful when a proper balance is needed between the spiritual and the earthly aspects of our being and finds broad application with many kinds of developmental delays and hesitations.

Notes

1 The reader who is newly encountering anthroposophic understandings and terminology will do well to explore what are often termed Steiner's basic books, including *Theosophy*, *An Outline of Esoteric Science*, and *How to Know Higher Worlds*. Building familiarity with the language and the specific vocabulary used in Anthroposophy is very useful, though as one works more and more into the processes described in the following chapters, it should be possible to gain a general understanding from the context and descriptions offered.

2 *Merriam-Webster*, s.v. "Materialism," accessed Jan. 25, 2017, http://www.merriam-webster.com/dictionary/materialism.

3 Older anthroposophic literature often refers to the "I" as the "ego," which was a stylistic choice made in translating the German word for "I," *ich*. But the word *ego* in anthroposophic literature indicates something very different from Freud's description of an ego, generally corresponding much more to an anthroposophic description of the feeling realm, which lives in the astral body and not the "I." To avoid confusion, we use "I" or ""I"-being" to indicate this individualized, spiritual core.

4 Temperament—commonly defined as innate characteristics of emotion and patterns of behavior already observable in newborn infants—has been broadly studied, particularly as to how it influences patterns of attachment, maternal postpartum depression, cognitive developmental status, and even language development.

5 This kind of spectrum thinking, placing imbalance at the ends of a spectrum, leads to moral understanding which no longer views good and evil as a twofold, black and white phenomenon, but as threefold: imbalance on one extreme, imbalance on the other, health in the middle. This is discussed in very broad spiritual dynamics in the Steiner, Nov. 21, 1919, *The Incarnation of Ahriman*.

6 See Selg, *Unborness*, pp. 34–35.

7 For a beautiful survey of the spiritual preparation that comes before conception and birth, see Selg, *Unbornness*.

8 Steiner, Aug. 26, 1906, *Founding a Science of the Spirit* (previous edition: *At the Gates of Spiritual Science*).

9 Ibid.

10 Steiner, May 28, 1907, *Rosicrucian Wisdom* (previous edition: *Theosophy of the Rosicrucian*).

11 Steiner, Oct. 22, 1906, *Original Impulses for a Science of the Spirit.*

12 Steiner, May 26, 1922, *The Human Soul in Relation to World Evolution.*

13 Steiner, June 25, 1924, *Education for Special Needs: The Curative Education Course.*

14 Steiner, May 28, 1907, *Rosicrucian Wisdom.*

15 Ibid.

16 Steiner, Aug. 26, 1906, *Founding a Science of the Spirit.*

17 Steiner, May 28, 1907, *Rosicrucian Wisdom.*

18 Steiner, Apr. 21, 1924, *Understanding Healing.*

19 Steiner, June 25, 1924, *Education for Special Needs.* Note: some quoted translations have been revised.

20 Steiner, Apr. 21, 1924, *Understanding Healing.*

21 For more exploration of this phenomenological approach, see Rohen, *Functional Morphology: The Dynamic Wholeness of the Human Organism*; and L. F. C. Mees, *Secrets of the Skeleton: Form in Metamorphosis.*

22 Steiner, June 13, 1921, *Education for Adolescents.*

23 Ibid.

24 Ibid.

25 Ibid.

26 Ibid.

27 Ibid.

28 Ibid.

29 Ibid.

30 Ibid.

31 Ibid.

32 Ibid.

33 Ibid.

34 Steiner, *The Invisible Man within Us: Pathology as a Basis for Therapy.*

35 Healthy ways to support a child through an inflammatory illness as well as discussions relating to the trade-offs of vaccinating for many classical childhood illnesses can be found in Glöckler and Goebel, *A Guide to Child Health: A Holistic Approach to Raising Healthy Children*; and Murphy, ed., *The Vaccination Dilemma.*

36 Steiner, May 26, 1922, *The Human Soul in Relation to World Evolution.*

37 Ibid.

38 Ibid.

39 Goddard Blythe, *The Well Balanced Child: Movement and Early Learning.*

40 See McAllen, *The Extra Lesson: Movement, Drawing and Painting Exercises to Help Children with Difficulties in Writing, Reading, and Arithmetic*; and Joep Eikenboom, *Foundations of the Extra Lesson.*

41 Steiner, June 30, 1924, *Education for Special Needs.*

42 Ibid.

43 Ibid.

44 Ibid.

45 Ibid.

46 Steiner, June 13, 1921, in *Education for Adolescents.*

47 Steiner, June 30, 1924, in *Education for Special Needs.*

48 Ibid.

49 Ibid.

50 Steiner and Wegman, ch. 5, "Plant, Animal, Human Being," *Fundamentals of Therapy*; alternate translation: *Extending Practical Medicine: Fundamental Principles Based on the Science of the Spirit.*

51 Ibid.

52 Steiner, Sep. 14, 1924, in *Pastoral Medicine: The Collegial Working of Doctors and Priests*; current edition: *Broken Vessels.*

53 Steiner and Wegman, ch. 5, *Extending Practical Medicine.*

54 Ibid.

55 Steiner, Aug. 24, 1919, *The Foundations of Human Experience* (previously available as *Study of Man*).

56 Ibid.

57 Ibid.

58 Ibid.

59 Ibid.

60 As part of Steiner's description of the "wish"—that which is working forward into the future—he indicated that this dynamic refining and releasing activity continues beyond the realm of the "I" and into the activity of the Spirit Self (the part of our astral body that has been completely transformed and refined by the "I"). Steiner explained that the "undertone of wish which accompanies our intentions" is the "first element of all that remains after death. It is something of this remainder which we feel when we say: we ought to have done it better; we wish we had done it better. In the wish, in the form in which I have described it to you, we have something which belongs to the Spirit Self." Rudolf Steiner, Aug. 24, 1919, *The Foundations of Human Experience.*

61 Steiner, June 30, 1924, *Education for Special Needs.*

62 Steiner, Feb. 20, 1924, *Eurythmy as Visible Speech.*

63 Steiner, Jul. 1, 1924, *Education for Special Needs.*

64 Ibid.

65 Steiner, Feb. 20, 1924, *Eurythmy as Visible Speech.*

66 Steiner, Feb. 21, 1924, ibid.

67 Steiner, Feb. 20, 1924, ibid.

68 For clarity the eurythmy vowel sound will now indicated as "I[ee]," so as to avoid possible confusion with the spiritual member of the human being, the "I."

69 Steiner, Feb. 20, 1924, *Eurythmy as Visible Speech.*

70 Steiner, Sep. 14, 1924, *Pastoral Medicine.*

71 Ibid.

72 Ibid.

73 Ibid.

74 Steiner, June 30, 1924, *Education for Special Needs.*

75 Steiner, Jul. 1, 1924, ibid.

76 Steiner, Feb. 20, 1924, *Eurythmy as Visible Speech.*

77 Steiner, Feb. 21, 1924, ibid.

78 Steiner, Jul. 1, 1924, *Education for Special Needs.*

79 Steiner, Feb. 20, 1924, *Eurythmy as Visible Speech* (emphasis added).

80 Steiner, Feb. 20 and 21, 1924, *Eurythmy as Visible Speech.*

81 Steiner, Jul. 2, 1924, *Education for Special Needs.*

82 Steiner, Feb. 21, 1924, *Eurythmy as Visible Speech.*

83 Steiner, June 13, 1921, *Education for Adolescents.*

84 Steiner, June 12, 1921, ibid.

85 Brothers Grimm, "Iron John," *Household Tales*, last modified Mar. 27, 2016, https://ebooks.adelaide.edu.au/g/grimm/g86h/chapter136.html.

86 Steiner and Wegman, ch. 7, "The Nature of Medicinal Actions," in *Extending Practical Medicine.*

87 Brothers Grimm, "Iron John." *Household Tales.*

88 Steiner, June 30, 1924, *Education for Special Needs.*

89 Brothers Grimm, "Iron John," *Household Tales.*

90 Steiner, Feb. 21, 1924, *Eurythmy as Visible Speech.*

91 Brothers Grimm, "Iron John," *Household Tales.*

92 Ibid.

93 Steiner, Feb. 21, 1924, *Eurythmy as Visible Speech.*

94 Brothers Grimm, "Iron John," *Household Tales.*

95 Ibid.

96 Ibid.

97 Steiner, Feb. 20, 1924, *Eurythmy as Visible Speech.*

98 Brothers Grimm, "Iron John," *Household Tales.*

99 Steiner, Feb. 20, 1924, *Eurythmy as Visible Speech.*

100 Steiner, June 27, 1924, *Education for Special Needs.*

101 Steiner, Jul. 4, 1924, ibid.

102 "Asberger's Disorder," DSM-IV Diagnostic Classifications, Autism Society, accessed Oct. 26, 2016, http://www.autism-society.org/dsm-iv-diagnostic-classifications/.

103 Ibid.

104 Ibid.

105 Steiner, June 30, 1924, *Education for Special Needs.*

106 Ibid.

107 Steiner, Jul. 4, 1924, ibid.

108 Steiner, Feb. 1, 1923, *The Invisible Man Within Us.*

109 Steiner, June 27, 1924, *Education for Special Needs.*

110 Ibid.

111 *Merriam-Webster*, s.v. "Kleptomania," accessed Oct. 26, 2016, http://www.merriam-webster.com/dictionary/kleptomania.

112 Steiner, June 27, 1924, *Education for Special Needs.*

113 Steiner, Jul. 15, 1924, *Faculty Meetings with Rudolf Steiner*, vol. 2.

114 Steiner, June 27, 1924, *Education for Special Needs.*

115 Steiner, Jul. 4, 1924, ibid.

116 Ibid.

117 Walter, case 29, *Abnormalities of Soul and Spiritual Development: Guidelines to an Understanding of Collected Case Histories with Indications by Rudolf Steiner.*

118 Steiner, Mar. 8, 1920, *Faculty Meetings with Rudolf Steiner*, vol. 1.

119 Steiner, Apr. 28, 1922, ibid.

120 Steiner, Jul. 15, 1924, *Faculty Meetings with Rudolf Steiner*, vol. 2.

121 Steiner, "note 6," *Education for Special Needs.*

122 Steiner, Apr. 28, 1920, *The Renewal of Education.*

123 Steiner, Feb. 4, 1919, *The Esoteric Aspect of the Social Question: The Individual and Society.*

124 Steiner, June 16, 1921, *Education for Adolescents.*

125 Steiner, Sep. 22, 1920, *Balance in Teaching.*

126 Ibid.

127 Ibid.

128 Steiner, June 13, 1921, *Education for Adolescents.*

129 Steiner, Dec. 7, 1905, *Esoteric Development.*

130 Steiner, Dec. 19, 1920, *Understanding Healing.*

131 Ibid.

132 Steiner, Jan. 2, 1914, *Esoteric Lessons: 1913–1923.*

133 Ibid.

134 Steiner, Dec. 7, 1905, "Inner Development," *Esoteric Development.*

135 Steiner, Sep. 2–5, 1906, *Founding a Science of the Spirit.*

136 Steiner, Dec. 19, 1920, *Understanding Healing.*

137 Steiner, Dec. 7, 1905, "Inner Development," *Esoteric Development.*

138 Steiner, Sep. 2–5, 1906, *Founding a Science of the Spirit.*

139 Steiner, Dec. 7, 1905, "Inner Development," *Esoteric Development.*

140 Ibid.

141 For interested readers, see Lipson, *Stairway of Surprise: Six Steps to a Creative Life*. It can be recommended as a highly accessible and inspirational guide to the six basic exercises.

142 Steiner, Sep. 3, 1919, *The Foundations of Human Experience.*

143 Steiner's description of the senses varied and evolved over time. At one point he described ten discrete senses, weaving touch as an additional sensing activity in amongst them. See Steiner, *Anthroposophy (A Fragment): A New Foundation for the Study of Human Nature*, written in 1910. With additional research and observation, Steiner expanded the scope of the senses to come to a full circle of twelve. While he lectured about the twelve senses multiple times, the ordering of the four lower senses was presented in different ways at different times. In lectures given at the founding of the first Waldorf school, the order given was balance, movement, life, and touch—with touch placed as the inmost sense. See Steiner, *The Foundations of Human Experience*, lectures given in 1919. Not long afterward he changed the placement of the touch sense, having at one point said that touch is actually part of all of the senses, and he ordered the senses as touch, balance, movement, life—with the life sense as the innermost sense. See Steiner, Aug. 8, 1920, *Spiritual Science as a Foundation for Social Forms*. For our exploration of the lower senses, we use this last ordering, as it has proved for the author to be clinically very helpful and particularly applicable in observing children.

144 Steiner, Aug. 8, 1920, *Spiritual Science as a Foundation for Social Forms.*

145 Ibid.

146 Ibid.

147 Ibid.

148 Ibid.

149 Ibid.

150 Steiner's description of a circle of twelve senses can additionally be broken into those senses relating to the will (the "lower" senses: touch, balance, movement, and life), those senses related to the feeling life (the "middle" senses: warmth, vision, taste, and smell), and those senses related more to thinking (the "higher" senses: hearing, work, thought, and sense of "I").

151 Steiner, Aug. 8, 1920, *Spiritual Science as a Foundation for Social Forms.* Emphasis added.

152 In the lecture in which Steiner laid out this progression inward through the "lower senses," he also described their higher spiritual correlate, the capacities that "stream into the soul." He went on: "Without the sense

of touch, people would have no feeling for God. What is felt by the sense of touch as roughness or smoothness, hardness or softness is the element flowing outward. What is turned back as soul phenomenon is the condition of permeation with cosmic substance, with *being* as such. It is precisely through the sense of touch that we ascertain the existence of the outer world.... What permeates all things and penetrates into us also, what holds and bears all of you—this all-pervading substance of God—enters consciousness and is the inwardly reflected experience of the sense of touch." He goes on to equate sense of balance with inner rest and feeling oneself as spirit, sense of movement with the experience of one's own free soul nature, and the sense of life with the feeling of wellbeing. Steiner, Aug. 8, 1920, *Spiritual Science as a Foundation for Social Forms.*

153 Temple Grandin has published many books on the experience of high-functioning autism and Asperger's syndrome, including *The Autistic Brain: Helping Different Kinds of Minds Succeed* and *Thinking in Pictures: My Life with Autism.*

154 Highly recommended explorations of the four lower senses include Henning Köhler, *Working with Anxious, Nervous, and Depressed Children: A Spiritual Perspective to Guide Parents*, and Sally Goddard Blythe, *The Well Balanced Child: Movement and Early Learning.*

155 Steiner, *The Invisible Man within Us.*

156 See the description of the "seed" meditation in Rudolf Steiner, *How to Know Higher Worlds: A Modern Path of Initiation.*

157 Steiner, Apr. 25, 1924, *Understanding Healing.*

158 Ibid.

159 Ibid.

160 Ibid.

161 Steiner, Feb. 6, 1923, in *Faculty Meetings with Rudolf Steiner*, vol. 2.

162 Eugen Kolisko was the first physician to work cooperatively with the faculty of a Waldorf school. He was part of the founding of the first Waldorf school, in Stuttgart, Germany, in 1919.

163 Steiner, Feb. 6, 1923, in *Faculty Meetings with Rudolf Steiner*, vol. 2.

164 Ibid.

165 Ibid.

166 Ibid.

167 Ibid.

168 Ibid.

169 Ibid.

170 Ibid.

171 Ibid.

172 Ibid.

173 Ibid.

174 Ibid.

175 Ibid.

176 This protection from the darker or scarier aspects of a story can, of course, be lost. It fades when a great deal of awareness is awoken in the child. This could be compared to young children walking on a log, losing confidence, and falling off when made overly aware of their body or they receive continuous feedback (positive or negative). Some fairy tales are certainly not appropriate until children are older (late kindergarten and some not until the early grades), but the truthfulness of the spiritual pictures in fairy tales can be an important experience for children and the adults who care for them.

177 Steiner, Feb. 6, 1923, *Faculty Meetings with Rudolf Steiner*, vol. 2.

178 Steiner, lectures of June 25 and June 26, 1924, *Education for Special Needs*.

179 Steiner, June 26, 1924, in *Education for Special Needs*. Emphasis added.

180 Ibid.

181 Steiner, Feb. 6, 1923, *Faculty Meetings with Rudolf Steiner*, vol. 2.

182 Steiner, Nov. 4, 1910, "Consciousness and Soul Life," *A Psychology of Body, Soul, and Spirit: Anthroposophy, Psychosophy, and Pneumatosophy*. Steiner asks, "What does our soul life consist of now?" He responds, "It consists of the stream flowing from the past into the future meeting another stream flowing from the future into the past. Since that meeting constitutes the soul life of the present moment, you can easily understand that the two streams come together or overlap, so to speak, within the soul; that overlap is consciousness. There is no other explanation for consciousness than this. That is how the soul participates in everything flowing from the past into the future, and from the future everything into the past. You can say, whenever you look into your soul life, that you are involved with an interpenetration of those two streams—what flows from the past into the future and the opposite flow of desires, interests, wishes, and so on. The two streams interpenetrate each other."

183 Steiner, Feb. 6, 1923, *Faculty Meetings with Rudolf Steiner*, vol. 2.

184 Ibid.

185 Steiner, Apr. 25, 1924, *Understanding Healing*.

186 Steiner, Aug. 22, 1919, *The Foundations of Human Experience*.

187 Related dietary indications are also given, using either the roots or the blossoms of a plant, respectively, for the polarity of "too much" sulfur and "not enough" sulfur. These are discussed in the next section.

188 Steiner, Feb. 6, 1923, *Faculty Meetings with Rudolf Steiner*, vol. 2.

189 Ibid.

190 Ibid.

191 Steiner, Nov. 30, 1923, *Mystery Knowledge and Mystery Centres*.

192 Ibid.

193 Steiner, Dec. 14, 1923, *Mystery Knowledge and Mystery Centres.*

194 Ibid.

195 Rudolf Steiner, Aug. 15, 1924, *True and False Paths in Spiritual Investigation.*

196 For a more complete overview of the seven-year changes, see Nancy Blanning, ed., *First Grade Readiness: Resources, Insights, and Tools for Waldorf Educators.*

197 See Nancy Foster, "Some Guidelines for First Grade Readiness," in Nancy Blanning, *First Grade Readiness: Resources, Insights, and Tools for Waldorf Educators.*

198 Schramm, *The Healing Power of Planetary Metals in Anthroposophic and Homeopathic Medicine.*

199 Steiner and Wegman, ch. 19, "Characteristic Illnesses," case 1, in *Extending Practical Medicine.*

200 Brothers Grimm, "Little Snow White," accessed on Oct. 21, 2016, http://www.pitt.edu/~dash/grimm053.html.

201 Brothers Grimm, "Little Snow White."

202 Ibid.

203 Ibid.

204 Ibid.

205 In the last chapter of Rudolf Steiner and Ita Wegman's *Extending Practical Medicine*, pyrite (iron sulfide) is described as a remedy for those illnesses in which there is an imbalance between the blood (linked to the sulfur component of pyrite) and the breathing system (the iron component).

206 We might contrast this with another Grimm fairy tale, that of Snow-White and Rose-Red. In that fairy tale we are given imaginations that are more contrasting, with Snow White being quieter, observant, and more retiring, while Rose-Red is active and exploring; there the polarity of the two girls builds the balance of nerve and blood. In the story of Snow White and the seven dwarfs ("Little Snow White"), we are taking a different journey—that from the head down into the metabolism.

207 Steiner's descriptions of the relation of the zodiac to the planetary movements and the twelve senses to the seven life processes support the placement of the life sense as the most inward of the senses, as opposed to the sense of touch. As Steiner presented the order of the lower senses in both ways (touch, balance, movement, life versus balance, movement, life, touch), we can be confident that both orderings bear spiritual truthfulness.

208 Steiner, Aug. 12, 1916, *The Riddle of Humanity: The Spiritual Background of Human History.*

209 Ibid.

210 Brothers Grimm, "Little Snow White."

211 Ibid.

212 Ibid.

213 Steiner, Aug. 12, 1916, *The Riddle of Humanity.*

214 Figure adapted from two of Steiner's chalkboard drawings from Aug. 12, 1916, *The Riddle of Humanity.*

215 Brothers Grimm, "Little Snow White."

216 Ibid.

217 Steiner described back pain as one of a complex of symptoms in a young woman in whom "the excessive inherent activity of the astral body causes too little of its forces to flow over into the physical and etheric body." Steiner and Wegman, ch. 19, "Characteristic Illnesses," case 1, *Extending Practical Medicine.*

218 See the descriptions of *Belladonna*, *Hyoscyamus*, and *Stramonium* for the maniacal constitution within appendix 2.

219 Brothers Grimm, "Little Snow White."

220 Ibid.

221 Ibid.

222 Ibid.

223 See descriptions of the "will to heal" in Steiner, lect. Jan. 8, 1924, *Understanding Healing.*

224 For more information about this process, see Steiner's descriptions of the consciousness soul and the development of the spirit self in *Theosophy* and other foundational writings.

225 Steiner, *Education for Special Needs: The Curative Education Course,* June 25, 1924.

226 This kind of boomerang movement can be experienced very beautifully when working as a group through the six basic exercises. If the time is taken to consciously work with each exercise for a full month, there is often a kind of natural evolution in which we begin to unfold the next meditative activity before we have even consciously transitioned from one to another, for example, control of actions flows over into a feeling of equanimity, which opens the door for positivity, and so on.

227 Steiner, *The Foundations of Human Experience,* Aug. 21, 1919.

228 Two very helpful guides are Michaela Strauss, *Understanding Children's Drawings: Tracing the Path of Incarnation*; and Audrey E. McAllen, *Reading Children's Drawings: The Person, House and Tree Motifs.*

229 This comment may seem strange, as a very young child is, of course, physically and functionally much more directly dependent on the support and protection of the outside world to live. Naturally, an infant is dependent on breast milk. So in very early childhood the connection with the outside is essential, though we should recognize that it is simultaneously so inherent as to almost be unconscious. With adolescence a child finds ever-greater skills of independent activity and self-sufficiency on a physical level while becoming keenly aware of the importance of social and emotional connection.

230 Steiner, June 22, 1924, *Karmic Relationships,* vol. 2.

231 Ibid.

232 Steiner, June 27, 1924, *Education for Special Needs.*

233 Ibid.

234 Steiner, June 28, 1924, ibid.

235 Steiner, June 27, 1924, ibid.

236 Ibid.

237 Steiner, June 28, 1924, ibid.

238 Steiner, June 27, 1924, ibid.

239 Ibid.

240 Ibid.

241 Ibid.

242 Ibid.

243 Rudolf Steiner, Jul. 5, 1924, ibid.

244 Ibid.

245 Steiner, ch. 7, "Changes in the Dream Life of the Esoteric Student," *How to Know Higher Worlds.*

246 Steiner, Jul. 5, 1924, *Education for Special Needs.*

247 Ibid.

248 Ibid.

249 Steiner, June 28, 1924, ibid.

250 Ibid.

251 Ibid.

252 Ibid.

253 Ibid.

254 Ibid.

255 Ibid.

256 Steiner, Feb. 6, 1923, *Faculty Meetings with Rudolf Steiner*, vol. 2.

257 Steiner, June 28, 1924, *Education for Special Needs.*

258 Ibid.

259 Ibid.

260 Ibid.

261 Steiner, June 27, 1924, ibid.

262 Ibid.

263 Ibid.

264 Brothers Grimm, "The Goose-Girl at the Well," in *Household Tales,* https://ebooks.adelaide.edu.au/g/grimm/g86h/chapter180.html (accessed Sept. 29, 2018).

265 Ibid.

266 Ibid.

267 Ibid.

268 Ibid.

269 Ibid.

270 Ibid.

271 Ibid.

272 Ibid.

273 Ibid.

274 Ibid.

275 Ibid.

276 Steiner, June 27, 1924, *Education for Special Needs.*

277 Steiner, June 28, 1924, ibid.

278 Steiner, Feb. 1, 1923, *The Invisible Man within Us.*

279 Steiner, June 15, 1921, *Education for Adolescents.*

280 Ibid.

281 Ibid.

282 Ibid.

283 Ibid.

284 Ibid.

285 Steiner, June 30, 1924, ibid.

286 Ibid.

287 Ibid.

288 Ibid.

289 Ibid.

290 Ibid.

291 Ibid.

292 Ibid.

293 Ibid.

294 Ibid.

295 Ibid.

296 Steiner, Mar. 8, 1920, *Faculty Meetings with Rudolf Steiner*, vol. 1.

297 "Diagnostic Criteria for Autism Spectrum Disorder," Centers for Disease Control and Prevention, accessed Oct. 29, 2016, https://www.cdc.gov/ncbddd/autism/hcp-dsm.html.

298 Ibid.

299 Ibid.

300 Adapted from Steiner's blackboard drawing, Aug. 8, 1920, *Spiritual Science as a Foundation for Social Forms.*

301 "Diagnostic Criteria for Autism Spectrum Disorder," Centers for Disease Control and Prevention, accessed Oct. 29, 2016, https://www.cdc.gov/ncbddd/autism/hcp-dsm.html.

302 Ibid.

303 Ibid.

304 Ibid.

305 Steiner, Mar. 22, 1910, *Macrocosm and Microcosm.*

306 Schoorel, ch. 1, "The Importance of the First Seven Years for the Rest of Life," *The First Seven Years: Physiology of Childhood.*

307 Selg, *I Am Different from You: How Children Experience Themselves and the World in the Middle of Childhood.* This book gives an excellent physiologic and pedagogical picture of this important change.

308 Steiner, Apr. 12, 1921, *Illness and Therapy: Spiritual-Scientific Aspects of Healing* (old edition: *Anthroposophical Spiritual Science and Medical Therapy: The Second Medical Course*).

309 Hilma Walter, *Abnormalities in Soul-Spiritual Development: Guidelines to an Understanding of Collected Case Histories with Indications by Rudolf Steiner* (Spring Valley, NY: Mercury Press, 2010). Other volumes by Walter, not yet translated into English, focus on the plant world (*Die Pflanzenwelt*), and the seven metals (*Die Sieben Hauptmetale*). Also, the writings of A. G. Degenaar, *Zur Anthroposophicen Medizin: Themen aus dem Gesamtwerke Rudolf Steiners* (Zeist, Netherlands: Privatdruck, 1989).

310 Steiner, Apr. 15, 1921, *Illness and Therapy.*

311 Steiner, June 30, 1924, *Education for Special Needs.*

312 Steiner, Jul. 1, 1924, *Education for Special Needs.*

313 Steiner, Apr. 1, 1920, *Introducing Anthroposophical Medicine* (Great Barrington, MA: SteinerBooks, 2010).

314 Steiner, Apr. 15, 1921, *Illness and Therapy.*

315 Ibid.

316 Von Zabern, *Compendium for the Remedial Treatment of Children, Adolescents and Adults in Need of Soul Care.*

317 Ibid.

318 Medical Section of the School of Spiritual Science et al., entry for "Levico," in *Vademecum of Anthroposophic Medicines,* 1st English ed., 2009 (Dornach, Switzerland: Medical Section of the School of Spiritual Science). Supplement to *Der Merkurstab: Journal of Anthroposophic Medicine,* 2009; 62 (5).

319 Steiner, Jul. 4, 1924, in *Education for Special Needs.*

320 Steiner and Ita Wegman, ch. 19, "Characteristic Illnesses," case 2, *Extending Practical Medicine.*

321 Steiner, June 30, 1922, in *Human Questions and Cosmic Answers: Man and His Relation to the Planets.*

322 Hilma Walter, case 1, "Grippe, Encephalitis, Poliomyeliti: Zur Pathogenese und Behandlung mit Krankengeschichten," cited under "Mercurius," in Hans Krüger, comp., Heilmittel Angaben Rudolf Steiners ["Remedy Indications from Rudolf Steiner"] (Dornach, Switzerland: Medizischen Sektion der Freien Hochschule für Geisteswissenschaft am Goetheanum, 1999/2000) (author's translation).

323 Ibid.; author's translation.

324 Medical Section of the School of Spiritual Science, Dornach, Switzerland, et al., "Mercurius vivus naturalis," in *Vademecum of Anthroposophic Medicines*. Please note that the European designation for level of 1 to 10 parts "Dilution" in this reference (e.g., D5) is equivalent to the "x" designation (e.g., 5x) which is more commonly used in North America. But the "D_" and "_x" designations can be used interchangeably.

325 Steiner, Dec. 22, 1923, *Mystery Knowledge and Mystery Centres.*

326 Steiner and Wegman, ch. 17, "Perceiving the Nature of Substances as a Basis of Pharmacognosy," *Extending Practical Medicine.*

327 Case "KG IV 131," cited under "Oxalis," in Hans Krüger, comp., Heilmittel Angaben Rudolf Steiners ["Remedy Indications from Rudolf Steiner"].

328 Case "KG V 99," cited under "Oxalis," in Hans Krüger, comp., *Heilmittel Angaben Rudolf Steiners.*

329 A. G. Degenaar, case 71, in "Krankheitsfälle und andere medizinische Fragen, besprochen mit Rudolf Steiner," cited under "Mercurius," in Hans Krüger, comp., *Heilmittel Angaben Rudolf Steiners.*

330 Steiner, Jan. 1, 1924, *Physiologisch-Therapeutisches auf Grundlage der Geisteswissenschaft* ["Physiology and Therapy on the Foundation of Spiritual Science"], accessed Oct. 26, 2016, Freie Verwaltung des Nachlasses Rudolf Steiners, http://fvn-rs.net/index.php?option=com_content&view=article&id=3221%3Azweiter-vortrag-dornach-1-januar-1924&catid=209%3Aga-314-physiologisch-therapeutisches-auf-grundlage&Itemid=15. Author's translation. Published in English: *Physiology and Healing: Treatment, Therapy, and Hygiene—Spiritual Science and Medicine.*

331 See von Zabern, *Compendium for the Remedial Treatment of Children, Adolescents, and Adults in Need of Soul Care.*

332 Steiner, Jan. 1, 1924, in Physiologisch-Therapeutisches auf Grundlage der Geisteswissenschaft, http://fvn-rs.net/index.php?option=com_content&view=article&id=3222:erster-vortrag-dornach-31-dezember-1923&catid=209:ga-314-physiologisch-therapeutisches-auf-grundlage&Itemid=15; author's translation.

333 Steiner, Apr. 1, 1920, *Introducing Anthroposophical Medicine.*

334 Steiner, June 25, 1924, *Education for Special Needs.*

335 Erik W. Baars, "The Effect of Hepar Magnesium D10 on Fibromyalgia Symptoms: A Pilot Study," *European Journal of Integrative Medicine* 2, no. 1 (2010): 15–21.

336 Erik W. Baars, "The Effect of Hepar Magnesium on Seasonal Fatigue Symptoms: A Pilot Study," *Journal of Alternative and Complementary Medicine* 14, no. 4 (2008): 395–402.

337 Steiner, Jul. 1, 1924, *Education for Special Needs.*

338 Ibid.

339 Steiner went on to describe *Hypophysis* as only one aspect of the boy's therapy, which needed to be matched with *Carbo animalis*: "For the child we are considering, pituitary gland must not however be used just in the way we use it for rickety children in whom we definitely want to induce dispersal. Here we have to call into action at the same time the opposite principle that works centripetally. You will accordingly need to find something which will have, while working together with pituitary gland, the tendency to build up the human organism out of this substance. Both *Carbo vegetabilis* and *Carbo animalis* are able to do this. You could therefore use *Carbo animalis*, alternating with the pituitary gland. The *Carbo animalis* will supply the form principle, and then in the *Hypophysis cerebri* you will have the organizing principle that tends to encourage *growth*" (from Steiner, Jul. 6, 1924, *Education for Special Needs*).

340 Steiner, Apr. 25, 1921, *Illness and Therapy.*

341 Steiner and Wegman, "Characteristic Illnesses," case 4, ch. 19, *Extending Practical Medicine.*

342 Steiner, Jul. 5, 1924, *Education for Special Needs.*

343 Heinz-Harmut Vogel, "Cuprum aceticum," *Finding Remedies: Spiritual Knowledge of Man and Nature,* vols. 1 and 2.

344 Schramm, "Zincum valerianicum" in *Heilmittel-Fiebel zur anthroposophischen Medizin.*

345 Steiner, Mar. 26, 1920, *Introducing Anthroposophical Medicine.*

346 Steiner, Apr. 18, 1921, *Illness and Therapy.*

347 Steiner, Dec. 23, 1923, *Mystery Knowledge and Mystery Centres.*

348 Steiner, Apr. 8, 1920, *Introducing Anthroposophical Medicine.*

349 Ibid.

350 Ibid.

351 Steiner indicated that there is an inverse relationship between substances as they are found in their natural form (as mineral, plant, animal, or human substance) and the therapeutic effect they can have within the human body as anthroposophic medicines. He also indicated that substances from the mineral kingdom work upon the "I"-organization, plants address the astral body, animal and organ preparations work on the etheric, and human substances (blood, insulin, antibodies) address the physical body.

352 Steiner, Apr. 4, 1920, *Introducing Anthroposophical Medicine.*

353 Steiner, Apr. 25, 1924, *Understanding Healing.*

354 Wolff, *Remedies for Typical Diseases: Concerning the Remedies Developed by Rudolf Steiner Using New Concepts and New Methods.*

355 "*Onopordon* compound" is the name that is often given for WALA-type preparations that contain the same basic ingredients as *Cardiodoron.*

356 Medical Section of the School of Spiritual Science, Dornach, Switzerland, et al., "Plumbum," *Vademecum of Anthroposophic Medicines.*

357 Henning M. Schramm, "Plumbum," *Heilmittel-Fibel zur anthroposophischen Medizin.*

358 Steiner, Apr. 17, 1921, *Illness and Therapy.*

359 Steiner, Jan. 4, 1924, *Understanding Healing.*

360 Steiner, Dec. 14, 1923, *Mystery Knowledge and Mystery Centres.*

361 Steiner, Jan. 4, 1924, *Understanding Healing.*

362 Medical Section of the School of Spiritual Science, Dornach, Switzerland, et al.,"Plumbum," *Vademecum of Anthroposophic Medicines.*

363 Husemann and Wolff, "The School Child and the School Physician's Guidance," *The Anthroposophical Approach to Medicine*, vol. 1.

364 Steiner and Wegman, ch. 20, "Typical Medicines," *Extending Practical Medicine.*

365 Steiner, Mar. 27, 1920, *Introducing Anthroposophical Medicine.*

366 Steiner and Ita Wegman, ch. 14, "The Therapeutic Way of Thinking," *Extending Practical Medicine.*

367 Ibid.

368 Steiner, Mar. 30, 1920, *Introducing Anthroposophical Medicine.*

369 Ibid.

370 Ibid.

371 Medical Section of the School of Spiritual Science, Dornach, Switzerland, et al., "Cichorium plumbo culta," *Vademecum of Anthroposophic Medicines.*

372 Steiner, Aug. 28, 1923, *The Healing Process.*

373 Steiner, Apr. 23, 1924, *Understanding Healing.*

374 Steiner, Jan. 9, 1924, ibid.

375 "Arlesheim Preparations List," 1920–1925, cited in "Argentum," Hans Krüger, comp., *Heilmittel Angaben Rudolf Steiners* ["Remedy Indications from Rudolf Steiner"]. Author's translation.

376 Steiner, Feb. 6, 1923, *Faculty Meetings with Rudolf Steiner*, vol. 2.

377 Steiner, Jul. 24, 1924, *The Healing Process* (old translation: *What Can the Art of Healing Gain Spiritual Science?*).

378 Steiner, Nov. 16, 1923, ibid.

379 Medical Section of the School of Spiritual Science, Dornach, Switzerland, et al., "Argentum," *Vademecum of Anthroposophic Medicines.*

380 Steiner and Wegman, ch. 13, "On the Nature of Illness and Healing," *Extending Practical Medicine.*

381 Husemann and Wolff, "The School Child and the School Physician's Guidance," *The Anthroposophical Approach to Medicine,* vol. 1.

382 Steiner, Mar. 27, 1920, *Introducing Anthroposophical Medicine.*

383 Steiner, June 27, 1924, *Education for Special Needs.*

384 Steiner, *The Invisible Man Within Us.*

385 Steiner, Apr. 8, 1920, *Introducing Anthroposophical Medicine.*

386 Case "KG III 101," cited under "Atropa Belladonna," Hans Krüger, comp., *Heilmittel Angaben Rudolf Steiners* ["Remedy Indications from Rudolf Steiner"].

387 Case "KG III 109," cited under "Atropa Belladonna," Hans Krüger, comp., *Heilmittel Angaben Rudolf Steiners* ["Remedy Indications from Rudolf Steiner"].

388 A. G. Degenaar, case 9, "Krankheitsfälle und andere medizinische Fragen, besprochen mit Rudolf Steiner," cited under "Atropa Belladonna," in Hans Krüger, comp., *Heilmittel Angaben Rudolf Steiners* ["Remedy Indications from Rudolf Steiner"].

389 Steiner, Aug. 28, 1923, *The Healing Process.*

390 "Aerztebesprechung," Aug. 11, 1922, cited under "Atropa Belladonna," Hans Krüger, comp., *Heilmittel Angaben Rudolf Steiners* ["Remedy Indications from Rudolf Steiner"].

391 Cases "KG II 26," "KG II 37," and "KG IV 10," cited under "Sulfur," Hans Krüger, comp., *Heilmittel Angaben Rudolf Steiners* ["Remedy Indications from Rudolf Steiner"].

392 Steiner and Wegman, ch. 13, "On the Nature of Illness and Healing," *Extending Practical Medicine.*

393 Steiner and Wegman, ch. 20, "Typical Medicines," *Extending Practical Medicine.*

394 Ibid.

395 Steiner, Jul. 5, 1924, *Education for Special Needs.*

396 Case "KG III 103" (another description of the boy presented in the curative course), also cases from an "Insert for Medical Section Members in Natura," 1928, page 57, and the "Arlesheimer Praeparate-Liste" 159, all cited under "Vaucheria," Hans Krüger, comp., *Heilmittel Angaben Rudolf Steiners* ["Remedy Indications from Rudolf Steiner"].

397 See the description in part 1, related to scarlet fever and measles as archetypal inflammatory illnesses for balancing an excessive spiritual stream and a dominant hereditary body, respectively.

398 Steiner, June 14, 1924, *Karmic Relationships*, vol. 7.

399 Steiner, discussion of Sept. 2, 1919, *Discussions with Teachers.*

400 Steiner, Jan. 2, 1924, *Physiologisch-Therapeutisches auf Grundlage der Geisteswissenschaft* ["Physiology and Therapy on the Foundation of

Spiritual Science, the Fourth Medical Course"]; accessed Oct. 26, 2016, Freie Verwaltung des Nachlasses Rudolf Steiners (http://fvn-rs.net/index.php?option=com_content&view=article&id=3222:erster-vortrag-dornach-31-dezember-1923&catid=209:ga-314-physiologisch-therapeutisches-auf-grundlage&Itemid=15).

401 Steiner and Wegman, ch. 19, "Characteristic Illnesses," case 5, *Extending Practical Medicine.*

402 Case "KG III 98" (also described in *Extending Practical Medicine*, "Characteristic Illnesses," case 4) cited under "Chamomilla," in Hans Krüger, comp., *Heilmittel Angaben Rudolf Steiners.*

403 Steiner and Ita Wegman, ch. 15, "The Method of Treatment," in *Extending Practical Medicine.*

404 Cases "KG III 31," "KG V 36," "KG V 127," cited under "Nicotiana Tabacum," in Hans Krüger, comp., *Heilmittel Angaben Rudolf Steiners*..

405 "Therapeutische und pharmakologish-pharmazeutische Erfahrungen," cited in "Bryophyllum," in Hans Krüger, comp., *Heilmittel Angaben Rudolf Steiners.*

406 Steiner, Mar. 25, 1920, in *Introducing Anthroposophical Medicine.*

407 Cases "KG II 37," "KG E I," "KG V 47," and "DG 144," cited under "Calcium," in Hans Krüger, comp., *Heilmittel Angaben Rudolf Steiners.*

408 Hilma Walter, case 16, in Der Krebs und seine Behandlung (Verein für Krebsforschung: Arlesheim, 1953), Hilma Walter, cases 27 and 93, in *Die Sieben Hauptmetalle* (Natura Verlag: Dornach, 1999) cited under "Calcium," in Hans Krüger, comp., *Heilmittel Angaben Rudolf Steiners.*

409 Steiner, Nov. 16, 1923, *The Healing Process.*

410 Ibid.

411 Rudolf Steiner, Jul. 6, 1924, *Education for Special Needs.*

412 Ibid.

413 Ibid.

414 Ibid.

415 See "Berberis/Apis comp.," "Berberis e fructibus comp.," "Berberis/Hypericum comp.," and other "Berbis" entries in Heinz-Hartmut Vogel, *Finding Remedies: Spiritual Knowledge of Man and Nature,* vols. 1 and 2.

416 Hilma Walter, case 22, in *Der Krebs und seine Behandlung*, cited under "Berberis vulgaris," in Hans Krüger, comp., *Heilmittel Angaben Rudolf Steiners.*

417 The description of Phosphorus as polar activity to those of Silica, Silver, and Calcium Carbonate can be found in Steiner, Nov. 16, 1923, *The Healing Process.* A discussion of Phosphorus and Sulfur as opposite to Arsenic, mediated by Stibium, is found in Steiner, Apr. 12, 1921, *Illness and Therapy.*

418 Steiner, Nov. 16, 1923, in *The Healing Process.*

419 Ibid.

420 Steiner, Apr. 12, 1921, *Illness and Therapy.*

421 "Doctor's Discussion 4, 1922, about Fever, KG DG Anhang," cited under "Phosphorus," Hans Krüger, comp., *Heilmittel Angaben Rudolf Steiners.*

422 Case "KG IV 46," cited under "Argentum," in Hans Krüger, comp., *Heilmittel Angaben Rudolf Steiners.*

423 Steiner and Wegman, ch. 13, "On the Nature of Illness and Healing," *Extending Practical Medicine.*

424 Steiner, Apr. 2, 1920, *Introducing Anthroposophical Medicine.*

425 Steiner, June 27, 1924, *Education for Special Needs.*

426 Steiner, Apr. 1, 1920, *Introducing Anthroposophical Medicine.*

427 Steiner, June 13, 1921, *Education for Adolescents.*

428 For additional information, see Holtzapfel, *The Human Organs: Their Functional and Psychological Significance*; the chapters "The Fourfold Organ System," "The Liver-Gall System and its Diseases," "The Renal System and its Diseases," "The Cardiovascular System and its Diseases," and "The Lungs and their Diseases" in Husemann and Wolff, eds., *The Anthroposophical Approach to Medicine,* vol. 2; Rudolf Treichler's chapter "The Relation of Physical Organs to Psychological Disorders" Husemann and Wolff, eds., *The Anthroposophical Approach to Medicine,* vol. 3; and Wolfgang Rißmann, "Therapy of Depression: Anthroposophical Medicines," *Der Merkurstab* Sep.–Oct. (2006): 407–413.

429 Steiner, Mar. 29, 1920, *Introducing Anthroposophical Medicine.*

430 Steiner, Apr. 2, 1920, ibid.

431 Steiner, Jul. 2, 1921, *Therapeutic Insights: Earthly and Cosmic Laws.*

432 Steiner and Wegman, ch. 7, "The Nature of Medicinal Actions," *Extending Practical Medicine.*

433 Steiner, Apr. 1, 1920, ibid.

434 Steiner, Apr. 9, 1920, ibid.

435 Steiner, Jul. 2, 1921, *Therapeutic Insights: Earthly and Cosmic Laws.*

436 Steiner, Mar. 26, 1920, *Introducing Anthroposophical Medicine.*

437 Steiner, Mar. 31, 1920, ibid.

438 Ibid.

439 Steiner, Mar. 29, 1920, ibid.

440 Steiner, Apr. 2, 1920, ibid.

441 Steiner, Jul. 2, 1921, *Therapeutic Insights.*

442 Ibid.

443 Steiner, June 13, 1924, *Agriculture.*

444 Steiner, June 24, 1924, *Education for Special Needs.*

445 Steiner, Mar. 31, 1920, *Introducing Anthroposophical Medicine.*

446 Steiner, Mar. 29, 1920, ibid.

447 Steiner, Mar. 31, 1920, ibid.

448 Steiner, Jul. 2, 1921, *Therapeutic Insights.*

449 Steiner, Nov. 16, 1923, *The Healing Process.*

450 Steiner, Jul. 21, 1924, ibid.

451 Steiner and Wegman, ch.. 14, "The Therapeutic Way of Thinking," *Extending Practical Medicine.*

452 Steiner and Wegman, ch. 19, "Characteristic Case Histories" cases 5 and 1; and ch. 10, "The Method of Treatment," *Extending Practical Medicine.*

453 Steiner, Mar. 31, 1920, in *Introducing Anthroposophical Medicine.*

454 Ibid.

455 Ibid.

456 Steiner, Mar. 22, 1920, Ibid.

457 Steiner, Oct. 3, 1922, *Spiritual Relations in the Human Organism.*

458 Steiner, Mar. 29, 1920, *Introducing Anthroposophical Medicine.*

459 Steiner, Jul. 2, 1921, *Therapeutic Insights.*

460 Wolff, *Remedies for Typical Diseases: Concerning the Remedies Developed by Rudolf Steiner Using New Concepts and New Methods.*

461 A. G. Degenaar, case 8, "Krankheitsfälle und andere medizinische Fragen, besprochen mit Rudolf Steiner," cited under "Hypericum," Hans Krüger, comp., *Heilmittel Angaben Rudolf Steiners* ["Remedy Indications from Rudolf Steiner"].

462 Steiner, Jan. 1, 1924, *Physiologisch-Therapeutisches auf Grundlage der Geisteswissenschaft* ["Physiology and Therapy on the Foundation of Spiritual Science, the Fourth Medical Course"] (accessed Oct. 26, 2016), Freie Verwaltung des Nachlasses Rudolf Steiners, http://fvn-rs.net/index.php?option=com_content&view=article&id=3222:erster-vortrag-dornach-31-dezember-1923&catid=209:ga-314-physiologisch-therapeutisches-auf-grundlage&Itemid=15 (author's translation).

463 Steiner, Mar. 26, 1920, *Introducing Anthroposophical Medicine.*

Bibliography

Blanning, Nancy (ed.). *First Grade Readiness: Resources, Insights, and Tools for Waldorf Educators.* Spring Valley, NY: Waldorf Early Childhood Association of North America, 2009.

Eikenboom, Joep. *Foundations of the Extra Lesson.* Fair Oaks, CA: Rudolf Steiner College, 2007.

Glöckler, Michaela, and Wolfgang Goebel. *A Guide to Child Health: A Holistic Approach to Raising Healthy Children.* Edinburgh: Floris Books, 2013.

Goddard Blythe, Sally. *The Well Balanced Child: Movement and Early Learning.* Stroud, UK: Hawthorn Press, 2005.

Grandin, Temple. *The Autistic Brain: Helping Different Kinds of Minds Succeed.* New York: Mariner Books, 2014.

———. *Thinking in Pictures: My Life with Autism.* New York: Vintage, 2006.

Holtzapfel, Walter. *The Human Organs: Their Functional and Psychological Significance.* Cornwall, UK: Lanthorn Press, 2002.

Husemann, Friedrich, and Otto Wolff. *The Anthroposophical Approach to Medicine*, vol. 1. Spring Valley, NY: Anthroposophic Press, 1982.

———. *The Anthroposophical Approach to Medicine,* vol. 2. Hudson, NY: Anthroposophic Press, 1987.

———. *The Anthroposophical Approach to Medicine,* vol. 3. Spring Valley, NY: Mercury Press, 2003.

Köhler, Henning. *Working with Anxious, Nervous, and Depressed Children: A Spiritual Perspective to Guide Parents.* Chatham, NY: Research Institute for Waldorf Education, 2001.

Lipson, Michael. *Stairway of Surprise: Six Steps to a Creative Life.* Great Barrington, MA: Anthroposophic Press, 2002.

McAllen, Audrey E. *The Extra Lesson: Movement, Drawing and Painting Exercises to Help Children with Difficulties in Writing, Reading, and Arithmetic.* Fair Oaks, CA: Rudolf Steiner College, 2004.

———. *Reading Children's Drawings: The Person, House and Tree Motifs.* Fair Oaks, CA: Rudolf Steiner College, 2004.

Mees, L. F. C. *Secrets of the Skeleton: Form in Metamorphosis.* Hudson, NY: Anthroposophic Press, 1995.

Murphy, Christine (ed.). *The Vaccination Dilemma.* Brooklyn, NY: Lantern Books, 2002.

Rohen, Johannes W. *Functional Morphology: The Dynamic Wholeness of the Human Organism.* Hillsdale, NY: Adonis Press, 2007.

Schoorel, Edmond. *The First Seven Years: Physiology of Childhood.* Fair Oaks, CA: Rudolf Steiner College, 2004.

Schramm, Henning. *The Healing Power of Planetary Metals in Anthroposophic and Homeopathic Medicine.* Great Barrington, MA: Lindisfarne Books, 2013.

———. *Heilmittel-Fiebel zur anthroposophischen Medizin.* Schauffhausen, Switzerland: Novalis Verlag, 1997.

Selg, Peter. *I Am Different from You: How Children Experience Themselves and the World in the Middle of Childhood.* Great Barrington, MA: SteinerBooks, 2011.

———. *Unborness: Human Pre-existence and the Journey toward Birth.* Great Barrington, MA: SteinerBooks, 2010.

Steiner, Rudolf. *Abnormalities of Soul and Spiritual Development: Guidelines to an Understanding of Collected Case Histories with Indications by Rudolf Steiner.* Chestnut Ridge, NY: Mercury Press, 2010.

———. *Agriculture.* Kimberton, PA: Bio-Dynamic Farming and Gardening Association, 1993.

———. *Anthroposophy (A Fragment): A New Foundation for the Study of Human Nature.* Hudson, NY: Anthroposophic Press, 1996.

———. *Balance in Teaching.* Great Barrington, MA: SteinerBooks, 2007.

———. *Balance in Teaching: Meditatively Acquired Knowledge of the Human Being.* Spring Valley, NY: Mercury Press, 1990.

———. *Broken Vessels: The Spiritual Structure of Human Frailty.* Great Barrington, MA: SteinerBooks, 2002.

———. *Course for Young Doctors: Meditative Contemplations and Instructions for Deepening the Art of Healing.* Spring Valley, NY: Mercury Press, 1994.

———. *Discussions with Teachers.* Hudson, NY: Anthroposophic Press, 1997.

———. *Education for Adolescents.* Hudson, NY: Anthroposophic Press, 1996.

———. *Education for Special Needs: The Curative Education Course.* London: Rudolf Steiner Press, 1998.

———. *The Esoteric Aspect of the Social Question: The Individual and Society.* London: Rudolf Steiner Press, 2001.

———. *Esoteric Development: Lectures and Writings.* Great Barrington, MA: SteinerBooks, 2003.

———. *Esoteric Lessons: 1913–1923.* Great Barrington, MA: SteinerBooks, 2011.

———. *Eurythmy as Visible Speech.* London: Rudolf Steiner Press, 1984.

———, and Ita Wegman. *Extending Practical Medicine: Fundamental Principles Based on the Science of the Spirit.* London: Rudolf Steiner Press, 1997.

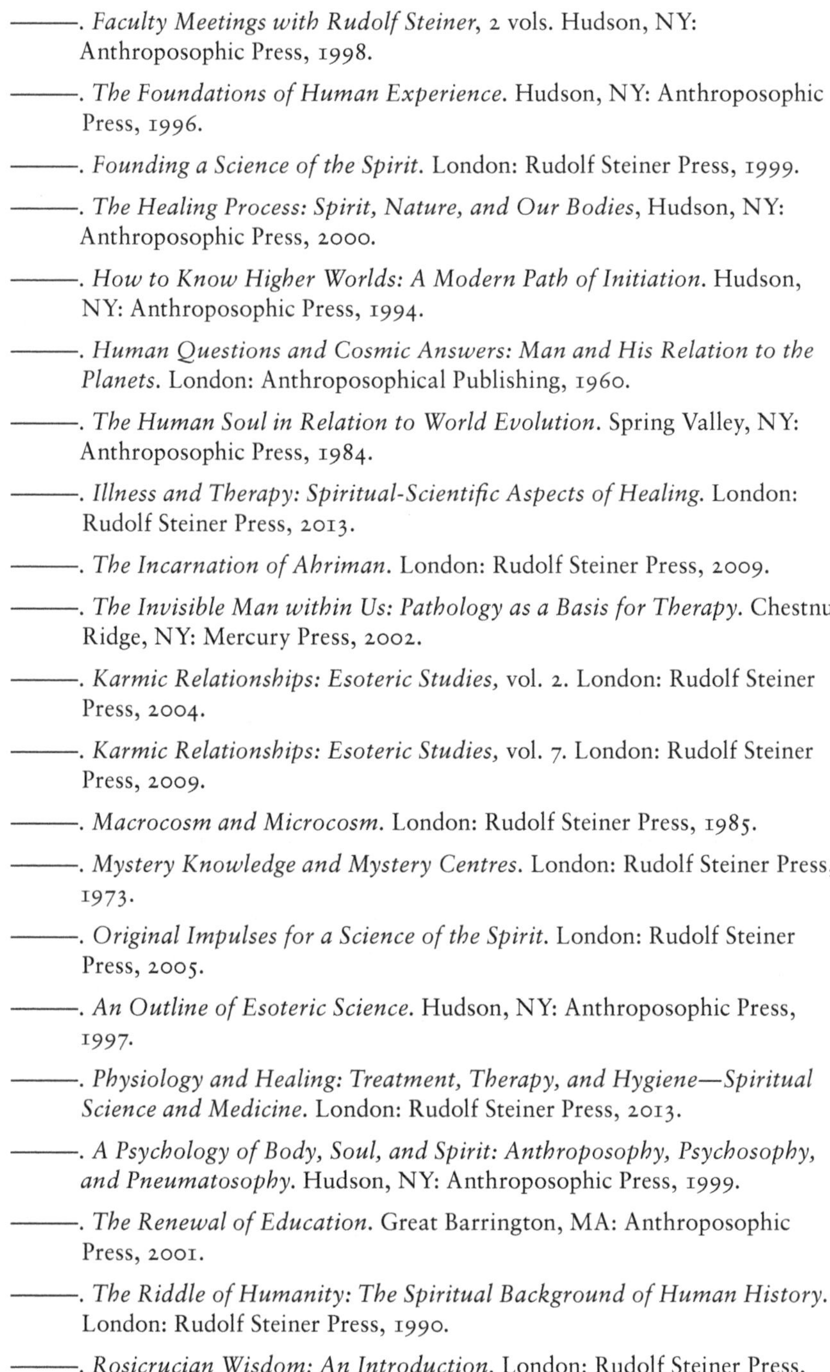

———. *Faculty Meetings with Rudolf Steiner*, 2 vols. Hudson, NY: Anthroposophic Press, 1998.

———. *The Foundations of Human Experience*. Hudson, NY: Anthroposophic Press, 1996.

———. *Founding a Science of the Spirit*. London: Rudolf Steiner Press, 1999.

———. *The Healing Process: Spirit, Nature, and Our Bodies*, Hudson, NY: Anthroposophic Press, 2000.

———. *How to Know Higher Worlds: A Modern Path of Initiation*. Hudson, NY: Anthroposophic Press, 1994.

———. *Human Questions and Cosmic Answers: Man and His Relation to the Planets*. London: Anthroposophical Publishing, 1960.

———. *The Human Soul in Relation to World Evolution*. Spring Valley, NY: Anthroposophic Press, 1984.

———. *Illness and Therapy: Spiritual-Scientific Aspects of Healing*. London: Rudolf Steiner Press, 2013.

———. *The Incarnation of Ahriman*. London: Rudolf Steiner Press, 2009.

———. *The Invisible Man within Us: Pathology as a Basis for Therapy*. Chestnut Ridge, NY: Mercury Press, 2002.

———. *Karmic Relationships: Esoteric Studies*, vol. 2. London: Rudolf Steiner Press, 2004.

———. *Karmic Relationships: Esoteric Studies*, vol. 7. London: Rudolf Steiner Press, 2009.

———. *Macrocosm and Microcosm*. London: Rudolf Steiner Press, 1985.

———. *Mystery Knowledge and Mystery Centres*. London: Rudolf Steiner Press, 1973.

———. *Original Impulses for a Science of the Spirit*. London: Rudolf Steiner Press, 2005.

———. *An Outline of Esoteric Science*. Hudson, NY: Anthroposophic Press, 1997.

———. *Physiology and Healing: Treatment, Therapy, and Hygiene—Spiritual Science and Medicine*. London: Rudolf Steiner Press, 2013.

———. *A Psychology of Body, Soul, and Spirit: Anthroposophy, Psychosophy, and Pneumatosophy*. Hudson, NY: Anthroposophic Press, 1999.

———. *The Renewal of Education*. Great Barrington, MA: Anthroposophic Press, 2001.

———. *The Riddle of Humanity: The Spiritual Background of Human History*. London: Rudolf Steiner Press, 1990.

———. *Rosicrucian Wisdom: An Introduction*. London: Rudolf Steiner Press, 2000.

———. *Spiritual Relations in the Human Organism.* Spring Valley, NY: Mercury Press, 1984.

———. *Spiritual Science as a Foundation for Social Forms.* Hudson, NY: Anthroposophic Press, 1986.

———. *Study of Man.* London: Rudolf Steiner Press, 2007.

———. *Theosophy: An Introduction to the Spiritual Processes in Human Life and in the Cosmos.* Hudson, NY: Anthroposophic Press, 1994.

———. *Therapeutic Insights: Earthly and Cosmic Laws.* Spring Valley, NY: Mercury Press, 1984.

———. *True and False Paths in Spiritual Investigation.* London: Rudolf Steiner Press, 1969.

———. *Understanding Healing: Meditative Reflections on Deepening Medicine through Spiritual Science.* London: Rudolf Steiner Press, 2013.

———. *What Can the Art of Healing Gain through Spiritual Science?* Spring Valley, NY: Mercury Press, 1986.

Steiner, Rudolf, and Ita Wegman. *Fundamentals of Therapy.* Spring Valley, NY: Mercury Press, 1999.

Strauss, Michaela. *Understanding Children's Drawings: Tracing the Path of Incarnation.* London: Rudolf Steiner Press, 2007.

Vogel, Heinz-Harmut. *Finding Remedies: Spiritual Knowledge of Man and Nature,* vols. 1 and 2. Bad Boll, Germany: Natur Mensch Medizin Verlag, 2000.

von Zabern, Bertram. *Compendium for the Remedial Treatment of Children, Adolescents and Adults in Need of Soul Care: Experiences and Indications from Anthroposophic Therapy.* Spring Valley, NY: Mercury Press, 2009.

Walter, Hilma. *Die Sieben Hauptmetalle.* Natura Verlag: Dornach, 1999.

Wolff, Otto. *Remedies for Typical Diseases: Concerning the Remedies Developed by Rudolf Steiner Using New Concepts and New Methods.* Spring Valley, NY: Mercury Press, 1996.

Index

Index

A Note from SteinerBooks

SteinerBooks is a 501 (c) 3 not-for-profit organization, incorporated in New York State since 1928 to promote the progress and welfare of humanity and to increase public awareness of Rudolf Steiner (1861–1925), the Austrian-born polymath writer, lecturer, spiritual scientist, philosopher, cosmologist, educator, psychologist, alchemist, ecologist, Christian mystic, comparative religionist, and evolutionary theorist, who was the creator of Anthroposophy ("human wisdom") as a path uniting the spiritual in the human being with the spiritual in the universe; and to this end publish and distribute books for adults and children, utilize the electronic media, hold conferences, and engage in similar activities making available his works and exploring themes arising from, and related to, them and the movement that he founded.

- We commission translations of books by Rudolf Steiner unpublished in English, as well as new translations for updated editions.
- Our aim is to make works on Anthroposophy available to all by publishing and distributing both introductory and advanced works on spiritual research.
- New books are publish for both print and digital editions to reach the widest possible readership.
- Recent technology also makes it efficient for us to make our previously out-of-print works available for the next generation.

SteinerBooks depends on our readers' financial support, which is greatly needed, appreciated, and tax-deductible. Please consider a donation by check or other means to SteinerBooks, 610 Main St., Great Barrington, MA 01230. We also accept donations via PayPal on our website. For more information about supporting our work, send email to friends@stcincrbooks.org or call 413-528-8233.

Printed in the USA
CPSIA information can be obtained
at www.ICGtesting.com
LVHW092044061123
762972LV00057B/1225

9 781584 209508